Prostate Cancer: Molecular Events and Therapeutic Modalities

Gautam Sethi • Milad Ashrafizadeh
Nasim Ebrahimi
Editors

Prostate Cancer: Molecular Events and Therapeutic Modalities

Springer

Editors
Gautam Sethi
Yong Loo Lin School of Medicine, Department of Pharmacology
National University of Singapore
Singapore, Singapore

Nasim Ebrahimi
Division of Genetics, Department of Cell and Molecular Biology and Microbiology, Faculty of Biological Science and Technology
University of Isfahan
Isfahan, Iran

Milad Ashrafizadeh
Shandong First Medical University and Shandong Academy of Medical Sciences
Department of Radiation Oncology, Shandong Cancer Hospital and Institute
Jinan, China

ISBN 978-981-97-4611-8 ISBN 978-981-97-4612-5 (eBook)
https://doi.org/10.1007/978-981-97-4612-5

This Springer imprint is published by the registered company Springer Nature Singapore Pte Ltd.
The registered company address is: 152 Beach Road, #21-01/04 Gateway East, Singapore 189721, Singapore

Preface

Urological cancers are responsible for high mortality and morbidity around the world. Prostate cancer is one of the leading causes of death in men, and currently, surgical resection, chemotherapy, and radiotherapy are utilized for the treatment of this disease. However, tumor cells can develop resistance to therapy, making surgical resection less relevant in advanced stages. Moreover, several risk factors for the pathogenesis of prostate cancer include environmental factors, physical activity, smoking, alcohol consumption, and genomic alterations. Therefore, understanding the underlying mechanisms involved in prostate cancer progression can provide new insights into its treatment. This book presents an introduction to the anatomy of prostate tissue, the pathogenesis of prostate cancer, and the epidemiology of prostate cancer. Then, the major biological mechanisms dysregulated in prostate cancer including proliferation, cell cycle, apoptosis, autophagy, metastasis, and epithelial–mesenchymal transition are covered in this book. In order to better understand the major molecular pathways involved in prostate cancer progression, we dedicated some chapters to evaluating the roles of major signaling pathways including Wnt, STAT3, lncRNAs, miRNAs, and circRNAs, among others. Understanding the dysregulation of biological and molecular mechanisms can contribute to the development of novel therapeutics for the treatment of prostate cancer. The genomic alterations accumulate during the progression of prostate cancer and therefore, highlighting their upregulation or downregulation along with interactions with other molecular pathways can improve the knowledge toward the genomic and epigenetic profiles of prostate cancer. The tumor microenvironment components show interaction in prostate cancer that can determine the biological profile of this disease. In order to further direct the future therapeutics for prostate cancer, some chapters were allocated to understand the role of new therapeutics including natural products, genetic tools, and nanoparticles for the treatment of prostate cancer. The natural products are biocompatible factors and have multi-targeting impact. They can affect different molecular pathways and biological mechanisms to eliminate prostate cancer. Moreover, genetic tools have been introduced for the treatment of prostate cancer. Furthermore, the development of nanostructures, especially biomimetic and stimuli-responsive nanoparticles can pave the way for the treatment of prostate cancer.

Singapore, Singapore Gautam Sethi
Jinan, China Milad Ashrafizadeh
Isfahan, Iran Nasim Ebrahimi

Contents

Part I
General Aspects

Chapter 1
Anatomy and Function of Prostate

Mehrdad Hashemi, Vahid Tavakolpour, Sima Orouei, Mina Alimohammadi, Saba Asadi, Zeinab Khazaei Koohpar, Behdokht Jamali, Kiavash Hushmandi, Rasoul Raesi, Maliheh Entezari, and Mitra Behroozaghdam

The original version of the chapter has been revised. A correction to this chapter can be found at https://doi.org/10.1007/978-981-97-4612-5_15

M. Hashemi · M. Entezari
Farhikhtegan Medical Convergence Sciences Research Center, Farhikhtegan Hospital Tehran Medical Sciences, Islamic Azad University, Tehran, Iran

Faculty of Advanced Science and Technology, Department of Genetics, Tehran Medical Sciences, Islamic Azad University, Tehran, Iran

V. Tavakolpour
Department of Stem Cells and Regenerative Medicine, Institute of Medical Biotechnology, National Institute of Genetic Engineering and Biotechnology (NIGEB), Tehran, Iran

S. Orouei
Department of Biology, Science and Research Branch, Islamic Azad University, Tehran, Iran

M. Alimohammadi
Department of Immunology, School of Medicine, Shahid Beheshti University of Medical Sciences, Tehran, Iran

S. Asadi · M. Behroozaghdam (✉)
Farhikhtegan Medical Convergence Sciences Research Center, Farhikhtegan Hospital Tehran Medical Sciences, Islamic Azad University, Tehran, Iran

Z. K. Koohpar
Faculty of Biological Sciences, Department of Cell and Molecular Biology, Tonekabon Branch, Islamic Azad University, Tonekabon, Iran

B. Jamali
Department of Microbiology and Genetics, Kherad Institute of Higher Education, Bushehr, Iran

K. Hushmandi
Department of Epidemiology, University of Tehran, Tehran, Iran

R. Raesi
Department of Nursing, Torbat Jam Faculty of Medical Sciences, Torbat Jam, Iran

Department of Health Services Management, Mashhad University of Medical Sciences, Mashhad, Iran

G. Sethi et al. (eds.), *Prostate Cancer: Molecular Events and Therapeutic Modalities*, https://doi.org/10.1007/978-981-97-4612-5_1

Abstract Since prostate carcinogenesis can be seen as the restoration of development in the adult prostate, understanding the complex process of prostate development is becoming increasingly important in both basic developmental biology studies and clinical prostate cancer research. Researchers have shown via the use of rodent animal models that androgen receptor (AR) signaling is the primary mediator of prostate development, with additional signaling pathways also playing critical roles. The scarcity of suitable fetal materials is largely to blame for the numerous unanswered questions surrounding human prostate biology. When it comes to producing seminal fluid to aid in reproduction, the functions of the prostate glands in humans and mice are very similar. Understanding the normal morphology and histology of the murine prostate is crucial for understanding alterations in genetically modified mice models, as there are notable variations between the murine and human prostates in terms of these aspects. The course of prostate cancer can vary greatly from patient to patient, and the illness itself has a long and storied past. There has been a tidal change in the way researchers and healthcare providers approach prostate cancer in the last several years. Deep sequencing's power has unearthed previously unknown cistromic and transcriptome information on prostate cancer.

Keywords Prostate biology · Prostate development · Prostate embryology · Prostate cancer

1.1 Introduction

A walnut-sized organ situated beneath the bladder of a human being is known as the prostate [1]. This area is the starting point for three fundamental health problems: prostatitis, benign prostatic hyperplasia (BPH), and prostate cancer. Furthermore, people pay more attention to it due to these problems than they would to an organ of this size. In addition, Andreas Vesalius published his observations of the male accessory glands in 1543, which means that anatomical images of the prostate have been published at least as far back as the mid-sixteenth century [2]. It has also been known for hundreds of years that testicular and prostatic function are related. In 1786, John Hunter's "Observations on the glands situated between the rectum and the bladder, called vesiculae seminales" wrote that "the prostate and Cowper's glands and those of the urethra which in the perfect male are soft and bulky with a secretion salty to the taste, in the castrated animal are small, flabby, tough and ligermentous and have little secretion" [3].

Additionally, a compound tubular-alveolar gland, the adult prostate is present in the vast majority of mammalian species [4]. Species vary greatly in their outward appearance. Anatomists and pathologists in the early-to-mid-twentieth century did a lot of the descriptive work on the prostate's development, from its origins in the hindgut to descriptions of the adult organ. Much later research revealed the molecular underpinnings of these characterizations. The human prostate and other animal models of human disease, such as rats and mice, are the primary foci of research in prostate biology. The results of animal studies must be evaluated with a thorough comprehension of the structural distinctions between human and rodent prostates.

More research in the field of cell lineage has illustrated that the whole urethra starts from the endoderm, and the prostate develops from the urogenital sinus (UGS) [5, 6]. Urogenital sinus epithelium (UGE) and urogenital sinus mesenchyme (UGM) are the two components that make up the UGS. According to recombinant tissue research, a fully grown prostate can be produced just by interacting with the UGM and the UGE [7, 8]. The role of androgens, which are released from the testes, in regulating prostate development was recognized early in [9]. At around 9 weeks of gestation in humans and E13–14 in mice, the fetal testes begin to manufacture testosterone. The 5α-reductase then converts testosterone into dihydrotestosterone, a more potent androgen [10]. An essential step in prostate induction is the androgen receptor (AR) pathway [11]. Another point worth noting is that epithelial prostatic budding occurs at roughly 9–10 weeks of gestation in humans [12] and at E17.5 in mice [13].

On top of that, prostate epithelial cells have elevated levels of Forkhead Box A1 (FOXA1), a pioneer gene in endoderm-derived epithelial cells [14]. One of the pioneer factors that FOXA1 can do is interact with closed chromatin, which loosens nucleosomes and makes it possible for AR to bind to DNA [15]. The most crucial finding is that mutations in FOXA1 disrupt prostate differentiation [16]. When it comes to prostate specification, NK3 homeobox 1 (NKX3-1) is just as absolutely important as AR. Two days before prostatic budding, NKX3-1 expression begins, which means that NKX3-1 may indicate the beginning of prostate organogenesis. Moreover, no other tissues of the male urogenital system have been exhibited to have NKX3-1, which is exclusive to the prostate epithelium. In mice, prostate development is affected by a functional NKX3-1 deficiency [17]. Furthermore, the master regulator inference technique, a computational system approach, has identified AR, FOXA1, and NKX3-1 as a driver for prostate organogenesis [18]. Reprogramming induced epithelial cells sourced from mouse fibroblasts into prostate tissue is another application of these master regulators. Grafting these reprogrammed prostate-like cells into a mouse model resulted in the right histological and molecular characteristics of the prostate [18].

1.2 Prostate Embryology and Postnatal Development

A mammalian embryo can alter its phenotypic from female to male during its early stages of development [1]. This trajectory is predetermined during conception in normally developing humans and is mirrored in the embryonic stage by the interplay of four absolutely necessary units: the fetal gonad, the urogenital sinus (UGS), the Wolffian and Müllerian ducts, and the urogenital sinus (US).

Moreover, in human embryos, the Wolffian ducts begin to form in 2–3 mm long embryos about 25–30 days after conception. In the early embryo, these ducts serve as pathways for waste elimination by the mesonephros, the organ responsible for kidney function. In addition, a definite kidney's acquisition of excretory function is necessary for the ducts to integrate into the genital system. As the female reproductive system develops, the genital tract components detach from the Wolffian duct, leaving just the ureters as a remnant of this developmental process. The Wolffian ducts remain in an ambisexual form, sometimes even until birth, in reptiles and birds whose mesonephros have a long excretory function. By the time a human embryo reaches 4–5 mm in length, the ducts that connect the hindgut (which later becomes the cloaca) to the mesonephros and gonad have enlarged and lumenized [1].

Furthermore, after the Wolffian ducts have developed for approximately 6 weeks of gestation, the Müllerian ducts begin to constitute. Between the gonadal and mesonephric portions of the urogenital ridge, a fissure is produced, which is bordered with epithelial cells. As it narrows, it forms a tube that, parallel to the Wolffian ducts, runs through the mesenchyme surrounding it. By the eighth week of gestation, the Müllerian ducts have progressed to the point where they form the Müllerian tubercle; nevertheless, they have not yet broken into the UGS. As the embryo develops into a sac of length between 7 and 9 mm, a structure called the urorectal septum forms, dividing the cloaca into the sac and the UGS. Part of the UGS that is below the Müllerian tubercle is a vaginal portion in females and a penile urethra in males; the higher portion is the urethra.

The androgens secreted by the fetal testis dictate the course of male sexual differentiation. If the testes are not present, the testicles are not functioning, or there is a mutation in the androgen receptor gene, the fetus will acquire a female phenotype since these hormones and receptors are not present. The male reproductive system undergoes an asymmetrical process of sexual differentiation, which includes the stability of the Wolffian ducts by androgens and the regression of the Müllerian duct system induced by Anti-Müllerian hormone expressed in the testicular Sertoli cells.

The second stage of male sexual development is regulated by testosterone, which is secreted by the Leydig cells of the developing testis. During this process, the tubules that link the testis to the mesonephros undergo modifications, giving rise to the vasa efferentia, the convoluted epididymal duct, and the vas deferens. Both the external genitalia and the UGS are masculinized by the androgenic stimulation. The penis, the labial-scrotal lobes, the prostate, and the prostatic utricle all develop during this time. At the location of the Müllerian tubercle, epithelial buds begin to develop laterally from the UGS walls in 50 mm embryos, marking the beginning of the rudimentary prostate. During the process of local mesenchymal control, the buds transform into solid branching cords. Then, these cords begin to establish a lumen, which eventually gives birth to a network of tubules and alveoli. Some of the apical cells seem to start secretory activity and undergo structural polarization as the lumen forms. A stroma with abundant smooth muscle develops in the organ, and a luminal layer of tall columnar secretory epithelium and a layer of flat basal epithelium border the ducts and acini [19]. The appearance, function, and expression of distinct cytokeratin classes (keratins 5 and 14 in basal cells, 8 and 18 in luminal cells) allow for their differentiation from one another [20].

The majority of our understanding of prostate development, especially the molecular aspects, relies heavily on data derived from investigations conducted on rats and mice. This kind of research is possible with these animals since their tissues are readily available and transgenic and gene knock-out models have recently been developed. It should be mentioned that Dorothy Price is one of several pioneers in the field who laid the groundwork for the basic profile of rodent prostate development [4, 21, 22]. While human prostatic embryogenesis follows a similar pattern to that of rodents, the timing is significantly faster in these animals. For instance, early prostatic buds appear a day or two after the UGS is present in rats (embryonic day 18) and mice (embryonic day 16). The historical records are greatly supplemented by newly published and richly illustrated accounts of the molecular and gross phenotypes of the developing urogenital tract in rats [23, 24].

The process of the prostate's growth and development starts during fetal development, when prostatic buds are formed from the UGS, and ends when a man reaches sexual maturity [25]. Approximately 10 weeks into a human fetus's gestation, this starts at 19 days in rats, 17 days in mice, and 12 days in humans [12, 26]. From the urogenital sinus epithelium (UGE) into the surrounding urogenital sinus mesenchyme (UGM), firm epithelial buds first emerge, marking the commencement of prostate morphogenesis [25]. Testicular androgens stimulate prostatic bud proliferation, which ultimately results in the formation of solid epithelial cell cords that migrate into the UGM according to a precise geographic pattern, thus establishing the lobar divisions of the prostate [13, 26–28]. Rodents have a little prostate with a few immature buds when they're born. After birth, these cells divide rapidly, especially at the tips [29], and the prostate canalizes itself from the urethra outward. At the same time, epithelial cells undergo phenotypic transitions between luminal and basal forms [30]. Conventional histologic sections fail to reveal the complex phenotype of prostatic basal cells, which, at least in rats, have processes that round the ducts [31, 32]. The proliferation and differentiation of UGM into interfascicular fibroblasts and prostatic smooth muscle occur simultaneously with epithelial development [33]. After birth, androgens trigger a process of differentiation in the epithelial cells, which includes the development of androgen receptors. These cells then start to produce secretory proteins that are particular to distinct lobes and species [34].

Most of the prostate's branch points form before the mouse reaches 15 days of age [35], and by 60 days of age, the prostate has grown and developed to its fullest extent [36]. The human prostate, on the other hand, doesn't expand much from birth until puberty, when it starts to expand in reaction to increased androgen levels. A gradual enlargement of the prostate follows, spread out over a number of years. Although androgens are primarily responsible for the maturation and expansion of the prostate, they are also essential for the preservation of a growth-quiescent adult organ. Prostatic enlargement and cancer are conditions linked to aging and a decline in serum androgen titers; they do not take place in young adult males when androgen levels are at their lifetime peak.

1.3 Anatomy of Prostate Tissue

In an effort to shed light on the formation of the middle and posterior lobes, which had been distinguished by previous researchers, Lowsley [26] used serial sections as anatomical models to describe the fetal human prostate lobes in 1912 [1, 37]. Lowsley classified five distinct sets of prostatic ducts that originated in the UGS and referred to them as lobes using fetal tissue taken at 3 months of gestation. The four parts were named the ventral lobe, two lateral lobes, and the central lobe. The ventral lobe, according to Lowsley, is created by four sets of epithelial buds originating from the anterior or ventral wall of the prostatic urethra. The bladder and the ejaculatory ducts were located beneath the urethral floor, and the middle lobe was constituted by around twelve tubules connected to the posterior urethra. Arising from the urethral sides and following the prostatic furrows, the biggest set of tubules is the paired left and right lateral tubules. On the caudal part of the urethra, the tubules gave birth to the posterior lobe through lateral and posterior growth; they were placed distal to the ejaculatory ducts. Even while most of the ducts expanded toward the bladder, as can be seen in the lateral lobe, a handful grew anteriorly.

A dispute on the terminology used to describe the prostate anatomy began with Lowsley's investigations and persisted for around 70 years. The fusion of his described lobes in an adult human makes dissection impossible to separate or identify them, leading to competing theories on the prostate's anatomical divisions [38–40]. The situation is further complicated because, according to morphological, histological, and physiological evidence, the different prostatic lobes are separable to varied degrees in the majority of animals, including certain other primates.

Moreover, John McNeal's terminology is currently the de jure standard for describing the human prostate [38]. According to McNeal, there are three main sections of the prostate, each with its own anatomy and histology. The organ is encased in a nonglandular fibromuscular stroma, and there are two glandular zones, the peripheral zone and the central zone, each with its own complicated ductal system that can be identified histologically. The central zone is a wedge-shaped area of glandular tissue that encircles the ejaculatory ducts and makes up the majority of the prostate's base. The gland was completed by the periphery zone. It expanded caudally to partially encircle the distal part of the urethra and encircled the majority of the central zone. McNeal included Lowsley's lateral lobes and a section of the posterior lobe in his peripheral zone classification, while Lowsley's middle lobe and some of the posterior lobe in his previous investigations were included in McNeal's central zone classification. A second, less extensive glandular area, the transition zone, was also discovered by McNeal to surround the prostatic urethra.

The human prostate gland, which is located behind the bladder, is anatomically characterized by its pyramidal shape. Both the penile urethra and the bladder are touched at its highest point [41, 42]. Right below the urinary bladder is where the prostate gland can be observed. The prostate encircles the prostatic urethra, a conduit via which urine leaves the bladder. A healthy prostate typically weighs about 15–20 g. There are two seminal vesicles at the base of the prostate. Each of the three histological zones consisting of peripheral, transition, and central, make up the human prostate, a singular gland. In most cases of prostate cancer, the disease begins in the peripheral zone, which encircles the prostate's outer segment distally. Approximately 70% of the typical prostate is made up of it [41]. Although it makes up just around 5% of the prostate, the transition zone is usually not noticeable in young men and is situated close to the prostatic urethra. The transition zone is typically noticeably larger in older men due to benign prostatic hyperplasia, a very frequent benign growth in transition zone tissue. Various degrees of benign prostatic hyperplasia are visible in the majority of specimens taken from radical prostatectomy procedures. Despite the high degree of overlap, there is strong evidence that tumors developing in the transition zone differ clinically and physiologically from those in the peripheral zone. Conical in shape, the central zone encompasses the area around the ejaculatory ducts and has its widest point at the prostate's base and its narrowest point at the verumontanum. The location is not the starting point for any illness, although cancer might indirectly affect it.

Luminal, basal, and neuroendocrine cells line the acini and ducts creating the human prostate glandular epithelium. In a significant number of instances, the acini will look papillary or undulating. The center zone has a much more noticeable papillary structure [41]. Near the cell base, columnar luminal cells have spherical nuclei and pale eosinophilic cytoplasm. The generation of seminal fluid is aided by a range of products secreted into the lumen by specialized cells known as luminal cells. One of these compounds is PSA, which is highly detectable by immunohistochemistry in luminal cells. Basal cells are characterized by their ovoid nuclei and barely perceptible cytoplasm; they are located alongside the basement membrane. From one prostate gland to the next, the amount of basal cells can vary widely. Even while they are typically visible in routine H&E sections, they really stand out when stained with immunohistochemistry for p63 (nuclear) and high-molecular-weight cytokeratins (cytoplasmic). Despite the unreliability of H&E sections, neuroendocrine cells can be consistently identified using immunohistochemistry for markers such as chromogranin and synaptophysin. The lumens of the acini often reveal eosinophilic corpora amylacea that are spherical and layered.

There is an enormous variety of smooth muscle cells mixed together with fibroblasts, blood arteries, nerves, and blood in the fibromuscular prostatic stroma. The prostate does not have any adipose tissue. When compared to the prostates of mice, where the fibromuscular stroma is much thinner, this one stands out significantly. Although skeletal muscle fibers are mostly located outside the prostate, they can also reach into its outer region [42].

The majority of tissue in most radical prostatectomies displays benign prostatic hyperplasia, as mentioned earlier, and many prostates removed for the treatment of prostate cancer exhibit varying degrees of this condition. This shows up as tissue nodules that are either mostly epithelial or entirely stromal, depending on the ratio of epithelium to stroma [42].

Many different types of epithelial and stromal modifications can be seen in the human prostate. Both basal cell hyperplasia and epithelial atrophy are very prevalent. Acute inflammation can range from localized to systemic, and even abscess development can occur, in addition to the prevalence of chronic inflammation. In benign prostatic hyperplasia, squamous metaplasia may be visible around the margins of infarcts, when tissues die due to compromised blood supply [42].

A series of smaller glands empties into the central lumen of the bilaterally tubular human seminal vesicles, which are lined by a columnar epithelium with eosinophilic cytoplasm. The epithelial cells contain the characteristic lipofuschin pigment, which is yellow in color. Degenerative atypia and hyperchromatic nuclei are possible. Prominent smooth muscle layers, one circular and one longitudinal, encircle the epithelium. Although seminal vesicle primary neoplasia is very uncommon, prostatic cancer invasion of one or both seminal vesicles is common and is accompanied by a considerably worse prognosis [41].

Another point to consider is that the rodent prostate is physically distinct from the human prostate in several ways. To put it another way, there are four separate lobular structures constituting the rodent prostate: the lateral lobe, the anterior lobe (also titled the coagulating gland), and the dorsal and ventral lobes [29]. On either side of the brain, you will find these lobes paired up. The distinctive ultimate shape of each lobe is a result of variations in lobe-specific branching morphogenesis [25].

Underneath the urine bladder on the back side of the urethra are the ventral lobes in mice and rats. Partially covering the ventral lobes and dorsally merging with the dorsal lobe, the lateral lobes are located directly below the coagulating glands and seminal vesicles [43, 44]. On top of that dollars located beneath the seminal vesicles and coagulating glands, the dorsal lobes are situated inferiorly and posteriorly to the urine bladder. The seminal vesicles are closely near to the anterior lobes, which are coagulating glands.

1.4 An Overview of Prostate Tissue: Physiology and Pathology

The prostate is about 20 g in weight, 3 cm in length (about the size of a walnut), and 1 g in diameter. The organ is responsible for producing one-third of the overall amount of seminal fluid [45]. The prostate gland is positioned in the male pelvis at the base of the penis. Immediately forward of the rectum and below the urine bladder is where you'll find it [45]. Although it may be confusing, the prostate really covers the back of the urethra. The interior lining of the prostate and the urethra are identical, hence terms like "prostatic urethra," "proximal urethra," and "posterior urethra" all refer to the same structure [46]. A quarter to a third of the semen comes from the fluid produced by the glandular tissue that makes up the prostate. The alkalinity and nutrients provided by this fraction of the semen that is located in the prostate help keep the pH of the sperm high. What remains of the seminal fluid is made by the seminal vesicles [45, 47, 48]. Androgens, specifically testosterone, are essential for the proper functioning of the prostate gland. Hormonal therapy, including testosterone deprivation, is highly effective for this reason. Intracellular androgen production is postulated in castrate-resistant cancers [49]. Cancer develops when normally functioning cells of the prostate gland, notably the basal cells in the periphery, undergo a mutation [50]. Digital rectal examination (DRE) palpable prostate tissue is the most typical site of prostate cancer detection in the peripheral zone [51].

The tissue giving rise to the prostate, the primitive urogenital sinus, develops as a caudal extension of the hindgut during development [45]. Moreover, the endodermal origin of the primitive urogenital sinus and its entirety, including the distal urethra, has been proven via lineage tracing [5]. On top of that at embryonic cloaca, the urogenital sinus and hindgut are originally fused into a single urinary tract. By 8 weeks of gestation in humans and 13.5 days postcoitum (dpc) in mice, the cloaca divides into separate urogenital and anorectal tracts [52]. It is interesting to note that this process was previously believed to happen by formation of a urorectal septum, but a new model has been suggested [53]. The primitive urogenital sinus (UGS) divides into the urogenital sinus B-Lymphoid Tyrosine Kinase (BLK) in the middle and the penile urethra at the caudal end; the bladder is situated at the rostral end of this sinus. In humans, the process of prostate development begins at approximately 10 weeks of gestation [12], but in mice, it begins at 17.5 days postconception [17, 54]. Afterward, during the gestational period and the prepubertal years, prostate organogenesis is influenced by circulating androgens and continues until the prostate reaches its full size at puberty. Particularly noteworthy is the publication of a comprehensive description of the anatomy of the mouse urogenital system during development [24].

Furthermore, organogenesis of the prostate can be conceptualized as a four-stage process. Males undergo prostate induction in the earliest stage of development, before epithelial budding, in response to developmental signals that are either directly or indirectly mediated by androgens. In addition, a system of ducts made of solid epithelial cords is formed as the urogenital sinus epithelium (UGE) buds into the surrounding urogenital sinus mesenchyme (UGM) in the second stage, following the determination of prostatic fate. This process begins with tissue outgrowth and branching morphogenesis. Androgen receptor (AR) function is essential to modulate epithelial outgrowth in this process, which entails paracrine communication from the UGM to the UGE. The mature ductal network is born in the third stage, which is characterized by ductal expansion and branching morphogenesis. While this process creates separate prostatic zones inside a unilobular organ in humans, it distributes the prostate into four sets of lobes in mice, each with its own unique pattern of ductal branching [13, 34]. The last step is cytodifferentiation, which produces functional glandular epithelium with completely differentiated cell types, and canalization, constituting the ductal lumen from the solid epithelial cords.

Moreover, multiple morphologically unique cell types create the adult prostate epithelium. In addition to secretory proteins such prostate-specific antigen (PSA; also known as KLK3, a member of the kallikrein family of serine proteases), tall columnar epithelial cells titled luminal cells express cytokeratins (CK; also known as Keratin (KRT)) 8 and 18 [55–57]. Below the luminal layer, on the basement membrane, there are nonsecretory basal cells that express p63 (Trp63), CK5, and CK14 [58, 59]. In contrast to the nearly universally high AR expression by luminal cells, basal cells in the prostates of both mice and humans show negligible or undetectable AR levels [60, 61]. Despite much conjecture, the question of whether intermediate cells constitute a functionally separate cell type is still unanswered. On occasion, cells in the basal layer will co-express luminal and basal markers in addition to other markers such as CK19 [57, 62, 63]. The last kind of cells to be discussed are the uncommon neuroendocrine cells. These cells are basally located, release hormones and neuropeptides, and often have a dendritic-like process connecting the glandular lumen [64].

Another factor to consider is that many other kinds of differentiated cells are seen in the prostate's mesenchymal compartment as well. As a good example, the embryonic UGM cells create a smooth muscle layer that encases the epithelium and contracts to help the prostate pump out its contents into the ejaculate [33]. Furthermore, there is a substantial number of fully developed fibroblasts in the adult prostate stroma. These fibroblasts release an extracellular matrix that forms a network of structural proteins, glycoproteins, and proteoglycans; it also mediates growth factor signaling [65]. Last but not least, the stroma also contains lymphatics, nerves, blood arteries, and immune cells; the latter two groups have been linked to prostate cancer and stem cell control.

In addition, a large body of research has focused on AR as a potential biomarker for prostate cancer and prostate development. Although AR is known to bind to androgen hormones, it is only after entering the nucleus that it can perform its transcription factor role [66]. Dihydrotestosterone, which is produced from testosterone by 5α-reductase, binds to AR immediately after sex determination. This activates the activation of several prostatic genes, including NKX3-1, FOXA1, PSA, and others. As a result, this process promotes the budding of the prostate, branching morphogenesis, and maturation [67]. The lack of prostatic buds in testicular feminization mutant (Tfm) mice, who have a genetic mutation in the AR locus, highlights the crucial involvement of AR [68]. A mouse model has shown that branching morphogenesis can be impaired by conditional deletion of AR in both smooth muscle cells and stromal fibroblasts [69], indicating that AR plays an extra crucial function in the subsequent ductal branching morphogenesis. Also, whereas female mice have a relatively low amount of circulating androgens, male mice have an abundance of AR and circulating androgens in their UGS, suggesting that the latter serve as a priming agent. The fact that both Tfm male mice and wild-type female mice can have their UGS induced to budding by exogenous dihydrotestosterone lends credence to this idea [70]. The process of prostate initiation and budding involves signals that are not dependent on androgens. When it comes to deciding which cells will become what kinds of cells, the Wingless-Related Integration Site (WNT) signaling pathway is among the most crucial [71]. In order to stimulate the transcription of WNT target genes, the nuclear β-catenin protein, which is encoded by the Catenin Beta 1 (CTNNB1) gene, forms a complex with members of the T-Cell Factor (TCF)/(LEF) Lymphoid Enhancer Factor family [72]. This translocation is essential for the classical WNT signaling pathway.

The WNT signaling pathway controls the self-renewal of prostate stem cells, the formation of the prostate, and the processes of prostatic budding and epithelial branching morphogenesis. There are more WNT ligands and the WNT upstream regulator R-spondin 3 in the male UGS compared to the female UGS, and they are all present in the lower urogenital tract throughout prostate development [73]. In the prostatic bud epithelium, the β-catenin and WNT/β-catenin-responsive downstream genes AXIN2 and LEF1 are found in close proximity to NKX3-1 and exhibit high levels of expression. In addition, the number of prostatic buds is decreased and NKX3-1 expression is inhibited when UGS explant cultures are treated with a WNT antagonist, such as DKK1. This suggests that WNT/β-catenin plays crucial roles in prostate specification and bud production [74]. The development of prostate buds and prostatic differentiation are both halted when β-catenin is conditionally deleted from the UGS of E15.5 mice. Curiously, even after inducing β-catenin deletion by tamoxifen treatment, rudimentary bud development may be achieved by pretreating the mouse E15.5 UGS with dihydrotestosterone for 24 h [74]. It can be inferred from this that β-catenin is necessary for the start of prostatic differentiation but is not necessary for the creation of the prostate gland itself. Supporting this result, the selective ablation of β-catenin in adult luminal epithelial cells in the prostate gland in Probasin-Cre mice does not alter glandular homeostasis [75].

Interestingly, there appears to be a subtle dosage effect of WNT signaling on the morphogenesis of branching in prostatic epithelial cells when cultured postnatal rat ventral prostates are treated with the WNT agonist WNT3A or the WNT antagonist DKK1 [76]. Another factor that contributes to the formation of a distinct branch pattern in prostate branching morphogenesis is the noncanonical WNT/calcium pathway. This pathway is involved in the activation of the Ca^{2+}-sensitive kinases CAMK2 and PKC by means of intracellular Ca^{2+} transients induced by noncanonical WNT ligands like WNT4, WNT5A, and WNT11 [77]. Although WNT5A is mostly expressed at the tips of the prostate, ex vivo studies reveal that treating the prostate with WNT5A controls the size and quantity of buds rather than their commencement [78].

The BMP signaling pathway plays an essential role in both the budding of the prostate and its subsequent development. Over the course of embryonic development (E14–birth), the male UGS expresses a high level of BMP4. There is a dose-dependent inhibition of prostate ductal budding by exogenous BMP4, and an increased number of duct tips is observed in the prostate of adult mice with BMP4 haplo-insufficient genotypes [79]. In order to maintain a normal number of ductal tips during prostate development, these data show that the BMP signal prevents prostate ductal budding. Furthermore, activin A expression is downregulated in the prostatic epithelium throughout development but increased in the adolescent years. The prostatic epithelium expresses follistatin and activin receptors at various locations. Follistatin, an activin-binding protein that suppresses TGFβ signaling, can enhance branching in vitro, while activin A can impede prostatic branching in cultures of prostate organs [80]. These observations, when considered collectively, indicate that the morphogenesis of prostatic ductal branching is adversely regulated by the TGFβ/BMP signaling system.

BMP signaling pathways synergistically determine prostate development/BMP signaling pathways synergistically determine prostate development. The expression of NKX3-1 becomes undetectable when β-catenin is conditionally knocked out in the UGS, whereas AR remains robustly expressed [75]. These findings suggest that WNT/β-catenin signaling is essential for prostate lineage specification, even in the presence of an active AR signaling pathway. Nevertheless, the classical WNT signaling pathway is not necessary for prostate development after prostatic lineage commitment is complete [75]. When AR is removed from AXIN2-expressing prostate cells in mice, the resulting prostates are underdeveloped and tiny, according to both in vitro and in vivo studies [81]. This proves that AR is required for WNT-responsive cells to function properly throughout the whole prostate growth process. In the LNCaP prostate cancer cell line, WNT3A treatment can enhance AR binding to the promoter regions of WNT target genes like Myelocytomatosis (MYC) and Cyclin (CYCLIN) D1. Furthermore, AR and β-catenin can be recruited to the promoter and enhancer regions of the AR target gene PSA [82]. The possibility that WNT/β-catenin could enhance AR expression by binding LEF1 to the AR promoter was also mentioned in another study [83]. Furthermore, the activation of WNT/β-catenin can trigger BMP signaling at the tips of prostatic bud, which in turn prevents improper budding of the prostate and, collectively, guarantees the start of prostate growth [84]. The transcriptional regulation of TGFβ2, TGFβ3, and BMP4 in prostate stromal cells is enhanced by β-catenin, and basal cell proliferation is suppressed by the active TGFβ pathway [84, 85]. One strategy to minimize prostatic regression is through the influence of the TGFβ and AR signaling pathways in the stroma on the WNT signaling pathway [86]. For prostate budding to occur, a harmony must be maintained between the WNT and TGFβ/BMP signaling pathways.

1.5 Prostate Cancer

The industrialized world has a significant health care burden with prostate cancer [87], which is the most frequent male cancer type in the United States [88], the majority of European countries [89], and the second most common cancer type in the globe [90]. There is a great deal of variation in the clinical course of prostate cancer. Cancer of the prostate is the fifth leading cause of cancer-related deaths globally [90], with some individuals suffering from slow-moving forms that never spread and others from extremely aggressive forms that metastasize quickly and are resistant to treatment. Patients whose disease starts out locally but eventually spreads to other parts of their body and becomes incurable fall somewhere in the middle [91]. Clinical, pathologic, molecular, and therapeutic characteristics pertaining to prostate cancer have recently been the focus of precision medicine methods, which are detailed in this Special Issue. Moreover, in a review study, Cimadamore and coworkers outline the novel tissue-based biomarkers for prostate cancer that were developed in 2021 [92]. Modern prostate cancer grading, AI and computational pathology benefits, immunohistochemistry and morphologic characteristics of aggressive prostate cancer variants, and molecular markers for disease aggressiveness and treatment response are all topics covered.

In its early stages, prostate cancer may not cause any noticeable symptoms at all. The disease tends to progress slowly and may not even need treatment. Nevertheless, the most common issue is that of nocturia, increased frequency of urine, and difficulty urinating, all of which can be caused by prostatic enlargement. Since bone metastatic illness most commonly occurs in the axis skeleton, patients with late stages of the disease may experience symptoms such as back discomfort and urine retention. The presence of abnormally high amounts of the glycoprotein prostate-specific antigen (PSA >4 ng/mL) in the blood is a diagnostic tool for several prostate malignancies. Tissue biopsies are now considered the gold standard for cancer diagnosis, yet higher PSA levels in healthy men have also been detected [93].

There is a strong correlation between a sedentary lifestyle and an increased risk of prostate cancer. The disparities in prostate cancer incidence rates that are seen on a global and ethnic scale are primarily linked to dietary variables [94, 95]. The majority of research efforts focus on determining which genes are involved in both the inherited and acquired forms of prostate cancer. Consequently, the relationship between environmental triggers for genetic alterations and their involvement in promoting tumor progression can be better understood through a thorough examination of prostate cancer epidemiology and assessment of risk factors. Better techniques for screening and preventing prostate cancer will be possible once more about the disease's origins and the variables that put men at risk are known [93].

Furthermore, lineage plasticity, in which neoplastic cells can adapt to their environment by switching between different lineages and phenotypic cell states, and the genomic heterogeneity of prostate cancer contribute to the disease's clinical variability [96]. An essential process in tumor development and treatment resistance is the epithelial-to-mesenchymal transition, which exemplifies lineage plasticity. An article by Papanikolaou and coworkers reviews the literature on prostate cancer and its aggressiveness, therapy resistance, and the molecular pathology of the epithelial-to-mesenchymal transition, outlining the pathways by which it develops, and also discusses possible therapeutic targeting opportunities [97].

On top of that, men with localized prostate cancer have a life expectancy of more than 10 years and a 99% chance of survival if the disease is detected early on [98, 99]. In order to live with slow-growing, sometimes even indolent, prostate cancer, most men with the disease must manage a personalized treatment plan. However, for a number of men, relapsed prostate cancer after a definitive treatment plan can be aggressive and, in rare instances, unresponsive to the current standard of care. Approximately 15% of men diagnosed with prostate cancer have locoregional metastases, while about 5% have distant metastases (frequently in multiple sites) [100]. A dismal five-year overall survival rate of 30% is observed in men diagnosed with late-stage prostate cancer (distant metastases) [100]. More than 400,000 people die each year from metastatic prostate cancer, and experts predict that number will double or even triple by 2040 [101]. Also, around the same number of men will be expected to deal with treatment-related morbidity for over 10 years following diagnosis [101]. The tumor microenvironment can provide a secondary place for the dormant metastasized prostate cancer cells to remain for an extended period. Hematogenous metastasis to the stroma of the bone marrow in the axial skeleton and/or locoregional lymph nodes are the main features of prostate cancer metastasis [102]. The majority of distant metastases (more than 80%) are located in bone [102]. In rare instances, distant visceral locations are linked to prostate cancer metastases. Metastatic prostate cancer (MPC) is a deadly disease, and androgen deprivation therapy (ADT) is ineffective against castration-resistant prostate cancer (CRPC), which will eventually develop in nearly all patients. The main reasons for PCa-related illness and death are these characteristics [102]. Once metastasized CRPC (mCRPC) develops into therapy- and castration-resistant prostate cancer (t-CRPC), the disease is considered advanced and no longer treatable [103, 104].

Even in the same patient, morphological heterogeneity in localized prostate cancer is common. Intertumoral heterogeneity refers to the presence of many tumor foci within the prostate organ. Genetic differences between these foci might lead to different levels of metastasis and treatment resistance [105]. The idea of a "dominant cancer lesion" is confronted by the genetic heterogeneity seen in localized prostate cancer, which can be primarily responsible for a patient's clinical course. Moreover, cancer cells inside a single focus might develop from a variety of ancestral cells that undergo individual transformations [106] or, in the case of intratumoral heterogeneity, from a single clone that undergoes transformation and diverges into numerous separate clones within a single focus [107]. Multiple sites of metastasis are characteristic of clonally derived prostate cancer; however, this tumor type can also contain subclones that differ in genetic makeup and molecular characteristics [108].

Future therapeutic options with existing targeted medicines and understanding the clinical picture of prostate cancer at diagnosis are both made more difficult by the heterogeneity of probable cancer driver genes. Current ADT capitalizes on prostate cancer's reliance on androgen receptor (AR) activity, which is essential for the differentiation and proliferation of prostate epithelial cells. The heterogeneity is thought to be increased by ADT and second-line treatments as well [109]. Ongoing or poststandard ADT prostate cancer progression may be influenced by tumor heterogeneity. The severity of the disease and its resistance to conventional treatment may be determined by genomic traits, based on molecular heterogeneity [110]. Figure 1.1 shows the prostate cancer stages.

1.6 Conclusion and Perspectives

Although both the human and mouse prostates serve a comparable reproductive function, the anatomical and histological details of the two are very different. Models involving all lobes and, sometimes, many lobes have been developed; however, there is no conclusive proof that any one lobe of the murine prostate is more representative of human prostate cancer. Another point to consider is that the human prostate and the mouse prostate are structurally and histologically distinct, there is substantial evidence that genetic lesions found in human prostate cancer can cause neoplasia or neoplastic development in the mouse prostate. This can happen either

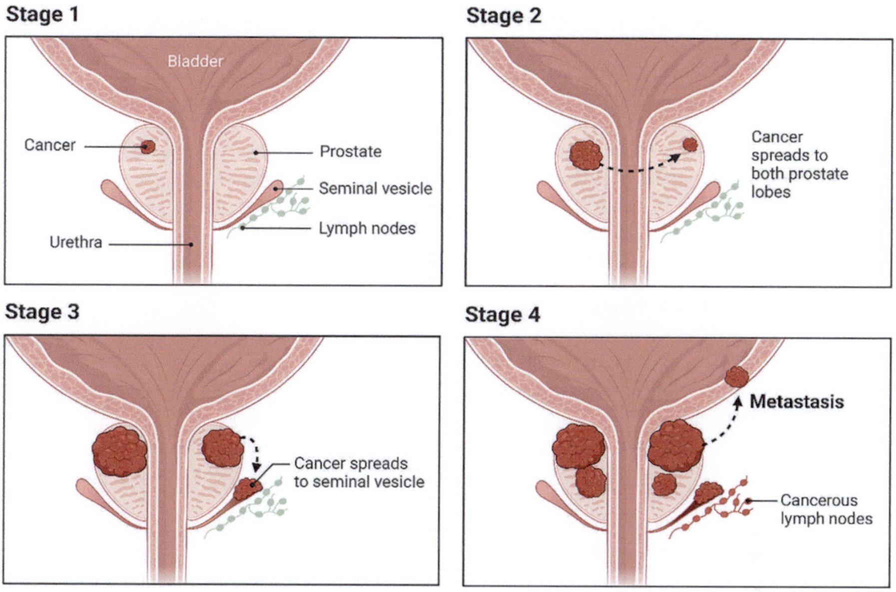

Fig. 1.1 The prostate cancer stages. In the advanced stages, prostate cancer starts to spread into other parts and the metastasis of cancer cells into lymph nodes is also observed (Biorender.com)

in isolation or in combination with other created lesions. When doing pathological investigation on genetically altered mice models, it is essential to constantly keep in mind the structural and anatomical distinctions between the human prostate and its rodent counterpart.

Conflict of Interest The authors declare no conflict of interest.

References

1. Aaron L, Franco OE, Hayward SW. Review of prostate anatomy and embryology and the etiology of benign prostatic hyperplasia. Urol Clin North Am. 2016;43(3):279–88.
2. Saunders JB, O'Malley C. The illustrations from the works of Andreas Vesalius of Brussels. San Francisco: Courier Corporation; 2013.
3. Geller J. Pathogenesis and medical treatment of benign prostatic hyperplasia. Prostate Suppl. 1989;2:95–104.
4. Price D, Williams-Ashman H, Young W. Sex and internal secretions. 3rd ed. Baltimore: Williams; 1961.
5. Seifert AW, Harfe BD, Cohn MJ. Cell lineage analysis demonstrates an endodermal origin of the distal urethra and perineum. Dev Biol. 2008;318(1):143–52.
6. Yu Y, Jiang W. Pluripotent stem cell differentiation as an emerging model to study human prostate development. Stem Cell Res Ther. 2020;11(1):285.

7. Cunha GR, et al. Epithelial-mesenchymal interactions in prostatic development. I. morphological observations of prostatic induction by urogenital sinus mesenchyme in epithelium of the adult rodent urinary bladder. J Cell Biol. 1983;96(6):1662–70.
8. Staack A, et al. Molecular, cellular and developmental biology of urothelium as a basis of bladder regeneration. Differentiation. 2005;73(4):121–33.
9. Feldman SC, Bloch E. Developmental pattern of testosterone synthesis by fetal rat testes in response to luteinizing hormone. Endocrinology. 1978;102(4):999–1007.
10. Berman DM, Tian H, Russell DW. Expression and regulation of steroid 5 alpha-reductase in the urogenital tract of the fetal rat. Mol Endocrinol. 1995;9(11):1561–70.
11. Lasnitzki I, Mizuno T. Prostatic induction: interaction of epithelium and mesenchyme from normal wild-type mice and androgen-insensitive mice with testicular feminization. J Endocrinol. 1980;85(3):423–8.
12. Kellokumpu-Lehtinen P, Santti R, Pelliniemi LJ. Correlation of early cytodifferentiation of the human fetal prostate and Leydig cells. Anat Rec. 1980;196(3):263–73.
13. Cunha GR, et al. The endocrinology and developmental biology of the prostate. Endocr Rev. 1987;8(3):338–62.
14. Gao N, et al. The role of hepatocyte nuclear factor-3 alpha (Forkhead Box A1) and androgen receptor in transcriptional regulation of prostatic genes. Mol Endocrinol. 2003;17(8):1484–507.
15. Zhao JC, et al. FOXA1 acts upstream of GATA2 and AR in hormonal regulation of gene expression. Oncogene. 2016;35(33):4335–44.
16. Adams EJ, et al. FOXA1 mutations alter pioneering activity, differentiation and prostate cancer phenotypes. Nature. 2019;571(7765):408–12.
17. Bhatia-Gaur R, et al. Roles for Nkx3.1 in prostate development and cancer. Genes Dev. 1999;13(8):966–77.
18. Talos F, et al. A computational systems approach identifies synergistic specification genes that facilitate lineage conversion to prostate tissue. Nat Commun. 2017;8:14662.
19. Shapiro E, Hartanto V, Lepor H. Quantifying the smooth muscle content of the prostate using double-immunoenzymatic staining and color assisted image analysis. J Urol. 1992;147(4):1167–70.
20. Josso N. Physiology of sex differentiation. A guide to the understanding and management of the intersex child. In: The intersex child. Basel: Karger; 1981. p. 1–13.
21. Price D. Normal development of the prostate and seminal vesicles of the rat with a study of experimental postnatal modifications. Am J Anat. 1936;60(1):79–127.
22. Price D. Comparative aspects of development and structure in the prostate. Natl Cancer Inst Monogr. 1963;12:1–27.
23. Staack A, et al. Mouse urogenital development: a practical approach. Differentiation. 2003;71(7):402–13.
24. Georgas KM, et al. An illustrated anatomical ontology of the developing mouse lower urogenital tract. Development. 2015;142(10):1893–908.
25. Marker PC, et al. Hormonal, cellular, and molecular control of prostatic development. Dev Biol. 2003;253(2):165–74.
26. Lowsley OS. The development of the human prostate gland with reference to the development of other structures at the neck of the urinary bladder. Am J Anat. 1912;13(3):299–349.
27. Timms BG, Mohs TJ, Didio LJ. Ductal budding and branching patterns in the developing prostate. J Urol. 1994;151(5):1427–32.
28. Kellokumpu-Lehtinen P. Development of sexual dimorphism in human urogenital sinus complex. Biol Neonate. 1985;48(3):157–67.
29. Sugimura Y, et al. Whole-mount autoradiography study of DNA synthetic activity during postnatal development and androgen-induced regeneration in the mouse prostate. Biol Reprod. 1986;34(5):985–95.
30. Hayward SW, et al. Epithelial development in the rat ventral prostate, anterior prostate and seminal vesicle. Acta Anat. 1996;155(2):81–93.

31. Hayward SW, Brody JR, Cunha GR. An edgewise look at basal epithelial cells: three-dimensional views of the rat prostate, mammary gland and salivary gland. Differentiation. 1996;60(4):219–27.
32. Soeffing WJ, Timms BG. Localization of androgen receptor and cell-specific cytokeratins in basal cells of rat ventral prostate. J Androl. 1995;16(3):197–208.
33. Hayward SW, et al. Stromal development in the ventral prostate, anterior prostate and seminal vesicle of the rat. Acta Anat. 1996;155(2):94–103.
34. Timms BG. Prostate development: a historical perspective. Differentiation. 2008;76(6):565–77.
35. Sugimura Y, Cunha GR, Donjacour AA. Morphogenesis of ductal networks in the mouse prostate. Biol Reprod. 1986;34(5):961–71.
36. Donjacour AA, Cunha GR. The effect of androgen deprivation on branching morphogenesis in the mouse prostate. Dev Biol. 1988;128(1):1–14.
37. Evatt EJ. A contribution to the development of the prostate in man. J Anat Physiol. 1909;43(4):314–21.
38. McNeal JE. Anatomy of the prostate and morphogenesis of BPH. Prog Clin Biol Res. 1984;145:27–53.
39. Franks LM. Benign nodular hyperplasia of the prostate; a review. Ann R Coll Surg Engl. 1953;14(2):92–106.
40. Tisell LE, Salander H. Anatomy of the human prostate and its three paired lobes. Prog Clin Biol Res. 1984;145:55–65.
41. Amin MB, Tickoo SK. Diagnostic pathology: genitourinary. Amsterdam: Elsevier; 2022.
42. Ittmann M. Anatomy and histology of the human and murine prostate. Cold Spring Harb Perspect Med. 2018;8(5):a030346.
43. Hayashi N, et al. Morphological and functional heterogeneity in the rat prostatic gland. Biol Reprod. 1991;45(2):308–21.
44. Roy-Burman P, et al. Genetically defined mouse models that mimic natural aspects of human prostate cancer development. Endocr Relat Cancer. 2004;11(2):225–54.
45. Toivanen R, Shen MM. Prostate organogenesis: tissue induction, hormonal regulation and cell type specification. Development. 2017;144(8):1382–98.
46. Abate-Shen C, Shen MM. Molecular genetics of prostate cancer. Genes Dev. 2000;14(19):2410–34.
47. Oates R. Evaluation of the azoospermic male. Asian J Androl. 2012;14(1):82–7.
48. Garraway IP, et al. Human prostate sphere-forming cells represent a subset of basal epithelial cells capable of glandular regeneration in vivo. Prostate. 2010;70(5):491–501.
49. Alukal JP, Lepor H. Testosterone deficiency and the prostate. Urol Clin North Am. 2016;43(2):203–8.
50. Lee SH, Shen MM. Cell types of origin for prostate cancer. Curr Opin Cell Biol. 2015;37:35–41.
51. Castillejos-Molina RA, Gabilondo-Navarro FB. Prostate cancer. Salud Publica Mex. 2016;58(2):279–84.
52. Hynes PJ, Fraher JP. The development of the male genitourinary system. I. The origin of the urorectal septum and the formation of the perineum. Br J Plast Surg. 2004;57(1):27–36.
53. Huang YC, Chen F, Li X. Clarification of mammalian cloacal morphogenesis using high-resolution episcopic microscopy. Dev Biol. 2016;409(1):106–13.
54. Lung B, Cunha GR. Development of seminal vesicles and coagulating glands in neonatal mice. I. The morphogenetic effects of various hormonal conditions. Anat Rec. 1981;199(1):73–88.
55. Liu AY, et al. Cell-cell interaction in prostate gene regulation and cytodifferentiation. Proc Natl Acad Sci USA. 1997;94(20):10705–10.
56. Verhagen AP, et al. Differential expression of keratins in the basal and luminal compartments of rat prostatic epithelium during degeneration and regeneration. Prostate. 1988;13(1):25–38.
57. Wang Y, et al. Cell differentiation lineage in the prostate. Differentiation. 2001;68(4-5):270–9.

58. Signoretti S, et al. p63 is a prostate basal cell marker and is required for prostate development. Am J Pathol. 2000;157(6):1769–75.
59. Verhagen AP, et al. Colocalization of basal and luminal cell-type cytokeratins in human prostate cancer. Cancer Res. 1992;52(22):6182–7.
60. Mirosevich J, et al. Androgen receptor expression of proliferating basal and luminal cells in adult murine ventral prostate. J Endocrinol. 1999;162(3):341–50.
61. El-Alfy M, et al. Localization of type 5 17beta-hydroxysteroid dehydrogenase, 3beta-hydroxysteroid dehydrogenase, and androgen receptor in the human prostate by in situ hybridization and immunocytochemistry. Endocrinology. 1999;140(3):1481–91.
62. De Marzo AM, et al. Stem cell features of benign and malignant prostate epithelial cells. J Urol. 1998;160(6):2381–92.
63. Xue Y, et al. Identification of intermediate cell types by keratin expression in the developing human prostate. Prostate. 1998;34(4):292–301.
64. Abrahamsson PA. Neuroendocrine cells in tumour growth of the prostate. Endocr Relat Cancer. 1999;6(4):503–19.
65. Tuxhorn JA, Ayala GE, Rowley DR. Reactive stroma in prostate cancer progression. J Urol. 2001;166(6):2472–83.
66. Cutress ML, et al. Structural basis for the nuclear import of the human androgen receptor. J Cell Sci. 2008;121(7):957–68.
67. Ekman P. The prostate as an endocrine organ: androgens and estrogens. Prostate Suppl. 2000;10:14–8.
68. Quigley CA, et al. Androgen receptor defects: historical, clinical, and molecular perspectives. Endocr Rev. 1995;16(3):271–321.
69. Lai KP, et al. Suppressed prostate epithelial development with impaired branching morphogenesis in mice lacking stromal fibromuscular androgen receptor. Mol Endocrinol. 2012;26(1):52–66.
70. Allgeier SH, et al. Androgenic regulation of ventral epithelial bud number and pattern in mouse urogenital sinus. Dev Dyn. 2010;239(2):373–85.
71. Logan CY, Nusse R. The Wnt signaling pathway in development and disease. Annu Rev Cell Dev Biol. 2004;20:781–810.
72. Li VS, et al. Wnt signaling through inhibition of β-catenin degradation in an intact Axin1 complex. Cell. 2012;149(6):1245–56.
73. Mehta V, et al. Atlas of Wnt and R-spondin gene expression in the developing male mouse lower urogenital tract. Dev Dyn. 2011;240(11):2548–60.
74. Kruithof-de Julio M, et al. Canonical Wnt signaling regulates Nkx3.1 expression and luminal epithelial differentiation during prostate organogenesis. Dev Dyn. 2013;242(10):1160–71.
75. Simons BW, et al. Wnt signaling though beta-catenin is required for prostate lineage specification. Dev Biol. 2012;371(2):246–55.
76. Wang BE, et al. Regulation of epithelial branching morphogenesis and cancer cell growth of the prostate by Wnt signaling. PLoS One. 2008;3(5):e2186.
77. Veeman MT, Axelrod JD, Moon RT. A second canon. Functions and mechanisms of beta-catenin-independent Wnt signaling. Dev Cell. 2003;5(3):367–77.
78. Huang L, et al. The role of Wnt5a in prostate gland development. Dev Biol. 2009;328(2):188–99.
79. Lamm ML, et al. Mesenchymal factor bone morphogenetic protein 4 restricts ductal budding and branching morphogenesis in the developing prostate. Dev Biol. 2001;232(2):301–14.
80. Cancilla B, et al. Regulation of prostate branching morphogenesis by activin A and follistatin. Dev Biol. 2001;237(1):145–58.
81. He Y, et al. An indispensable role of androgen receptor in Wnt responsive cells during prostate development, maturation, and regeneration. Stem Cells. 2018;36(6):891–902.
82. Schweizer L, et al. The androgen receptor can signal through Wnt/beta-Catenin in prostate cancer cells as an adaptation mechanism to castration levels of androgens. BMC Cell Biol. 2008;9:4.

83. Li Y, et al. LEF1 in androgen-independent prostate cancer: regulation of androgen receptor expression, prostate cancer growth, and invasion. Cancer Res. 2009;69(8):3332–8.
84. Mehta V, et al. Beta-catenin (CTNNB1) induces Bmp expression in urogenital sinus epithelium and participates in prostatic bud initiation and patterning. Dev Biol. 2013;376(2):125–35.
85. Wei X, et al. Spatially restricted stromal Wnt signaling restrains prostate epithelial progenitor growth through direct and indirect mechanisms. Cell Stem Cell. 2019;24(5):753–68.
86. Placencio VR, et al. Stromal transforming growth factor-beta signaling mediates prostatic response to androgen ablation by paracrine Wnt activity. Cancer Res. 2008;68(12):4709–18.
87. Tzelepi V. Prostate cancer: pathophysiology, pathology and therapy. Cancer. 2022;15(1):46.
88. Siegel RL, et al. Cancer statistics, 2022. CA Cancer J Clin. 2022;72(1):7–33.
89. Dyba T, et al. The European cancer burden in 2020: incidence and mortality estimates for 40 countries and 25 major cancers. Eur J Cancer. 2021;157:308–47.
90. Sung H, et al. Global cancer statistics 2020: GLOBOCAN estimates of incidence and mortality worldwide for 36 cancers in 185 countries. CA Cancer J Clin. 2021;71(3):209–49.
91. Johansson JE, et al. Natural history of early, localized prostate cancer. JAMA. 2004;291(22):2713–9.
92. Cimadamore A, et al. Prostate cancer in 2021: novelties in prognostic and therapeutic biomarker evaluation. Cancer. 2021;13(14):3471.
93. Rawla P. Epidemiology of prostate cancer. World J Oncol. 2019;10(2):63–89.
94. Chan JM, Gann PH, Giovannucci EL. Role of diet in prostate cancer development and progression. J Clin Oncol. 2005;23(32):8152–60.
95. Willis MS, Wians FH. The role of nutrition in preventing prostate cancer: a review of the proposed mechanism of action of various dietary substances. Clin Chim Acta. 2003;330(1-2):57–83.
96. Thankamony AP, et al. Lineage plasticity in cancer: the tale of a skin-walker. Cancer. 2021;13(14):3602.
97. Papanikolaou S, et al. Cell plasticity and prostate cancer: the role of epithelial-mesenchymal transition in tumor progression, invasion, metastasis and cancer therapy resistance. Cancer. 2021;13(11):2795.
98. Wasim S, Lee SY, Kim J. Complexities of prostate cancer. Int J Mol Sci. 2022;23(22):14257.
99. Rebello RJ, et al. Prostate cancer. Nat Rev Dis Primers. 2021;7(1):9.
100. Siegel RL, Miller KD, Jemal A. Cancer statistics, 2018. CA Cancer J Clin. 2018;68(1):7–30.
101. Sandhu S, et al. Prostate cancer. Lancet. 2021;398(10305):1075–90.
102. Berish RB, et al. Translational models of prostate cancer bone metastasis. Nat Rev Urol. 2018;15(7):403–21.
103. Virgo KS, et al. Second-line hormonal therapy for men with chemotherapy-Naïve, Castration-Resistant Prostate Cancer: American Society of Clinical Oncology Provisional Clinical Opinion. J Clin Oncol. 2017;35(17):1952–64.
104. Ritch CR, Cookson MS. Advances in the management of castration resistant prostate cancer. BMJ. 2016;355:i4405.
105. Boyd LK, Mao X, Lu YJ. The complexity of prostate cancer: genomic alterations and heterogeneity. Nat Rev Urol. 2012;9(11):652–64.
106. Cooper CS, et al. Analysis of the genetic phylogeny of multifocal prostate cancer identifies multiple independent clonal expansions in neoplastic and morphologically normal prostate tissue. Nat Genet. 2015;47(4):367–72.
107. Boyd LK, et al. High-resolution genome-wide copy-number analysis suggests a monoclonal origin of multifocal prostate cancer. Genes Chromosomes Cancer. 2012;51(6):579–89.
108. Berglund E, et al. Spatial maps of prostate cancer transcriptomes reveal an unexplored landscape of heterogeneity. Nat Commun. 2018;9(1):2419.
109. Shoag J, Barbieri CE. Clinical variability and molecular heterogeneity in prostate cancer. Asian J Androl. 2016;18(4):543–8.
110. Espiritu SMG, et al. The evolutionary landscape of localized prostate cancers drives clinical aggression. Cell. 2018;173(4):1003–13.

Chapter 2
Epidemiology, Risk Factors and Histopathological Profile of Prostate Cancer

Mehrdad Hashemi, Farnaz Azizi, Niloofar AbolfathyNajmabady, Samira Moradi, Munes Ghorbanalinia, Sima Orouei, Behdokht Jamali, Rasoul Raesi, Faramarz Khosravi, Maliheh Entezari, Mina Alimohammadi, Kiavash Hushmandi, and Mitra Behroozaghdam

Abstract An estimated 366,000 men lose their lives to prostate cancer every year, while an additional 1.6 million men receive a prostate cancer diagnosis. The current level of evidence regarding several dietary, lifestyle, and genetic variables linked to the risk of prostate cancer is reviewed in this review. Among male cancers, prostate

---

M. Hashemi · M. Entezari
Farhikhtegan Medical Convergence Sciences Research Center, Farhikhtegan Hospital Tehran Medical Sciences, Islamic Azad University, Tehran, Iran

Faculty of Advanced Science and Technology, Department of Genetics, Tehran Medical Sciences, Islamic Azad University, Tehran, Iran

F. Azizi · M. Ghorbanalinia · F. Khosravi · M. Behroozaghdam (✉)
Farhikhtegan Medical Convergence Sciences Research Center, Farhikhtegan Hospital Tehran Medical Sciences, Islamic Azad University, Tehran, Iran

N. AbolfathyNajmabady · S. Orouei
Department of Biology, Science and Research Branch, Islamic Azad University, Tehran, Iran

S. Moradi
Hormozgan University of Medical Sciences, Bandar Abbas, Hormozgan, Iran

B. Jamali
Department of Microbiology and Genetics, Kherad Institute of Higher Education, Bushehr, Iran

R. Raesi
Department of Nursing, Torbat Jam Faculty of Medical Sciences, Torbat Jam, Iran

Department of Health Services Management, Mashhad University of Medical Sciences, Mashhad, Iran

M. Alimohammadi
Department of Immunology, School of Medicine, Shahid Beheshti University of Medical Sciences, Tehran, Iran

K. Hushmandi
Department of Epidemiology, University of Tehran, Tehran, Iran

G. Sethi et al. (eds.), *Prostate Cancer: Molecular Events and Therapeutic Modalities*, https://doi.org/10.1007/978-981-97-4612-5_2

cancer ranks second in incidence and fifth in mortality rates globally. Early stages of prostate cancer may not cause any symptoms at all, and the disease tends to progress slowly, so regular monitoring may be all that's needed to catch it early. There is a substantial correlation between age and prostate cancer incidence and fatality rates, with the greatest incidence observed in males aged 65 and up. When compared to white men, African-American men experience a higher incidence rate and a more aggressive form of prostate cancer. A lower risk of prostate cancer can be achieved by reducing consumption of high-fat meals, increasing consumption of vegetables and fruits, and increasing exercise, yet there is currently no data on how to prevent this disease. African-American men and men with a family history of the disease should undergo screening at the age of 45.

Keywords Prostate cancer · Diet · Smoking · Mortality · Incidence

2.1 Introduction

The last 10 years have seen tremendous improvement in the treatment of prostate cancer [1]. Newly diagnosed cases of prostate cancer are mostly localized (80% of all cases), with a small percentage of cases being progressed or metastatic [2]. Moreover, survival rates range from 26% to 30% at 5 years, which is significantly lower than the extremely high rates seen in localized disease [3]. The extreme sensitivity of prostate cancer cells to androgen pathway modification is a feature exclusive to this malignancy [4, 5]. In addition, metabolites of testosterone promote the proliferation of prostate cancer cells, whereas castration and other hormonal manipulations can cause the death of prostate cancer cells [6]. Therefore, androgen deprivation is the foundation of the first line of defense against metastatic prostate cancer. This is done by reducing the amount of testosterone in the blood to a level below 50 ng/dL, therefore cutting off the cells' main source of energy for growth [7]. In most situations, there are no early or initial symptoms. However, in later stages, you may experience symptoms including exhaustion from anemia, discomfort in your bones, paralysis from spinal metastases, or renal failure from blockages in both ureters.

It should be mentioned that medications or surgical castrations, which make up androgen deprivation therapy (ADT), have long been the mainstay of treatment for individuals with metastatic prostate cancer. There is a stage called castration resistance that some men experience. It's when their prostate cancer cells figure out how to avoid ADT and keep growing even when testosterone levels are low. People diagnosed with castration-resistant prostate cancer (CRPC) often don't make it past the first 2 or 4 years after the diagnosis because the illness progresses so quickly [8, 9]. Docetaxel treatment significantly improved survival rates compared to placebo in multiple landmark randomized controlled trials (RCTs) (TAX-327 and SWOG 9916) that were completed between 2004 and 2005 for patients with metastatic CRPC (mCRPC). In two recent landmark trials that examined hormone-sensitive disorders, chemohormonal therapy was compared to ADT alone, while STAMPEDE and CHAARTED focused on chemotherapy and androgen deprivation therapy, respectively [10, 11]. Furthermore, studies have demonstrated that patients with hormone-sensitive prostate cancer who get abiraterone acetate + prednisone alongside ADT have a higher likelihood of survival compared to those who receive ADT alone [12, 13]. These trials, which have shown a statistically significant improvement in OS in every single one, have changed the way we think about handling metastatic prostate cancer. Survival benefits with innovative medications before and after docetaxel-based treatment in the castration-resistant scenario have been demonstrated in multiple key randomized controlled studies (RCTs) since 2010 and practically every year thereafter. The FDA has authorized six new medicines for the treatment of metastatic and non-metastatic (M0) CRPC, each with its own distinct mechanism of action, based on the results of these studies: sipuleucel-T, abiraterone acetate, enzalutamide, cabazitaxel, radium-223, and apalutamide. Apalutamide and enzalutamide were recently approved for the treatment of metastatic CRPC (M0) after two randomized controlled studies (RCTs)—SPARTAN and PROSPER—demonstrated a significant improvement in metastasis-free survival (MFS) [14, 15]. Prior to this research, no medications have been approved for M0 CRPC.

Although PSA testing for screening is still debatable, transrectal ultrasound-guided (TRUS) prostate tissue biopsies and prostate-specific antigen (PSA) testing are the mainstays of diagnosis [16, 17]. Modern methods of diagnosis encompass MRI imaging, PIRADS scoring, exosome testing, genetic analysis, the "4K" test, PCA3 urine testing, Prostate Health Index (PHI) scoring, MRI-TRUS fusion guided biopsies, and free and total PSA levels [18]. Cancer that has not spread beyond the prostate is said to be confined and may be treatable [19]. Furthermore, an enormous variety of targeted therapies, including bisphosphonates, hormone treatment, chemotherapy, radiopharmaceuticals, immunotherapy, focused radiation, and pain medicines, can be employed when the illness has progressed to other parts of the body or beyond the prostate. The degree of malignancy, tumor histology, age, and any comorbid health issues all play a role in the final prognosis [20]. Figure 2.1 shows the natural history of prostate cancer.

2.2 Epidemiology of Prostate Cancer

Prostate cancer is the main reason of cancer-related deaths and incidence throughout the world [21, 22]. There is a remarkable disparity in the incidence and mortality rates of prostate cancer across different regions. To better understand the epidemiology of prostate cancer, it is helpful to look at trends in the disease's occurrence and mortality rates over different populations and time periods. This will help elucidate the role that personal risk factors and screening habits play in this epidemic.

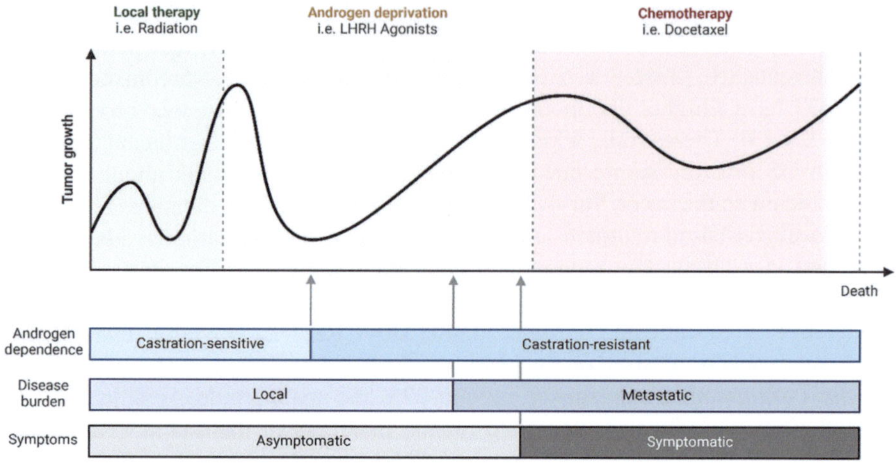

Fig. 2.1 The natural history of prostate cancer (Biorender.com)

2.2.1 *Incidence*

About 1.6 million new instances of prostate cancer were reported in 2015, making it the most frequent cancer among men worldwide [23]. Furthermore, it has been demonstrated that developed nations have an alarmingly high prostate cancer rate. In countries with a low-middle sociodemographic index, the possibility of a prostate cancer diagnosis by the age of 79 is one in 47, while in countries with a high sociodemographic index, it is one in six [23]. With an expected 180,890 new cases identified in 2016, prostate cancer remains the top cause of cancer incidence in the US [24].

Additionally, there is a lot of variance in prostate cancer incidence around the world. Based on two studies in this field, the age-adjusted incidence rates for men residing in their native countries had the lowest rate, while those of African-American men in the US had the highest rate [21, 24]. Disparities in diagnostic rigor caused by PSA screening practice contribute to the observed disparity in incidence rates among populations. Nevertheless, there is evidence that lifestyle variables may play a role in disease risk, as there was regional variance in prostate cancer incidence before PSA screening was introduced. It is worth mentioning that investigations on migration also provide credence to the idea that people's way of life has a part. As an example, men whose home countries have lower rates of prostate cancer tend to have higher rates of both the disease's incidence and death when they relocate to nations with higher rates of both [25, 26].

The influence of PSA screening on the epidemiology of prostate cancer is demonstrated by patterns of change in incidence rates over time on a global scale. To put it another way, the world's age-adjusted incidence rates have risen globally during the previous 40 years. It is worth mentioning that this rising tendency has coincided with the adoption of PSA screening in specific areas, such as Australia, Europe, and the US. Take the United States as a good example. It was in the early 1990s, when PSA screening was first used at the population level, that prostate cancer incidence peaked. There has been a change in the stage of diagnosis due to the introduction of PSA screening; now, more men are diagnosed with localized disease. Also, men are getting their diagnoses earlier due to the prostate cancer lead time, which is predicted to be 3–10 years [27]. On top of that one such negative effect of PSA screening is the rise in the number of malignancies that are overdiagnosed, meaning they would not have been clinically noticeable or caused death if screening hadn't been done [28, 29]. On the other hand, PSA testing is still not generally used, therefore there have been areas where incidence rates have increased, such as Japan and a few other nations in Eastern Europe and Asia [30]. Furthermore, environmental and lifestyle variables, which will be covered later in this chapter, may potentially impact the incidence of prostate cancer, according to the trend in these places.

2.2.2 *Survival*

Even though prostate cancer is quite common, a significant number of instances are only discovered when the cancer has already spread within the prostate region. With a prostate cancer diagnosis, the 5-year survival rate for American males is close to 98%. Moreover, a 5-year survival rate of 83% was recorded in the Eurocare 5 study, which followed men diagnosed with prostate cancer between 2003 and 2007 [31]. In Eastern European countries, the survival rate was 76%, whereas in Southern and Central European countries, it was 88%. While survival rates have gone up across the board in Europe, they've been steadily rising in Eastern European nations [32].

The second biggest cause of cancer mortality among males in the USA is prostate cancer, even though science has made a lot of strides in recent decades to uncover the molecular pathways and risk factors linked with the disease [31]. Finally, the rule of thumb for all malignancies is that the sooner they are detected, the better the chances of successfully treating them and keeping people disease-free. However, since most prostate cancers progress slowly and indolently (known as "low-risk" tumors), men can safely endure active surveillance or careful waiting instead of getting rapid treatment, which would involve potential side effects.

2.2.3 *Mortality*

With 366,000 fatalities and 6.3 million disability-adjusted life years in 2015, prostate cancer is distinguished as the fifth most prominent cause of cancer-related deaths worldwide [23]. Although death rates vary less than incidence levels among nations, there are clear disparities in death patterns between wealthy and poor areas. Moreover, the fatality rates from prostate cancer are the most significant in the Caribbean and Middle and Southern Africa, while they are lowest in Eastern and

South-Central Asia. On top of that an estimated 26,120 men would lose their lives to cancer in the US in 2016, with prostate cancer ranking second [24]. While the exact causes of the decline in prostate cancer deaths in the United States and other Westernized nations remain unknown, it is intriguing to note that this trend has occurred. One probable explanation for the drop in death rates in these nations is the widespread use of prostate-specific antigen (PSA) screening, which allows for early diagnosis and treatment. On the other side, prostate cancer mortality rates have been higher in regions where screening is less common, like Africa [33]. This needs further studies to figure out why there are such big differences in prostate cancer deaths across different regions.

Another point to consider is that alterations in the death rate are induced by variations in both the occurrence of prostate cancer and the survival rate of patients. The incidence-to-mortality ratio varies remarkably from one region to another; for example, it is 10:1 in North America, 2:1 in Australia, and nearly equal in some Caribbean and African countries (1.2:1). One possible explanation for these discrepancies is that nations with PSA screening tend to diagnose more slow-growing malignancies [34, 35] and, on the other hand, countries with lower diagnostic intensity tend to have disease symptoms manifest later. This disease's high prevalence reflects the enormity of the burden produced by prostate cancer. In addition, prostate cancer accounts for 25% of all prevalent malignancies due to its high incidence and extended survival rate, making it the most common cancer type in the 5-year period [21]. The number of men living with a prostate cancer diagnosis exceeds four million globally; 2.7 million of these guys reside in the US alone [36]. The distribution of resources for men receiving treatment or monitoring for this condition is noticeably affected by this.

2.3 Risk Factors of Prostate Cancer

Older age, being African-American, and having a positive family history of prostate cancer are the only known risk factors for the overall incidence of prostate cancer. Newer evidence of hereditary susceptibility to prostate cancer has come from genome-wide association studies (GWAS). There are over 180 verified genetic risk loci in populations with a varied range of ethnic backgrounds [37, 38]. The likelihood of developing total prostate cancer appears to rise with increasing stature, according to the available data [39]. Although these characteristics cannot be changed, they show potential processes in prostate cancer development and could be used to stratify those at risk of getting the disease.

Numerous aspects of personal biology and lifestyle affect the likelihood of getting prostate cancer and the probability of surviving the disease, as proven in epidemiologic studies of this disease. Moreover, our present knowledge of risk factors suggests approaches to identify high-risk individuals and employ behavior change to decline the disease burden, however many mysteries remain regarding the origin of this widespread disease. On top of that prostate cancer, presents with a wide range of symptoms and characteristics. Although some men experience a more aggressive type of prostate cancer, the majority of men experience a more slow-growing or benign condition. This disease's underlying etiology reflects the clinical heterogeneity as well. Several risk variables have distinct relationships with mild disease and deadly disease [40]. As a result, distinguishing between risk factors for prostate cancer in its early stages and those for more advanced or deadly forms is crucial in the field of prostate cancer epidemiology.

Since PSA screening may affect the observed relationships between risk factors and prostate cancer, it is of significant importance to take it into account when evaluating evidence for prostate cancer risk factors in epidemiologic research. On the one hand, prostate cancer risk factors may influence the disease at every stage of its pathogenesis, from initial cancer development to metastases and ultimately death. Therefore, clinical aspects of the disease, including tumor grade or stage, may influence the link between a factor and prostate cancer risk [41]. The biological basis for the idea that the risk factors for less aggressive prostate cancer would vary from those for more aggressive prostate cancer is strong. On top of that, PSA testing could be misleading because men who screen regularly are generally healthy, which has nothing to do with the likelihood that they will get prostate cancer. Examining how much data is derived from PSA screening is essential for assessing prostate cancer epidemiology research.

Racially and ethnically, there are noticeable disparities in the rates of prostate cancer and mortality. One example is the racial disparity in prostate cancer incidence rates in the US; Black men have three times the risk of white men. A further 2.4 times higher rate of prostate cancer-related mortality occurs among black men in the US compared to white men [24]. Asian/Pacific Islanders, American Indian/Alaskan Native, and Hispanic men have a reduced incidence and mortality rate of prostate cancer compared to non-Hispanic white men [24]. To find out what's causing these differences, more research is required. Disparities in life expectancy may, at least in part, be attributable to variations in diagnostic modalities and ease of access to care [42]. It is possible that inherited variables contribute to racial and ethnic disparities in prostate cancer incidence rates, since there are variations in the frequency of several genetic risk loci for the disease among different groups of people [43].

Furthermore, a high correlation between a personal or family history of prostate cancer and an increased risk of developing the disease has been discovered in genetic investigations. To express it another way, having a father or brother diagnosed with prostate cancer increases a man's risk of prostate cancer by two to three times compared to a man without a positive family history, and by nearly nine times for males with both [44]. The risk of fatal prostate cancer has also been found to be associated with this. The chance of dying from prostate cancer is two times higher for men whose father or brother had the disease compared to men whose cancer was detected in a family without a history of the disease [45]. A high heritability estimate of 57% is supported by additional evidence from twin studies, which demonstrate that shared genetic variables account for a significant portion of familial aggregation of prostate cancer [46, 47]. Approximately one-third of the heritability can be explained by the over 105 prostate cancer risk loci that have been validated across several studies [37, 48]. The fact that most germline risk loci have weak associations with prostate cancer [49, 50], which could indicate that hereditary factors play a role early on in the development of prostate cancer, is intriguing.

In general, prostate cancer risk is significantly higher in older men. It is uncommon for men under the age of 40 to develop prostate cancer. Similar to other epithelial malignancies, the incidence rate of prostate cancer spikes sharply beyond the age of 55. Both in less developed and more developed parts of the world, this pattern is reflected in the prostate cancer rates [21]. In addition, ten percent of American men with prostate cancer diagnoses in 2012 were younger than 55 years old; prostate cancer that develops in younger men may have a different cause and presentation than older men [51]. As a result of detecting prostate cancer before symptoms appear, the PSA screening procedure adds approximately 10 years to the detection time. Since PSA screening became standard practice in the US, the median age of diagnosis for prostate cancer has risen, and it is now 66 years old [24].

2.3.1 Smoking

There is a tremendous public health concern regarding the link between smoking and malignancies, particularly prostate cancer. There is "suggestive" evidence that smoking enhances the chance of dying from prostate cancer, advanced disease, and less-well-differentiated cancer, based on the most recent report from the US Surgeon General in 2014 [52]. To put it another way, with 5366 men diagnosed with prostate cancer followed prospectively for 22 years and 524 deaths from the disease recorded, HPFS was the biggest study to investigate this subject. Once relevant confounders were taken into account, the risk of prostate cancer mortality was 60% greater for men who smoked compared to those who never smoked (HR 1.61; 95% CI: 1.11–2.32) [53]. Subsequent adjustments for prostate cancer grade and stage did not reduce the high connection for current smoking. A weakening of this correlation, however, points to a potential mediating role for stage and grade in the smoking-related impact on prostate cancer mortality. Compared to nonsmokers, current smokers report fewer PSA tests, which may delay cancer diagnosis and treatment for smokers. Tobacco use may also affect the death rate from prostate cancer by altering the patient's reaction to treatment. Patients with prostate cancer who smoke had poorer results after radiotherapy, androgen deprivation therapy (ADT), and radical prostatectomy compared to nonsmokers in multiple investigations [54–57].

In addition, evidence from multiple studies on immigrants from low-risk developing nations to high-risk industrialized countries suggests that dietary factors play a significant role in the development of prostate cancer. To explain further, these studies demonstrated that the transition to a "westernized" lifestyle was associated with an increase in prostate cancer incidence. Environmental factors likely play a significant role, since studies have revealed that African Americans have a prostate cancer incidence rate that is 40 times higher than that of Africans, and that Chinese men living in the USA have an incidence rate that is 16 times higher than that of men in China [58, 59]. Numerous studies have linked specific meals to an increased risk of disease, while others have shown no such link.

Moreover, dangerous animal fat prostate mortality is positively correlated with the per capita consumption of meat, fat, and dairy items, according to multiple ecological studies [60, 61]. A recent case-control research in men and women younger than 60 years old indicated that a high total fat diet was linked to a significantly higher risk of prostate cancer [62]. A number of hypothesized molecular pathways link consumption of saturated animal fats to an increased risk of prostate cancer have been identified: (1) enhancing androgen-induced prostate cancer; (2) elevating lipid-related reactive oxygen species (ROS) and leukotrienes and prostaglandins levels; and (3) elevating insulin growth factor, basal metabolism, and tumor multiplicity [31].

Furthermore, excessive consumption of saturated animal fat, which is high in calories, has been found to promote the proliferation of prostate cancer cells by elevating circulating androgen levels [63, 64]. Even more so, vegetarians and those on low-fat or high-fat diets had lower levels of testosterone post-prandial, according to randomized cross-over studies [65]. Lastly, a number of studies have shown that testosterone levels are decreased by changing lipid levels in response to a low-fat diet [66, 67].

The levels of reactive oxygen species (ROS) and oxidative stress are both amplified in a fatty diet, which means that excess fat is attacking cells and damaging their DNA. In addition, studies in mice have shown that lipid metabolism and its metabolite play a role and that dietary fat significantly affects the progression of prostate cancer. Case in point: some research found no correlation between Western diet and tumor growth or survival in mice, while other studies found that low-fat corn-oil diets slowed the growth of cancer cells in mice, implying that the kind and quantity of fat are key factors [68].

Corn oil contains a high concentration of linoleic acid, an omega-6 fatty acid, which may have a carcinogenic effect. A number of pro-inflammatory prostaglandins (PG) are formed from arachidonic acid, a linoleic acid metabolite. These include PGE2, which promotes cell proliferation, and 5-hydroxyeicosatetraenoic acid, which is more abundant in aggressive prostate cancer, and is produced by the action of 5-lipoxygenase. Less omega-6 fatty acid consumption is associated with a lower risk of cancer. Unlike omega-6 fatty acids, which promote inflammation, omega-3 fatty acids have been shown to inhibit the progression of cancer [69].

Meat of red color research has linked the use of meat in the diet to an increased risk of prostate cancer, specifically by connecting the rate of cancer incidence and mortality to the amount of meat consumed per capita [70]. A greater risk of prostate cancer was associated with weekly consumption of five or more servings of processed meat, according to research by Rohrmann and colleagues [71]. No correlation was found between a high red meat intake and an elevated prostate risk in males of African-American descent. Red meat consumed by individuals who cooked it at high temperatures, however, raised the incidence of non-advanced prostate cancer by 20% [72]. An aromatic hydrocarbon and a carcinogenic heterocyclic amine can be formed when food is cooked at higher temperatures (125–300 °C) [73, 74]. Lipid peroxidation and DNA damage due to free radical generation can be induced by N-nitroso compounds that are formed when meat is grilled or barbecued [75, 76].

Some foods that contain calcium include milk and other dairy products. Many studies have found an increased risk of prostate cancer in men who regularly consume dairy products [77–79]. The risk of prostate cancer is increased in males who consume calcium supplements or dairy products. Researchers found that the risk of prostate cancer increased in correlation with calcium intake of more than 2000 mg daily. The Health Professional Follow-Up Study meticulously analyzed the protein, calcium, and animal product consumption of 47,885 male participants [79]. Extremely high calcium consumption was linked to 5861 cases of prostate cancer detected after a 24-year follow-up [80].

Garden Veggies: There has been mixed research on the effects of dietary fat on prostate cancer risk, but there is significant evidence that eating brassica vegetables (such as broccoli, brussels sprouts, cauliflower, cabbage, and turnips) lowers that risk. A number of phytochemicals, including indole-3-carbinol, phenyethyl isothiocyanate, and sulforaphane, are responsible for the anticancer effects of crucifers [81]. Researchers in the United States have found that eating a lot of broccoli may reduce the risk of prostate cancer [82]. Other investigations, however, have failed to find that brassica crops have any anticancer properties [83, 84].

Soy products for dietary purposes with green tea: Asian countries have a far lower prostate cancer incidence rate than North American ones. This disparity has sparked curiosity about the possible chemo-preventive effects of soy and green tea, two staples of Asian diets. Prostate cancer risk is lower in people who drink soy and green tea, according to research [85, 86]. As an example, catechins in green tea and isoflavones in soybeans both decrease metastasis [87, 88] and several stages of carcinogenesis [89, 90]. Less IGF-1 is produced by green tea polyphenols as well [91, 92].

Lycopene supplements and tomatoes: Garlic appears to lower prostate cancer risk. Among their many health benefits is the high concentration of lycopene, an antioxidant and cancer preventive [93, 94]. In addition to interacting with androgen receptors, lycopene counteracts dihydrotestosterone's actions and blocks the activation of insulin growth factor (IGF-I) via Akt, GSK3β, and tyrosine phosphorylation of GSK3 [95].

Both eating tomato products and getting enough lycopene were linked to a lower incidence of prostate cancer [41]. Given the Health Professional Follow-Up Study, eating 2–3 cups of tomato sauce weekly reduces the incidence of prostate cancer [79]. Only when combined with selenium and vitamin E was lycopene able to decrease prostate cancer incidence in the Lady transgenic mice model, as shown by Venkateswaran and Klotz [96].

Lycopene, however, failed to show any therapeutic advantage in an open phase II trial of advanced prostate cancer [97]. The findings of two further small-scale epidemiological investigations were in line with this. Research into the possible link between tomato consumption and prostate cancer risk has to be conducted.

On top of that the effects of weight across different stages of life have been the subject of further research. Except for a single study in a multiethnic cohort, there doesn't seem to be any correlation between weight gain between early adulthood (about 18 or 21 years old) and the risk of prostate cancer in middle age [98]. Men with prostate cancer who dropped weight at the time of diagnosis and a few months later had a lower chance of recurrence, but men who gained weight following prostatectomy were more likely to experience recurrence [99]. Prevention measures for prostate cancer can be better informed by further research into the mechanisms that underlie the correlations between obesity and weight change.

2.3.2 Height

There is substantial evidence for advanced illness and some indication that a higher stature may raise the risk of prostate cancer in general. There was a 1.09 (95% CI: 1.06–1.12) relative risk of prostate cancer overall and a 1.12 (95% CI: 1.05–1.19) related risk of advanced prostate cancer per 10 cm of height, according to a meta-analysis of 58 studies [100]. Comparing results from before and during the PSA period revealed similar patterns. A higher risk of advanced or fatal prostate cancer was associated with a higher height in the Health-Professionals Follow-up Study but no such association was found for total prostate cancer [101]. Nonetheless, there was no correlation between stature and the likelihood of developing complete or advanced prostate cancer in a prospective trial with a multiethnic group [98]. Height is not a modifiable risk factor, but understanding its impact on prostate cancer helps shed light on the disease's biology. The fact that adult height is a reflection of exposure to growth hormones like insulin-like growth factor 1 (IGF-1) in childhood may explain this correlation. Although there is no correlation between birth weight and prostate cancer risk, the fact that the prostate grows rapidly and matures during adolescence raises the possibility that this developmental period is the etiologically significant one [100].

2.3.3 Physical Activity

The incidence of prostate cancer, especially in advanced and deadly forms, is moderately inversely related to physical activity. Moreover, among males aged 65 and up in the HPFS cohort, the risk of advanced prostate cancer was 77% lower in the highest quintile of vigorous activity [102]. Men in the CPS-II cohort who were very active for fun were 31% less likely to develop aggressive prostate cancer than men in the control group who were not as active for fun [103]. On the other hand, the EPIC cohort found no correlation between leisure activity and advanced prostate cancer risk, but an inverse connection between occupational activity and risk [104].

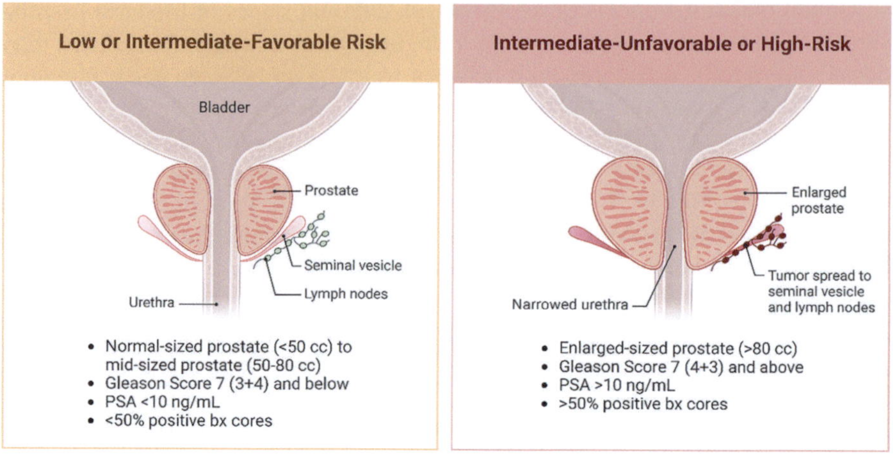

Fig. 2.2 The prostate cancer risk assessment (Biorender.com)

Men in the reference group might be as active as 25 MET hours per week, but the EPIC cohort had far greater activity levels.

2.3.4 *Coffee*

The epidemiology of prostate cancer has looked at coffee a lot, but most of the research has looked at total prostate cancer and found nothing. It should be mentioned that researchers discovered an inverse correlation when looking at the probability of fatal or advanced disease [105–107]. Also, Discacciati and colleagues found an inverse correlation with high-grade (Gleason 8–10) disease and an RR of 0.89 (95% CI: 0.82–0.97) for total prostate per three cups/day of coffee in their meta-analysis [108]. Furthermore, there may be underlying mechanisms linking coffee consumption to the advancement of prostate cancer among the many physiologically active chemicals found in coffee. For instance, as one of the most powerful antioxidant dietary components, coffee has been associated in both animal and observational studies with enhanced glucose metabolism and insulin secretion. Figure 2.2 shows the prostate cancer risk assessment.

2.4 Histopathological Profile of Prostate Cancer

In addition to the extraprostatic expansion of glands, histological evidence of perineural invasion, collagenous micronodules, and glomeruloid intraglandular projections inside the prostate are histologically thought to be diagnostic of prostatic carcinoma [109, 110]. Moreover, ectopic benign prostatic glands have been discovered in numerous anatomic sites outside the prostate, including the testis, epididymis, bladder, penile urethra, seminal vesicles, root of the penis, subvesical space, retrovesical space, pericolonic fat and submucosa, perirectal fat, urachal remnant, and spleen [111]. While the presence of prostatic glands outside the prostate is typically indicative of malignancy, it is useful to be aware of the wide variety of possible locations.

Prostate cancer is characterized by perineural invasion. The majority of cases, ranging from 84% to 94% according to the literature, involve perineural invasion of the whole prostate gland [112, 113]. Although only 11% of instances in a screening sample with smaller lower-stage tumors exhibited perineural invasion, over 25% of cases in needle core biopsy do [114]. For small or minimal amounts of carcinoma (<1 mm in maximum dimension) in needle biopsy tissue, the diagnostic value of perineural invasion is reduced to less than 2% due to the occurrence dropping to as low as 2% in this context [115, 116]. On the other hand, cancer cannot be conclusively diagnosed just by looking for prostatic glands close to a nerve. It is possible for benign prostatic glands to surround or touch nerves [117]. To differentiate between benign and malignant perineural epithelium, one should look at the cytologic characteristics of the epithelial cells surrounding a nerve.

In addition, as an uncommon reaction to invasive prostate cancer, collagenous micronodules (or mucinous fibroplasia) are tiny clusters of hyalinized stroma [109, 118, 119]. They are frequently linked to an abundance of mucin production, albeit this is not always the case. In addition to being mostly collagenous and paucicellular, the micronodules do include a small number of elongated fibroblastic nuclei. True nodules, masses with a lobule or two, or even streaks and threads of collagenous tissue inside mucinous pools can all be formed by collagen. The micronodules might be found in the glandular lumina or in the stroma surrounding adenocarcinomatous glands. Unfortunately, collagenous micronodules are only detected in a small percentage of carcinoma needle biopsies (1%–2%) [115, 118, 120] and a much higher percentage (13–22%) of carcinomas in whole glands in radical prostatectomy specimens [118, 121], so their diagnostic utility is somewhat limited. They are linked to adenocarcinomas with Gleason patterns 3 or 4 [122].

In prostatic adenocarcinoma, acini can develop glomerulations, which are epithelial clumps resembling renal glomeruli [109]. It is believed that carcinoma is the only tumor type that exhibits this pattern of epithelial development within the lumen [123]. The reason behind this is clearly manifest, since they only appear in 3–15% of adenocarcinoma needle biopsies and 5% of radical prostatectomies, glomerulations do not provide a very strong diagnostic picture [120, 123]. When examined under a microscope, glomeruloid bodies reveal cancerous glands that range in size from tiny to medium, with tufts that are either spherical or ball-shaped. In most cases, the glomeruloid bodies make up only a small percentage of the cancer. All things considered, they stand for a superior Gleason pattern 4 [124].

Furthermore, it is possible to consider lymphovascular space invasion by prostatic epithelial cells as a hallmark of a cancer diagnosis. Needle's core tissue is an unusual place to locate this. In 5–53% of subjects undergoing radical prostatectomy,

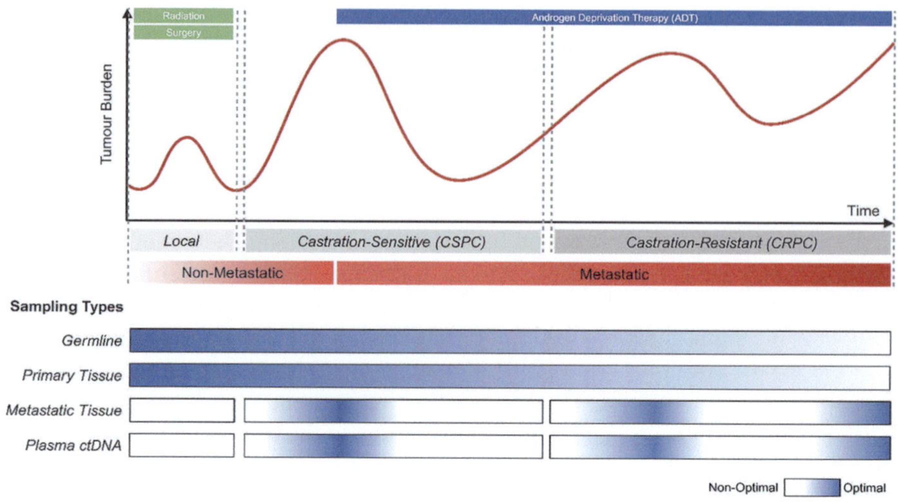

Fig. 2.3 The treatment landscape of prostate cancer (Biorender.com)

lymphovascular invasion is discovered. There is an association between greater grade, volume, and stage of intraprostatic lymphovascular invasion and an increased chance of biochemical failure, distant metastases, and overall survival following radical prostatectomy [125, 126]. To differentiate between real lymphovascular invasion and other possible causes such as benign gland displacement into lymphovascular spaces, cancer pressing on vascular spaces, or false separation of malignant glands from stroma [127], immunohistochemistry for endothelial cells with antibodies to CD31 or podoplanin (D2–40) may be necessary. Figure 2.3 shows the treatment procedure for prostate cancer.

2.5 Conclusion and Perspectives

After lung cancer, prostate cancer is the second most frequent malignancy among men. Biomarkers like PSA that have a positive correlation with prostate cancer diagnosis have changed the way this illness is studied epidemiologically. Actually, the incidence of prostate cancer in the United States has doubled since the late 1980s, when PSA tests and biopsies were first introduced. Other countries, especially those of a Western kind, also saw an uptick. The significant overdiagnosis and the harsh treatment side effects warned against the use of PSA as a screening program, while it turned out to be beneficial in reducing mortality from prostate cancer. Moreover, prevalence rates fluctuate among racial groupings, with African-American men having the greatest rates, which is perhaps the most striking data about prostate cancer incidence and mortality. This disparity could be explained by biological and social variables; however, researchers are still trying to determine which genes could be at play and how they interact with their surroundings. On top of that recent advances in genomic technology have made it possible to examine epigenetic and genetic alterations in human prostate cancer for the first time. By combining this data with specific functional tests, we were able to pinpoint key signaling pathways that play a supporting role in the development and progression of prostate cancer.

Conflict of Interest The authors declare no conflict of interest.

References

1. Ritch C, Cookson M. Recent trends in the management of advanced prostate cancer. F1000Res. 2018;7:1513.
2. Li J, Siegel DA, King JB. Stage-specific incidence rates and trends of prostate cancer by age, race, and ethnicity, United States, 2004-2014. Ann Epidemiol. 2018;28(5):328–30.
3. Steele CB, et al. Prostate cancer survival in the United States by race and stage (2001-2009): findings from the CONCORD-2 study. Cancer. 2017;24:5160–77.
4. Marques RB, et al. Bypass mechanisms of the androgen receptor pathway in therapy-resistant prostate cancer cell models. PLoS One. 2010;5(10):e13500.
5. Harris WP, et al. Androgen deprivation therapy: progress in understanding mechanisms of resistance and optimizing androgen depletion. Nat Clin Pract Urol. 2009;6(2):76–85.
6. Huggins C, Hodges CV. Studies on prostatic cancer. I. The effect of castration, of estrogen and androgen injection on serum phosphatases in metastatic carcinoma of the prostate. CA Cancer J Clin. 1972;22(4):232–40.
7. Leslie SW, et al. Prostate cancer. In: StatPearls. Treasure Island: StatPearls Publishing; 2024.
8. Patrikidou A, et al. Who dies from prostate cancer? Prostate Cancer Prostatic Dis. 2014;17(4):348–52.
9. Omlin A, et al. Improved survival in a cohort of trial participants with metastatic castration-resistant prostate cancer demonstrates the need for updated prognostic nomograms. Eur Urol. 2013;64(2):300–6.
10. Sweeney CJ, et al. Chemohormonal therapy in metastatic hormone-sensitive prostate cancer. N Engl J Med. 2015;373(8):737–46.
11. James ND, et al. Addition of docetaxel, zoledronic acid, or both to first-line long-term hormone therapy in prostate cancer (STAMPEDE): survival results from an adaptive, multiarm, multistage, platform randomised controlled trial. Lancet. 2016;387(10024):1163–77.
12. Fizazi K, et al. Abiraterone plus prednisone in metastatic, castration-sensitive prostate cancer. N Engl J Med. 2017;377(4):352–60.
13. James ND, et al. Abiraterone for prostate cancer not previously treated with hormone therapy. N Engl J Med. 2017;377(4):338–51.
14. Smith MR, et al. Apalutamide treatment and metastasis-free survival in prostate cancer. N Engl J Med. 2018;378(15):1408–18.
15. Hussain M, et al. PROSPER: a phase 3, randomized, double-blind, placebo (PBO)-controlled study of enzalutamide (ENZA) in men with nonmetastatic castration-resistant prostate cancer (M0 CRPC). Alexandria: American Society of Clinical Oncology; 2018.
16. Harvey CJ, et al. Applications of transrectal ultrasound in prostate cancer. Br J Radiol. 2012;85(1):S3–17.
17. Sadeghi-Nejad H, et al. Controversies in transrectal ultrasonography and prostate biopsy. Ultrasound Q. 2006;22(3):169–75.

18. Sivaraman A, Bhat KRS. Screening and detection of prostate cancer-review of literature and current perspective. Indian J Surg Oncol. 2017;8(2):160–8.
19. Wilt TJ, et al. Radical prostatectomy versus observation for localized prostate cancer. N Engl J Med. 2012;367(3):203–13.
20. Loriot Y, Massard C, Fizazi K. Recent developments in treatments targeting castration-resistant prostate cancer bone metastases. Ann Oncol. 2012;23(5):1085–94.
21. Ferlay J, et al. Cancer incidence and mortality worldwide: sources, methods and major patterns in GLOBOCAN 2012. Int J Cancer. 2015;136(5):E359–86.
22. Pernar CH, et al. The epidemiology of prostate cancer. Cold Spring Harb Perspect Med. 2018;8(12):a030361.
23. Fitzmaurice C, et al. Global, regional, and national cancer incidence, mortality, years of life lost, years lived with disability, and disability-adjusted life-years for 32 cancer groups, 1990 to 2015: a systematic analysis for the global burden of disease study. JAMA Oncol. 2017;3(4):524–48.
24. Howlader N, et al. SEER cancer statistics review, 1975-2013. Bethesda: National Cancer Institute; 2016.
25. Shimizu H, et al. Cancers of the prostate and breast among Japanese and white immigrants in Los Angeles County. Br J Cancer. 1991;63(6):963–6.
26. Yu H, et al. Comparative epidemiology of cancers of the colon, rectum, prostate and breast in Shanghai, China versus the United States. Int J Epidemiol. 1991;20(1):76–81.
27. Etzioni R, et al. Impact of PSA screening on the incidence of advanced stage prostate cancer in the United States: a surveillance modeling approach. Med Decis Mak. 2008;28(3):323–31.
28. Etzioni R, et al. Overdiagnosis due to prostate-specific antigen screening: lessons from U.S. prostate cancer incidence trends. J Natl Cancer Inst. 2002;94(13):981–90.
29. Ciatto S, et al. Determining overdiagnosis by screening with DRE/TRUS or PSA (Florence pilot studies, 1991-1994). Eur J Cancer. 2005;41(3):411–5.
30. Jemal A, et al. Global patterns of cancer incidence and mortality rates and trends. Cancer Epidemiol Biomarkers Prev. 2010;19(8):1893–907.
31. Rawla P. Epidemiology of prostate cancer. World J Oncol. 2019;10(2):63–89.
32. De Angelis R, et al. Cancer survival in Europe 1999-2007 by country and age: results of EUROCARE-5-a population-based study. Lancet Oncol. 2014;15(1):23–34.
33. Chu KC, Tarone RE, Freeman HP. Trends in prostate cancer mortality among black men and white men in the United States. Cancer. 2003;97(6):1507–16.
34. Johansson JE, et al. Natural history of early, localized prostate cancer. JAMA. 2004;291(22):2713–9.
35. Albertsen PC, Hanley JA, Fine J. 20-year outcomes following conservative management of clinically localized prostate cancer. JAMA. 2005;293(17):2095–101.
36. Howlader N. Seer cancer statistics review. Bethesda: National Cancer Institute; 2008. http://seer.cancer.gov/csr/1975_2008/
37. Eeles RA, et al. Identification of 23 new prostate cancer susceptibility loci using the iCOGS custom genotyping array. Nat Genet. 2013;45(4):385–91.
38. Al Olama AA, et al. A meta-analysis of 87,040 individuals identifies 23 new susceptibility loci for prostate cancer. Nat Genet. 2014;46(10):1103–9.
39. MacInnis RJ, English DR. Body size and composition and prostate cancer risk: systematic review and meta-regression analysis. Cancer Causes Control. 2006;17(8):989–1003.
40. Jahn JL, Giovannucci EL, Stampfer MJ. The high prevalence of undiagnosed prostate cancer at autopsy: implications for epidemiology and treatment of prostate cancer in the Prostate-specific Antigen-era. Int J Cancer. 2015;137(12):2795–802.
41. Giovannucci E, et al. Risk factors for prostate cancer incidence and progression in the health professionals follow-up study. Int J Cancer. 2007;121(7):1571–8.
42. Taksler GB, Keating NL, Cutler DM. Explaining racial differences in prostate cancer mortality. Cancer. 2012;118(17):4280–9.

43. Haiman CA, et al. Characterizing genetic risk at known prostate cancer susceptibility loci in African Americans. PLoS Genet. 2011;7(5):e1001387.
44. Hemminki K, Czene K. Attributable risks of familial cancer from the family-cancer database. Cancer Epidemiol Biomarkers Prev. 2002;11(12):1638–44.
45. Brandt A, Sundquist J, Hemminki K. Risk for incident and fatal prostate cancer in men with a family history of any incident and fatal cancer. Ann Oncol. 2012;23(1):251–6.
46. Lichtenstein P, et al. Environmental and heritable factors in the causation of cancer–analyses of cohorts of twins from Sweden, Denmark, and Finland. N Engl J Med. 2000;343(2):78–85.
47. Mucci LA, et al. Familial risk and heritability of cancer among twins in nordic countries. JAMA. 2016;315(1):68–76.
48. Hoffmann TJ, et al. A large multiethnic genome-wide association study of prostate cancer identifies novel risk variants and substantial ethnic differences. Cancer Discov. 2015;5(8):878–91.
49. Pomerantz MM, Freedman ML. Genetics of prostate cancer risk. Mt Sinai J Med. 2010;77(6):643–54.
50. Shui IM, et al. Prostate cancer (PCa) risk variants and risk of fatal PCa in the National Cancer Institute Breast and Prostate Cancer Cohort Consortium. Eur Urol. 2014;65(6):1069–75.
51. Salinas CA, et al. Prostate cancer in young men: an important clinical entity. Nat Rev Urol. 2014;11(6):317–23.
52. Agarwal SK. Smoking and its relationship with cancer. J Cancer Res Rev Rep. 2021;3(2):1–9.
53. Kenfield SA, et al. Smoking and prostate cancer survival and recurrence. JAMA. 2011;305(24):2548–55.
54. Pantarotto J, et al. Smoking is associated with worse outcomes in patients with prostate cancer treated by radical radiotherapy. BJU Int. 2007;99(3):564–9.
55. Oefelein MG, Resnick MI. Association of tobacco use with hormone refractory disease and survival of patients with prostate cancer. J Urol. 2004;171(6):2281–4.
56. Joshu CE, et al. Cigarette smoking and prostate cancer recurrence after prostatectomy. J Natl Cancer Inst. 2011;103(10):835–8.
57. Pickles T, et al. The effect of smoking on outcome following external radiation for localized prostate cancer. J Urol. 2004;171(4):1543–6.
58. Chu LW, et al. Prostate cancer incidence rates in Africa. Prostate Cancer. 2011;2011:947870.
59. Hsing AW, Tsao L, Devesa SS. International trends and patterns of prostate cancer incidence and mortality. Int J Cancer. 2000;85(1):60–7.
60. Howell MA. Factor analysis of international cancer mortality data and per capita food consumption. Br J Cancer. 1974;29(4):328–36.
61. Armstrong B, Doll R. Environmental factors and cancer incidence and mortality in different countries, with special reference to dietary practices. Int J Cancer. 1975;15(4):617–31.
62. Aronson WJ, et al. Growth inhibitory effect of low fat diet on prostate cancer cells: results of a prospective, randomized dietary intervention trial in men with prostate cancer. J Urol. 2010;183(1):345–50.
63. Venkateswaran V, Klotz LH. Diet and prostate cancer: mechanisms of action and implications for chemoprevention. Nat Rev Urol. 2010;7(8):442–53.
64. Pauwels EK. The protective effect of the Mediterranean diet: focus on cancer and cardiovascular risk. Med Princ Pract. 2011;20(2):103–11.
65. Fleshner N, Zlotta AR. Prostate cancer prevention: past, present, and future. Cancer. 2007;110(9):1889–99.
66. Hämäläinen E, et al. Diet and serum sex hormones in healthy men. J Steroid Biochem. 1984;20(1):459–64.
67. Rosenthal MB, et al. Effects of a high-complex-carbohydrate, low-fat, low-cholesterol diet on levels of serum lipids and estradiol. Am J Med. 1985;78(1):23–7.
68. Lloyd JC, et al. Fish oil slows prostate cancer xenograft growth relative to other dietary fats and is associated with decreased mitochondrial and insulin pathway gene expression. Prostate Cancer Prostatic Dis. 2013;16(4):285–91.

69. Berquin IM, et al. Modulation of prostate cancer genetic risk by omega-3 and omega-6 fatty acids. J Clin Invest. 2007;117(7):1866–75.
70. Gibson TM, et al. Epidemiological and clinical studies of nutrition. Semin Oncol. 2010;37(3):282–96.
71. Rohrmann S, et al. Meat and dairy consumption and subsequent risk of prostate cancer in a US cohort study. Cancer Causes Control. 2007;18(1):41–50.
72. Major JM, et al. Patterns of meat intake and risk of prostate cancer among African-Americans in a large prospective study. Cancer Causes Control. 2011;22(12):1691–8.
73. Sinha R, et al. Heterocyclic amine content of pork products cooked by different methods and to varying degrees of doneness. Food Chem Toxicol. 1998;36(4):289–97.
74. Kazerouni N, et al. Analysis of 200 food items for benzo[a]pyrene and estimation of its intake in an epidemiologic study. Food Chem Toxicol. 2001;39(5):423–36.
75. Sinha R, et al. Meat and meat-related compounds and risk of prostate cancer in a large prospective cohort study in the United States. Am J Epidemiol. 2009;170(9):1165–77.
76. Tappel A. Heme of consumed red meat can act as a catalyst of oxidative damage and could initiate colon, breast and prostate cancers, heart disease and other diseases. Med Hypotheses. 2007;68(3):562–4.
77. Gao X, LaValley MP, Tucker KL. Prospective studies of dairy product and calcium intakes and prostate cancer risk: a meta-analysis. J Natl Cancer Inst. 2005;97(23):1768–77.
78. Koh KA, et al. Dairy products, calcium and prostate cancer risk. Br J Cancer. 2006;95(11):1582–5.
79. Gupta S. Prostate cancer chemoprevention: current status and future prospects. Toxicol Appl Pharmacol. 2007;224(3):369–76.
80. Wilson KM, et al. Calcium and phosphorus intake and prostate cancer risk: a 24-y follow-up study. Am J Clin Nutr. 2015;101(1):173–83.
81. Singh SV, et al. Sulforaphane-induced cell death in human prostate cancer cells is initiated by reactive oxygen species. J Biol Chem. 2005;280(20):19911–24.
82. Joseph MA, et al. Cruciferous vegetables, genetic polymorphisms in glutathione S-transferases M1 and T1, and prostate cancer risk. Nutr Cancer. 2004;50(2):206–13.
83. Giovannucci E, et al. A prospective study of cruciferous vegetables and prostate cancer. Cancer Epidemiol Biomarkers Prev. 2003;12(12):1403–9.
84. Stram DO, et al. Prostate cancer incidence and intake of fruits, vegetables and related micronutrients: the multiethnic cohort study (United States). Cancer Causes Control. 2006;17(9):1193–207.
85. Fujiki H, et al. Cancer inhibition by green tea. Mutat Res. 1998;402(1-2):307–10.
86. Nakachi K, et al. Influence of drinking green tea on breast cancer malignancy among Japanese patients. Jpn J Cancer Res. 1998;89(3):254–61.
87. Fotsis T, et al. Genistein, a dietary ingested isoflavonoid, inhibits cell proliferation and in vitro angiogenesis. J Nutr. 1995;125(3):790s–7s.
88. Zhu BH, et al. Epigallocatechin-3-gallate inhibits growth of gastric cancer by reducing VEGF production and angiogenesis. World J Gastroenterol. 2007;13(8):1162–9.
89. Beltz LA, et al. Mechanisms of cancer prevention by green and black tea polyphenols. Anti Cancer Agents Med Chem. 2006;6(5):389–406.
90. Handayani R, et al. Soy isoflavones alter expression of genes associated with cancer progression, including interleukin-8, in androgen-independent PC-3 human prostate cancer cells. J Nutr. 2006;136(1):75–82.
91. Hastak K, et al. Ablation of either p21 or Bax prevents p53-dependent apoptosis induced by green tea polyphenol epigallocatechin-3-gallate. FASEB J. 2005;19(7):789–91.
92. Adhami VM, et al. Oral consumption of green tea polyphenols inhibits insulin-like growth factor-I-induced signaling in an autochthonous mouse model of prostate cancer. Cancer Res. 2004;64(23):8715–22.
93. van Breemen RB, Pajkovic N. Multitargeted therapy of cancer by lycopene. Cancer Lett. 2008;269(2):339–51.

94. Erdman JW Jr, Ford NA, Lindshield BL. Are the health attributes of lycopene related to its antioxidant function? Arch Biochem Biophys. 2009;483(2):229–35.
95. Liu X, et al. Lycopene inhibits IGF-I signal transduction and growth in normal prostate epithelial cells by decreasing DHT-modulated IGF-I production in co-cultured reactive stromal cells. Carcinogenesis. 2008;29(4):816–23.
96. Venkateswaran V, et al. A combination of micronutrients is beneficial in reducing the incidence of prostate cancer and increasing survival in the Lady transgenic model. Cancer Prev Res. 2009;2(5):473–83.
97. Schwenke C, et al. Lycopene for advanced hormone refractory prostate cancer: a prospective, open phase II pilot study. J Urol. 2009;181(3):1098–103.
98. Hernandez BY, et al. Relationship of body mass, height, and weight gain to prostate cancer risk in the multiethnic cohort. Cancer Epidemiol Biomarkers Prev. 2009;18(9):2413–21.
99. Joshu CE, et al. Weight gain is associated with an increased risk of prostate cancer recurrence after prostatectomy in the PSA era. Cancer Prev Res. 2011;4(4):544–51.
100. Zuccolo L, et al. Height and prostate cancer risk: a large nested case-control study (ProtecT) and meta-analysis. Cancer Epidemiol Biomarkers Prev. 2008;17(9):2325–36.
101. Möller E, et al. Body size across the life course and prostate cancer in the health professionals follow-up study. Int J Cancer. 2016;138(4):853–65.
102. Giovannucci EL, et al. A prospective study of physical activity and incident and fatal prostate cancer. Arch Intern Med. 2005;165(9):1005–10.
103. Patel AV, et al. Recreational physical activity and risk of prostate cancer in a large cohort of U.S. men. Cancer Epidemiol Biomarkers Prev. 2005;14(1):275–9.
104. Johnsen NF, et al. Physical activity and risk of prostate cancer in the European Prospective Investigation into Cancer and Nutrition (EPIC) cohort. Int J Cancer. 2009;125(4):902–8.
105. Zhong S, et al. Coffee consumption and risk of prostate cancer: an up-to-date meta-analysis. Eur J Clin Nutr. 2014;68(3):330–7.
106. Cao S, et al. Coffee consumption and risk of prostate cancer: a meta-analysis of prospective cohort studies. Carcinogenesis. 2014;35(2):256–61.
107. Lu Y, et al. Coffee consumption and prostate cancer risk: an updated meta-analysis. Cancer Causes Control. 2014;25(5):591–604.
108. Discacciati A, Orsini N, Wolk A. Coffee consumption and risk of nonaggressive, aggressive and fatal prostate cancer–a dose-response meta-analysis. Ann Oncol. 2014;25(3):584–91.
109. Baisden BL, Kahane H, Epstein JI. Perineural invasion, mucinous fibroplasia, and glomerulations: diagnostic features of limited cancer on prostate needle biopsy. Am J Surg Pathol. 1999;23(8):918–24.
110. Humphrey PA. Histopathology of prostate cancer. Cold Spring Harb Perspect Med. 2017;7(10):a030411.
111. Humphrey PA. Prostate pathology. Chicago: American Society for Clinical Pathology; 2003.
112. Bostwick DG. Gleason grading of prostatic needle biopsies. Correlation with grade in 316 matched prostatectomies. Am J Surg Pathol. 1994;18(8):796–803.
113. Byar DP, Mostofi FK. Carcinoma of the prostate: prognostic evaluation of certain pathologic features in 208 radical prostatectomies. Examined by the step-section technique. Cancer. 1972;30(1):5–13.
114. Bismar TA, et al. Multiple measures of carcinoma extent versus perineural invasion in prostate needle biopsy tissue in prediction of pathologic stage in a screening population. Am J Surg Pathol. 2003;27(4):432–40.
115. Thorson P, et al. Minimal carcinoma in prostate needle biopsy specimens: diagnostic features and radical prostatectomy follow-up. Mod Pathol. 1998;11(6):543–51.
116. Epstein JI. Diagnostic criteria of limited adenocarcinoma of the prostate on needle biopsy. Hum Pathol. 1995;26(2):223–9.
117. Ali TZ, Epstein JI. Perineural involvement by benign prostatic glands on needle biopsy. Am J Surg Pathol. 2005;29(9):1159–63.

118. Bostwick DG, Wollan P, Adlakha K. Collagenous micronodules in prostate cancer. A specific but infrequent diagnostic finding. Arch Pathol Lab Med. 1995;119(5):444–7.
119. McNeal JE, et al. Mucinous differentiation in prostatic adenocarcinoma. Hum Pathol. 1991;22(10):979–88.
120. Varma M, et al. Morphologic criteria for the diagnosis of prostatic adenocarcinoma in needle biopsy specimens. A study of 250 consecutive cases in a routine surgical pathology practice. Arch Pathol Lab Med. 2002;126(5):554–61.
121. Kaleem Z, et al. Prostatic adenocarcinoma with atrophic features: a study of 202 consecutive completely embedded radical prostatectomy specimens. Am J Clin Pathol. 1998;109(6):695–703.
122. Kim MJ, et al. Collagenous micronodules in prostate cancer revisited: are they solely associated with Gleason pattern 3 adenocarcinomas? Int J Clin Exp Pathol. 2015;8(4):3469–76.
123. Pacelli A, et al. Prostatic adenocarcinoma with glomeruloid features. Hum Pathol. 1998;29(5):543–6.
124. Epstein JI, et al. The 2014 International Society of Urological Pathology (ISUP) consensus conference on gleason grading of prostatic carcinoma: definition of grading patterns and proposal for a new grading system. Am J Surg Pathol. 2016;40(2):244–52.
125. Magi-Galluzzi C, et al. International Society of Urological Pathology (ISUP) Consensus Conference on Handling and Staging of Radical Prostatectomy Specimens. Working group 3: extraprostatic extension, lymphovascular invasion and locally advanced disease. Mod Pathol. 2011;24(1):26–38.
126. Fajkovic H, et al. Validation of lymphovascular invasion is an independent prognostic factor for biochemical recurrence after radical prostatectomy. Urol Oncol. 2016;34(5):233.
127. Kryvenko ON, Epstein JI. Histologic criteria and pitfalls in the diagnosis of lymphovascular invasion in radical prostatectomy specimens. Am J Surg Pathol. 2012;36(12):1865–73.

Part II
Molecular Mechanisms

Chapter 3
Prostate Cancer and Inflammation

Mehrdad Hashemi, Vahid Tavakolpour, Reza Morovatshoar, Ali Samadpour, Pezhman Shafiei Asheghabadi, Hasti Hadadian, Ali Bandsariyan, Zivar Ghasemi, Sima Orouei, Niloofar AbolfathyNajmabady, Mahdieh Bahrami Arz Aghdas, Shima Hajimazdarany, Behdokht Jamali, Rasoul Raesi, and Najma Farahani

Abstract All phases of carcinogenesis are accelerated by inflammation, which makes people more prone to developing cancer. To create an inflammatory tumor microenvironment (TME), cancer cells and neighboring stromal and inflammatory

The original version of the chapter has been revised. A correction to this chapter can be found at https://doi.org/10.1007/978-981-97-4612-5_15

M. Hashemi
Farhikhtegan Medical Convergence Sciences Research Center, Farhikhtegan Hospital Tehran Medical Sciences, Islamic Azad University, Tehran, Iran

Faculty of Advanced Science and Technology, Department of Genetics, Tehran Medical Sciences, Islamic Azad University, Tehran, Iran

V. Tavakolpour
Department of Stem Cells and Regenerative Medicine, Institute of Medical Biotechnology, National Institute of Genetic Engineering and Biotechnology (NIGEB), Tehran, Iran

R. Morovatshoar
Molecular Medicine Research Center, Hormozgan Health Institute, Hormozgan University of Medical Sciences, Bandar Abbas, Iran

A. Samadpour
Faculty of Science, Department of Biology, Mashhad Branch, Islamic Azad University, Mashhad, Iran

P. S. Asheghabadi · M. B. A. Aghdas · S. Hajimazdarany · N. Farahani (✉)
Farhikhtegan Medical Convergence Sciences Research Center, Farhikhtegan Hospital Tehran Medical Sciences, Islamic Azad University, Tehran, Iran

A. Bandsariyan · H. Hadadian
Faculty of Medicine, Medical Genetics Group, Hormozgan University of Medical Sciences, Bandar Abbas, Iran

Z. Ghasemi
Cellular and Molecular Biology Group, Tehran Medical Branch, Islamic Azad University, Tehran, Iran

G. Sethi et al. (eds.), *Prostate Cancer: Molecular Events and Therapeutic Modalities*, https://doi.org/10.1007/978-981-97-4612-5_3

cells participate in coordinated reciprocal interactions. Transmembrane cells are extremely malleable; they undergo constant phenotypic and functional changes. Moreover, it is common for inflammation to accompany the onset and advancement of cancer. Because the cells that cause inflammation in cancer are not susceptible to the fast development of drug resistance, addressing inflammation offers a promising approach to cancer prevention and treatment. The risk of cancer and its progression can be accelerated by tumor-extrinsic inflammation, which can be brought on by a variety of causes such as bacterial and viral infections, autoimmune illnesses, obesity, cigarette smoking, asbestos exposure, and heavy alcohol consumption. On the other hand, cancer-initiating mutations can cause cancer-intrinsic or cancer-elicited inflammation, which recruits and activates inflammatory cells and contributes to malignant progression. Inflammations, whether internal or external, can depress the immune system, making it an ideal environment for tumor growth. This review establishes a connection between inflammation and the progression of cancer.

Keywords Inflammation · Cancer · Interleukin-10 · Aspirin · Inflammatory factors

3.1 Introduction

When tissues are damaged by trauma, such as physical trauma, ischemia injury (when blood flow to an organ is inadequate), infection, or exposure to pollutants, the body reacts by inflammatory processes. To put it another way, inflammation triggers immunological reactions and cellular changes, which in turn lead to tissue repair and new cell development at the site of injury. The persistence of the inflammatory process or the failure of specific regulatory mechanisms responsible for shutting it down can lead to chronic inflammation. Cell mutation and proliferation can occur when these inflammatory reactions become persistent, frequently establishing conditions that are favorable to the development of cancer. Those with cancer confront a "perfect storm" of difficulties. Not only is this relevant for when cancer first starts, but it becomes even more crucial as the disease progresses. To activate these mutations within the cell, a significant number of signaling pathways play an important role in generating epigenetic modifications on the cell surface. Consequently, it is crucial to always treat the inflammatory causes [1].

Cells of both the innate and adaptive immune systems are activated, recruited [1], and put into action during inflammation, an ancient and developed process [2].

S. Orouei · N. AbolfathyNajmabady
Department of Biology, Science and Research Branch, Islamic Azad University, Tehran, Iran

B. Jamali
Department of Microbiology and Genetics, Kherad Institute of Higher Education, Bushehr, Iran

R. Raesi
Department of Nursing, Torbat Jam Faculty of Medical Sciences, Torbat Jam, Iran

Department of Health Services Management, Mashhad University of Medical Sciences, Mashhad, Iran

Inflammation promotes repair, regeneration, and remodeling, and although it was initially highlighted for its key role in host defense against infections, it is equally important for maintaining tissue homeostasis [3]. Inflammation and the immune system have been the subject of an explosion of studies examining cancer's development, progression, and treatment during the last several decades. In cancer research, the current paradigm is shifting from a "cancer cell-centric" to a more comprehensive approach. This new paradigm places cancer cells inside the tumor microenvironment (TME), which consists of stromal cells, fibroblasts, vascular cells, inflammatory immune cells, and more. Any kind of inflammation, whether it's a chronic inflammatory disease or tumor-elicited smoldering inflammation, alters the tumor microenvironment (TME), namely the receptivity of tumor and stromal cells to change. So, this is what we know about the immunological inflammatory pathways at work during carcinogenesis at the moment: Immunosurveillance and immunological modulation of tumor heterogeneity are two mechanisms by which the immune system might inhibit tumor growth. Concurrently, pro-tumorigenic inflammation is a cancer promoter because it inhibits antitumor immunity, changes the tumor microenvironment (TME) to be more tumor-permissive, and directs signals and activities that promote tumors onto cancer cells and epithelial cells. A wide range of immunotherapies, biological treatments, anticancer antibodies, cancer vaccines, and armored anticancer immune cells are all part of the immune system research that aims to uncover new mechanisms underlying potential cancer cures and prevention. It is now well-established that the immune system can be both pro- and antitumorigenic throughout the entire carcinogenesis process [4–8]. The immune system's ability to fight tumors is an inherent defense mechanism that generally activates in reaction to abnormal cells like malignant ones. On top of that, cancer immunotherapies that successfully reroute or hyperactivate the immune system to recognize, restrict, and kill cancer cells are among the most encouraging recent advances in cancer immunology. Cancer vaccines, immunosuppressive cell neutralization, oncolytic virus treatment, immunological "checkpoint" blockage, and synthetic biology using bi-specific antibodies or cells with "chimeric antigen receptors" (CAR) are all examples of such methods [2].

Moreover, studies of tumor microenvironment heterogeneity from an immunological perspective have also been heavily emphasized due to the recent success and tremendous potential of cancer immunotherapies. Cancer prognosis, sensitivity to conventional and immunotherapies, and future mechanistic insights can be informed by immunological signatures such as gene expression, cell type infiltration, and others, sometimes down to the single cell level [9–13]. Tumors that lack cellular and gene expression features favorable for antitumor action mainly by T cells are referred to as immunologically "cold," "infiltration-excluded," "T cell excluded," and most significantly, "immunological desert" and "non-inflamed" [14]. On the contrary, tumors with high levels of infiltrating T cells and increased presence of other components required for antitumor immune function are being called immunologically "hot" or "inflamed" tumor microenvironments. This language fails to take into consideration the existence of a second functional arm of the immune system that is pro-tumorigenic in cancer, even though it is helpful for defining cancers that may react to immune-mediated therapy. There, the immune system has a specific function, commonly known as "cancer-promoting inflammation," in the beginning, development, and progression of tumors. Tumors can still attract other immune cells, such as macrophages, monocytes, neutrophils, or innate lymphoid cells (ILC), and upregulate inflammatory mediators, even if tumors do not have a noticeable infiltration of T cells or their functional activation. At the same time, a large amount of epidemiological research has linked immune responses to inflammation and tissue repair to an increment in tumor incidence, development, and progression. On top of that many cancers have been found to have a decreased incidence and mortality rate when using nonsteroidal anti-inflammatory drugs (NSAIDs) like aspirin for "non-specific" inflammation inhibition [15, 16]. Another example is the reduction of the risk of lung cancer development when using canakinumab for "specific" cytokine inhibition [17]. Furthermore, cancer is more likely to occur at the same spot when there is persistent inflammation that is specific to an organ [18].

3.2 Inflammation in Cancer

To manifest the functions and processes of inflammation in cancer, one must first comprehend the temporal and environmental factors that initiate and sustain inflammation. Infection, persistent inflammation, or autoimmunity at the same tissue or organ location precedes about 15–20% of cancer instances [18, 19]. In such instances, inflammation is constituted and preexists tumor growth, both of which are cancerous. Some of the most common conditions that can increase the risk of colorectal cancer, liver cancer, gastritis caused by Helicobacter, and bladder inflammation caused by Schistosoma are inflammatory bowel disorders (IBD), chronic hepatitis, gastritis caused by Schistosoma, and bladder inflammation [20].

In addition to genetic predisposition, several environmental variables increase the risk of cancer by triggering chronic inflammation, which might be mild or moderate in intensity. Inflammation could be present before or after tumor growth in this scenario. In terms of the host, these variables can be systemic or organ- and site-specific. Inhalation of asbestos, secondhand smoke, and cigarette smoke, for instance, is known to aggravate airway and lung inflammation, which in turn increases the risk of mesothelioma and lung cancer [21, 22]. Conversely, liver, pancreatic, colon, breast, and other malignancies can be accelerated or increased risk due to low-grade inflammation caused by obesity, hyperglycemia, and excessive lipid accumulation, which is typically systemic in nature [23, 24]. It is possible to see type II diabetes, which has long been thought of as a separate cancer risk factor, as a component of the inflammation and tissue damage caused by obesity that ultimately leads to cancer. In light of the alarming rise of obesity in developed nations, it is crucial to understand how this condition and the inflammation it causes encourage tumor growth if we are to find effective treatments for the metabolic disorders that are ravaging our society. Breast cancer metastasis into the lungs can be accelerated by neutrophil activation and their extracellular trap formation function, which can occur even in the late stages of tumor development due to bacterial product-induced inflammation, obesity, and cigarette smoke [25].

In addition, injury to tissues, cell proliferation in response to that injury, and subsequent tissue repair are the hallmarks of chronic inflammation. The reversible change in a cell type known as "metaplasia" is often associated with cell proliferation in this situation. Since "dysplasia," a problem of cellular proliferation resulting in abnormal cell creation, is typically discovered next to the neoplasm site, it is considered the preceding event of carcinoma [26].

Furthermore, there are various forms of inflammation contributing to the development and advancement of cancer, each with its own unique source, mechanism, consequence, and degree of intensity [18]. To explain further, gastric cancer and mucosa-associated lymphoid tissue lymphoma are both linked to persistent Helicobacter pylori infection. The risk of hepatocellular carcinoma (HCC) is increased by hepatitis B (HBV) or C (HCV) virus infections, while the risk of bladder cancer is connected to infections with Schistosoma species and colon cancer to infections with Bacteroides species, respectively [27, 28]. As a normal component of host defense, the inflammatory response that starts in response to an infection aims to eliminate the pathogen before tumors develop. A tumorigenic pathogen, on the other hand, can evade the host's immune system and set up a chronic infection that causes low-grade inflammation. On the other hand, one microbial preparation is now used to treat bladder cancer, and in the 1890s, Coley utilized it to treat cancer with some success by inducing acute inflammation [29]. Although chronic inflammation promotes bladder carcinoma, the exact mechanism by which this cancer is more vulnerable to acute inflammation remains unclear. Inflammation as a cancer treatment tool? The answer to this critical question should shed light on that. The immune system becoming dysregulated or autoimmune is another source of chronic inflammation that occurs before tumors grow. The incidence of colorectal cancer is substantially elevated in cases of inflammatory bowel disease, for instance [30].

On the other hand, psoriasis and other chronic inflammatory illnesses may actually lower cancer risk, rather than increase it [31]. In contrast to diseases like psoriasis or rheumatoid arthritis, which do not substantially promote carcinogenesis, it is unclear what makes inflammatory bowel disease (IBD) or chronic hepatitis tumor-promoting. Potentially linked to environmental and dietary carcinogens that never reach the skin or joints is their impact on the gastrointestinal tract and liver. It is notable that environmental exposure is another potential cause of chronic inflammation. An increased risk of lung cancer is related to chronic obstructive pulmonary disease (COPD), which can be precipitated by irritants such as particulate matter from cigarette smoke [32]. Moreover, tobacco smoke promotes tumor growth and lung cancer in mice through inflammatory pathways [22]. Although they do not exhibit any overt mutagenesis activity, asbestos and silica particles inhaled can also cause lung cancer [22]. Nevertheless, these particles have the ability to cause inflammation by influencing the inflammasome's processing of pro-interleukin-1β (IL-1β) [33], which could explain how they cause tumors to form. It is noteworthy that hepatocellular carcinoma can develop due to persistent inflammation, which can be caused by obesity, which already increases the risk of cancer by 1.6 times [34]. Chronic inflammation promoting tumor growth can also result from the accumulation of damaged DNA and senescent cells [35, 36].

When tumors begin to form, a new kind of inflammation begins. An innate inflammatory response is established by the majority of solid cancers, which leads to the development of a microenvironment that is favorable to tumor growth [19]. Aside from cell-autonomous proliferation, oncogenes like Rat Sarcoma (RAS) and Myelocytomatosis (MYC) family members trigger a transcriptional program that changes the tumor microenvironment by bringing in leukocytes and lymphocytes, expressing chemokines and cytokines that promote tumors, and turning on an angiogenic switch [37, 38]. At some time, the blood supply to any solid tumor will become inadequate, and the tumor will starve to death. At the center of the tumor, this causes cells to die and release inflammatory mediators such IL-1 and HMGB1 [39]. The subsequent inflammatory reaction stimulates the process of neo-angiogenesis and supplies the cancer cells that manage to survive with extra growth factors that are made by newly recruited immune and inflammatory cells [27].

In addition, some malignancies, such as lung cancer, secrete chemicals that trigger inflammation; one such molecule is versican, an extracellular matrix component that activates macrophages via Toll-like receptor (TLR) 2 [40]. Some have called tumors "wounds, which never heal" owning to the constant cell renewal and proliferation caused by inflammation linked with tumors [41]. This inflammation primarily serves as a countermeasure to the body's natural processes of wound healing and tissue regeneration. In adult animals, not even dominant oncogenes like v-Src or K-Ras may cause cancer unless there is damage and then tissue regeneration [42, 43].

Not to mention, cancer treatment can start an inflammatory response that is strongly linked to tumors. Massive necrosis of cancer cells and adjacent tissues caused by radiation and chemotherapy sets off an inflammatory response similar to that of a wound-healing response [44]. On the one hand, therapy-induced inflammation can promote tumor growth by mimicking necrosis [39, 45], and on the other hand, it can improve tumor antigen cross-presentation and induce an antitumor immune response [46]. Therefore, the overall effect is debatable. What follows is a discussion of the latter and why it is important.

It is worth noting that chronic inflammation does not, however, precede the development of most malignancies and specific tumors. Intestinal inflammation is the precursor to approximately 2% of colorectal cancer cases, but inflammatory bowel disease (IBD) increases the risk of colitis-associated cancer (CAC) [47]. However, there are qualitative and quantitative differences in inflammatory cell recruitment, as well as increased expression of specific cytokines and chemokines in primary tumors and metastatic lesions, according to bulk transcriptional studies and other robust methods that investigate the cellular heterogeneity, accurate cell type identification and imaging, and cell-to-cell differential transcriptomics that make up the tumor microenvironment [14, 48]. The “CRC immunoscore” developed by the Galon group has shown that specific chemokines, cytokines, and myeloid cell subsets are associated with a poor prognosis in colorectal cancer (CRC) [49, 50]. This score will likely be refined and extended to include other types of tumors. Moreover, preclinical animal models using neutralization or genetic inactivation techniques show that inhibiting inflammatory responses in these “non-inflammatory” malignancies slows tumor development and progression. A concept called “tumor-elicited (associated) inflammation” (TEI) was coined because tumors that were once thought of as “non-inflammatory” actually recruit immune cells and boost the expression of inflammatory mediators in order to aid tumor growth and alter the tumor microenvironment (TME) to their advantage [18, 51]. On the other hand, TEI inducers in “sterile” tumors and those abundant in microbes may differ [19, 52]. For instance, in colorectal cancer (CRC), myeloid cells associated with tumors produce IL-23 and IL-23-dependent tumor-initiating inflammation (TII) when the protective intestinal barrier at the tumor site deteriorates early oncogene-induced [51]. On the other hand, recognizing oncogenic transformation, metabolic changes, cell death, or hypoxia may be the primary inflammatory triggers in cancers that are not connected with mucosal surfaces [19, 53].

When cancer patients undergo anticancer treatments like chemotherapy, radiation, or immunotherapies, a new kind of inflammation known as therapy-induced inflammation emerges. This type of inflammation is not present in intact tumors but is an important side effect of these treatments. Present immunotherapies are based on the premise that treatment activates the immune system within the tumor [54]. Stimulating antitumor immune responses through this technique can work in tandem with conventional cancer treatments. The production of IL-1α and other immunostimulatory cytokines can be stimulated in certain instances by the release of damage-associated molecular patterns (DAMPs) such as ATP and HMGB1 from tumor cells that are dying. This, in addition to an uptick in tumor neo-antigen production, has the potential to either inhibit the immune system or stimulate the formation of new T cells that fight tumors [55]. The overall result, however, may vary depending on the tumor type and the specific cytotoxic or radiotherapy regimen used, which in turn will alter the anticancer immune cells’ activation and function [56]. Cell death through necrosis may also be more immunostimulatory since many cancers lack apoptotic cell death [57, 58]. The immunosuppressive effects of therapies and the discharge of dead cell material from tumors are important to note, as is the fact that they often cause an inflammatory response similar to that seen after natural tissue damage, which in turn leads to wound healing and tissue restoration. In this case, myeloid cells and fibroblasts in the tumor microenvironment, as well as other cells, would produce cytokines and growth factors including TNF, Epidermal Growth Factor (EGF), IL-6, Wnt ligands, and others upon detection of dying tumor cells. Reduced therapeutic efficacy could be the result of these growth factors acting as cell extrinsic anti-apoptotic/generally anti-cell death signals. One important component of cancer therapy resistance is paracrine EGF family ligand synthesis, which can be induced by macrophages or fibroblasts [59]. Cancer stem cell phenotypic enforcement may involve other STAT3-activating cytokines such as IL-22, IL-11, and IL-6. Cancer stem cells are less metabolically active and proliferative, making them resistant to several types of chemotherapy and radiation. One example of the non-immune metabolic significance of inflammatory cells in therapeutic resistance is the fact that pancreatic tumors become resistant to gemcitabine when myeloid cells are recruited to the tumor more effectively and produce pyrimidine nucleotides [60]. Inflammatory signaling that targets residual tumor cells is a major driver of treatment resistance [61, 62], and cytokines like IL-17 can directly act on CRC cancer cells to give them resistance to 5-FU, a first-line anti-CRC treatment [63].

Furthermore, myelodysplastic syndrome [64], different metastatic cancers [25, 65], and the translocation of inflammatory microbial products all contribute to systemic inflammation and tumor promotion, which is likely an underappreciated mechanism. Chemotherapies can also damage normal tissues, especially in the intestine. All things considered, therapy-induced inflammation does not appear until after treatment has begun, yet it may be crucial in deciding whether or not the therapy is effective. To better understand how tumor progression affects the tumor microenvironment (TME), it is necessary to identify the precise signals that cause inflammation throughout tumor formation.

When normally functioning cells get a mutation that puts them on the path to becoming tumors by giving them an advantage over their neighbors in terms of growth and survival, this process is titled tumor initiation. Nevertheless, it usually takes at least four or five mutations for a cancer to develop [66, 67]. In cancers that develop within quickly renewed epithelia (such as skin and intestines cancers), oncogenic mutations must take place in either transient amplifying cells or long-lived stem cells, as the elimination of differentiated cells occurs so quickly between mutations. It is also crucial that each mutation is passed on to the cell's descendants. On the other hand, hepatocytes and other differentiated epithelial cells can acquire oncogenic mutations; these cells can proliferate and survive long enough to take more blows from mutations.

An inflammatory milieu may promote the growth of mutant cells and raise mutation rates, according to some research. The production of DNA damage and genomic instability can be induced by reactive nitrogen intermediates (RNI) and reactive oxygen species (ROS) released by activated inflammatory cells. Nevertheless, it remains uncertain if reactive oxygen species (ROS) and reactive nitrogen species (RNI) generated and discharged by macrophages and neutrophils (primarily in the context of acute inflammation) have enough half-life to permeate the extracellular matrix, penetrate epithelial cells, traverse their cytoplasm, reach the nucleus, and interact with DNA packaged into chromatin. On the other hand, inflammatory cells can promote the buildup of reactive oxygen species (ROS) in nearby epithelial cells by releasing cytokines such as tumor necrosis factor-α. Tumor initiation's primary drivers, then, have been argued to be immune-mediated pathways or environmental and dietary mutagens [68]. Cancer cells and inflamed, non-dysplastic epithelium in CAC both have p53 mutations, likely produced by oxidative damage; this shows

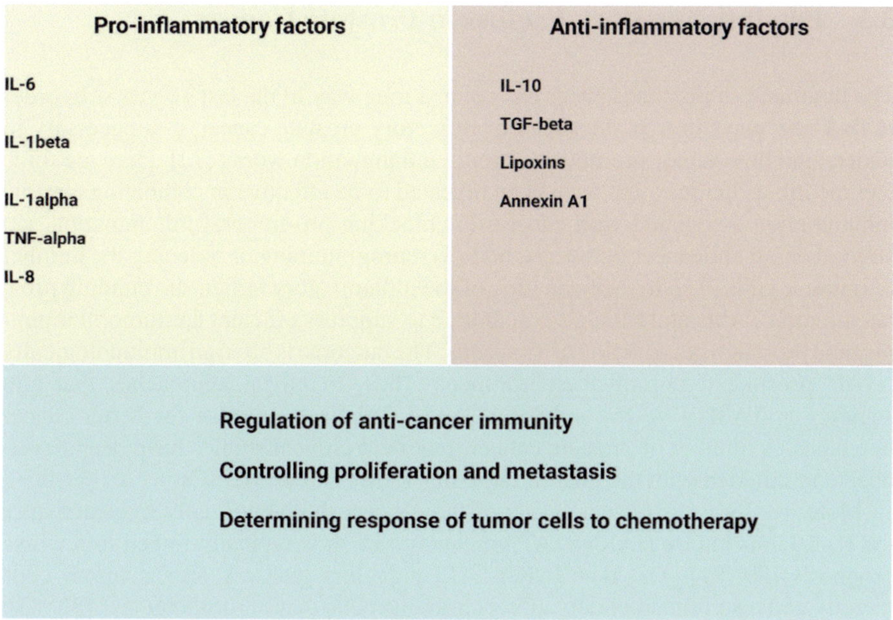

Fig. 3.1 The anti-inflammatory and pro-inflammatory factors in cancer (Biorender.com)

that prolonged inflammation causes genomic alterations [69]. Colonic irritant dextran sodium sulfate (DSS) can cause chronic inflammation, which in turn can cause DNA damage and the development of colonic adenomas [70]. As a standalone carcinogen, DSS, however, is not very dangerous [71].

When a tumor begins as a single started cell and progresses through the stages of promotion, it becomes a fully formed primary tumor. The initial expansion of a tumor is dependent on mechanisms mediated by inflammation, which enhance cell proliferation and decrease cell death. Most known tumor promoters, such as phorbol esters, are strong inflammatory inducers, and inflammation has many beneficial effects on cancer through tumor promotion [27]. Both early and late stages of tumor growth can be affected by inflammation-induced tumor promotion, which can activate pre-malignant lesions that had lain dormant for a long time. Inflammation promotes tumors in a variety of ways, including, but not limited to, accelerated proliferation and survival and the so-called angiogenic switch, which reawakens a small, dormant tumor to get blood flow for its next growth phase [27]. Below, we will go over the mechanisms that cause inflammation to promote tumors. Figure 3.1 shows the inflammatory factors in cancer.

3.3 Pro-inflammatory Factors in Prostate Cancer

The treatment of prostate cancer has come a long way in the last 10 years. In order to find new ways to treat advanced or refractory prostate cancer, it is necessary to understand how tumor-promoting chronic inflammation works [72]. Here are three therapeutic techniques that have been revealed to be effective in combating chronic inflammation associated with cancer: (1) blocking pro-tumoral inflammation, (2) strengthening anticancer pathways, and (3) reprogramming or reducing the number of immune cells [73]. In the formation of the inflammatory milieu surrounding prostate tumors, TAMs and MDSCs collaborate to suppress efficient antitumoral immunity and promote the induction of Treg cells. The outcome is often an immunologically "cold" prostate tumor microenvironment. Thus, treatment approaches that aim squarely at TAMs [74–76] and MDSCs [77–79] show promise for better cancer outcomes. A number of prostate cancer treatment clinical studies have been developed and initiated with the goal of targeting TAMs and/or MDSCs.

Moreover, prostate cancer is one of the cancers that abnormally hyperactivates the IL-6/Janus kinase (JAK)/STAT3 pathway, which is typically linked to a worse prognosis [80, 81]. The IL-6/JAK/STAT3 signaling pathway affects tumor cells directly and also fundamentally affects immune cells that infiltrate tumors [82, 83]. Antitumor immunity is likely downregulated upon STAT3 activation in immune cells because this protein negatively affects dendritic cells, effector T cells, natural killer cells, and neutrophils [84]. Also, STAT3 controls TAMs, MDSCs, Tregs, and Th17 cells in a beneficial way [85, 86]. An extremely immunosuppressive tumor microenvironment is thus a result of the IL-6/JAK/STAT3 pathway. Inhibiting IL-6 reduced inflammation of the prostate and cancer progression in a Pten-deficient mouse model of prostate cancer [87]. The Food and Drug Administration has authorized the use of the anti-IL-6 monoclonal antibody cetuximab (CNTO328) in the treatment of multicentric Castleman's disease [88]. Mice with androgen-dependent prostate cancer xenograft model prevented castration-resistant development when IL-6 was inhibited by siltuximab [89]. Siltuximab was found to have no significant clinical benefit in patients with metastatic Castration-Resistant Prostate Cancer (CRPC) who exhibited a dramatic increase in plasma IL-6 levels after treatment, according to phase 2 clinical trials (NCT00433446, NCT00385827). These trials also confirmed the poor prognosis linked to elevated IL-6 levels at baseline [90, 91]. Early on in the course of the disease, IL-6 blocking may be helpful, since analysis of specimens taken during a radical prostatectomy in a phase 1 trial showed that siltuximab therapy decreased levels of phosphorylated STAT3 and mitogen-activated protein kinases [92]. The oral anthelminthic medication niclosamide, which is another FDA-approved treatment, works by interacting with signaling pathways such as Wnt/β-catenin, STAT3, NF-κB, and Notch. Hence, it may have wide-ranging therapeutic uses for the treatment of disorders besides parasitic ones, such as metabolic disorders, infections, and cancer [93]. Through STAT3 and/or NF-κB signaling, niclosamide reduces inflammation that is generated by macrophages [94]. Also, in prostate cancer cells, niclosamide was found to be a strong inhibitor of androgen receptor splice variation 7 (AR-V7) [95]. The effects of niclosamide in combination with enzalutamide or abiraterone on patients with metastatic CRPC are now being studied in clinical trials (NCT03123978, NCT02807805). A mouse model of prostate cancer showed that antisense oligonucleotide, an alternative method of decreasing cellular STAT3, enhanced antitumor immunity, and inhibited immunosuppressive MDSCs were successful in eradicating the tumors [96].

Moreover, the ability of both IL-1β and IL-1α to promote tumor growth and metastasis is demonstrated in their roles in the evolution of prostate cancer [97, 98]. Beyond that, IL-1α and IL-1β have the ability to transform AR+ PCa cells into AR- PCa cells, leading to CRPC and treatment resistance [99]. The ability of IL-1α to form PSMA/PSA prostate clones through interaction with IL-6 has been documented [100]. Two members of the E26 Transformation-Specific (ETS) family, epithelium-specific ETS (also known as E26 transformation-specific) and ESE1 (also known as E74-like factor or ELF3), are linked to prostate cancer and poor patient outcomes; IL-1β can activate them via the NF-κB pathway [101]. Endothelin 1 (ET-1) and matrilysin 1, which are involved in the progression of PCa, can be induced by IL-1β as well [102, 103]. According to 64, it was also found that IL-1β might boost PCa growth by inducing IL-8 through the Mitogen-Activated Protein Kinase (MAPK) pathway. There is a negative correlation between Gleason score and the expression of the particular receptor antagonist IL-1RA. The ability of IL-1α and IL-1β to be inhibited has been shown in studies [104]. There is a lot of evidence that IL-1RA can decrease tumor-mediated inflammation and invasion, according to multiple studies [104, 105].

In addition, inhibiting the CSF-1 receptor significantly decreases TAMs and enhances cytotoxic CD8+ T cells in animal models, suggesting that CSF-1 is an important component in TAM survival [106]. Based on reports, irradiated prostate cancers have elevated CSF-1 levels, which in turn boost tumor-infiltrating TAMs and MDSCs, which may reduce the radiotherapy's effectiveness in a mouse model of prostate malignancies [107]. In prostate cancer cells produced by Androgen Deprivation Therapy (ADT), cytokines such as CSF-1 are expressed, which can lead to a rise in the infiltration of M2 TAM and, ultimately, castration-resistant cancer progression [108]. In tenosynovial giant cell tumor, the FDA-approved CSF-1 receptor inhibitor pexidartinib (PLX3397) demonstrates a strong tumor response [109]. By lowering the pro-tumorigenic effects of TAMs in mouse xenograft models, pexidartinib added to docetaxel increased treatment effectiveness in CRPC [110]. Pexidartinib in conjunction with radiation treatment and ADT is now being studied in a clinical trial for patients with localized prostate cancer (NCT02472275).

It is noteworthy that oral immunomodulatory drug tasquinimod (ABR-215050) binds to the inflammatory protein S100A9, which allegedly influences tumor-suppressing myeloid cell accumulation and function, MDSCs, and M2-like TAMs [111, 112]. Phase 3 randomized trial subjects with metastatic CRPC who had not previously received chemotherapy (n = 1245) were given either tasquinimod or a placebo. The trial's NCT number is 01234311. Despite no improvement in overall survival, tasquinimod considerably increased radiographic progression-free survival relative to placebo (HR0.64, 95% CI 0.54–0.75) [113]. An essential function of Bruton tyrosine kinase (BTK) is to polarize T2 TAMs and to aid in B cell growth. An FDA-approved inhibitor of BTK, ibrutinib, restores antitumor immune responses that are dependent on T cells and may slow the growth of solid tumors [114, 115]. In order to determine whether ibrutinib is effective against localized prostate cancer, a clinical trial is underway (NCT02643667). Numerous recent investigations have zeroed in on immunometabolism, with a special emphasis on how immune cells' internal metabolic pathways undergo alterations that impact their activity [116]. It was found that antitumor immunity relies on the tryptophan metabolic enzyme indoleamine 2,3-dioxygenase (IDO) [117]. Activation of regulatory T cells (Tregs) and monocyte-derived suppressor cells (MDSCs) occurs when IDO is overexpressed, and this is a common finding in many cancer types [118, 119]. Novel cancer therapies have thus been developed using inhibitors of IDO's enzyme activity and effector actions [120, 121]. A phase 2 clinical trial (NCT01560923) employed the IDO1 pathway inhibitor indoximod in conjunction with Sipuleucel-T to treat individuals with metastatic CRPC.

Furthermore, monocyte chemoattractant protein (MCP)-1, or CCL2, is an effective chemokine that attracts monocytes from the peripheral blood and plays a significant role in the recruitment of these cells to areas of inflammation and malignancies [122, 123]. Among prostate cancer patients, CCL2 expression is elevated in bone metastases, where it promotes tumor growth and advancement [124, 125]. In Vertebral-Cancer of the Prostate (VCaP) xenograft model mice, carlumab (CNTO888), a CCL2 monoclonal antibody, reduced tumor development and TAM infiltration. Therefore, CCL2 regulates TAMs, which in turn promotes prostate cancer growth [126]. Moreover, in mice with prostate cancer xenograft model, the tumor burden was dramatically reduced when carlumab was coupled with docetaxel to inhibit CCL2. This reduction was compared to docetaxel alone [127]. In the clinical trial (NCT00992186), carlumab was not able to successfully block serum CCL2 levels and did not demonstrate any antitumor action when used alone in patients with metastatic CRPC [128].

Additionally, SDF-1, or CXCL12, is a potent chemotactic for lymphocytes and myeloid cells (such as TAMs and MDSCs) [129, 130]. Tumorigenesis, angiogenesis, metastasis, and tumor progression are all significantly impacted by CXCL12 and its receptor, CXCR4 [131]. Bone metastases in prostate cancer are strongly correlated with CXCR4 protein expression [132]. Since CXCR4 signaling pathway in prostate cancer cells primarily regulates tumorigenic potential [133], plerixafor (AMD3100) or CTE9908 inhibition of CXCR4 considerably decreased bone metastasis in prostate cancer model mice [134]. In animals modeled by MYC-induced prostate tumors, plerixafor reduced inflammation-mediated tumor growth via the CXCL12-CXCR4/CXCR7 signaling axis [135]. To improve docetaxel's effectiveness in prostate cancer, plerixafor blocks tumor-stroma interactions via the CXCL12/CXCR4 pathway [136]. Plerixafor has numerous potential uses, including autologous transplantation in patients with multiple myeloma or non-Hodgkin's lymphoma, but it is also approved for use in a number of other cancers and immunological diseases [137].

3.4 Anti-inflammatory Factors in Prostate Cancer

With respect to prostate cancer, there is a wide range of anti-inflammatory factors that have been identified, playing a prominent role in modulating the tumor microenvironment and potentially impacting disease progression. These factors can influence various aspects of inflammation, immunity, and tumor biology.

Interleukin-10 (Il-10) By acting on immune cells to dampen the antitumor immune response [138, 139], IL10 contributes to boosting cancer aggressiveness and is best researched as an anti-inflammatory, immune-suppressive cytokine [140, 141]. Patients with prostate cancer who have high levels of IL10 serum are more likely to have a poor prognosis [142] and higher Gleason scores [143]. One possible source of IL10 production is the tumor cells themselves [144, 145], while another is the tumor elicitation of immune cells that infiltrate the tumor and create IL10 [146, 147]. The antitumor immune response is inhibited by IL10, which inhibits the activity of myeloid (macrophage and dendritic cell) and T effector cells [147]. IL10 also increases myeloid cell PDL1 (CD274) expression [148]. By binding to T cells' inhibitory receptor PD1, PDL1 renders the cell inactive and impedes the antitumor immune response of host T cells [149, 150].

On the other hand, Stearns and colleagues found that IL10 directly affects prostate cancer cells in the early 2000s [151, 152]. Moreover, prostate cancer cell lines treated with IL10 had an upregulation of TIMP1 [151] and a downregulation of MMP1 and MMP2 production [153]. Although the exact role of IL10 in regulating TIMP1 and MMP1/MMP2 expression in prostate cancer progression remains unclear, it is known that higher levels of Tissue Inhibitors of Metalloproteinases (TIMPs) and Matrix Metalloproteinases (MMPs) are linked to more advanced stages of the disease [154]. Since the Stearns group's published studies, no one has investigated the direct effects of IL10 on prostate cancer.

Furthermore, in tumor biopsies taken from patients who have developed resistance to Enzalutamide (ENZ), Bishop et al. discovered that PDL1 is mostly elevated on prostate cancer cells, not on tumor immune infiltrating cells [155]. For this reason, we set out to determine whether IL10 directly stimulates the in vitro production of NE-associated proteins and PDL1 in prostate cancer cells. We evaluated the impact of IL10, IL6, and ENZ on various AR-dependent and AR-independent prostate cancer cells. We also tested IL10 and IL6 for their capacity to regulate AR activity in lymph node carcinoma of the prostate (LNCaP) cells that had an AR-regulated Green Fluorescent Protein (GFP) reporter stably transduced into them [156]. In vitro, researchers discovered that prostate cancer cells treated with IL10 exhibited increased surface PDL1 protein expression and NE-like trait development. What this means for the future of IL10-based prostate cancer treatments is unclear.

Tumor growth factor-beta (TGF-B) in the early stages of prostate cancer, TGF-β mostly inhibits cell proliferation, but as the disease progresses, it takes on pro-oncogenic and pro-metastatic characteristics [157–159]. The normal prostate's stromal cells release TGF-β, which has a strong inhibitory effect on epithelial cell proliferation [160, 161]. Unchecked cell proliferation and a crucial role in carcinogenesis are caused by prostate tumor cells becoming resistant to the growth-inhibitory actions of TGF-β [162]. Research has demonstrated that in prostate cancer, an increase in tumor aggressiveness is associated with a decrease in TGF-β type II receptor expression [3, 98]. There may be other factors besides the loss of TGFβ receptors and other components of TGF-β signaling that contribute to tumor cells' resistance to TGFβ's growth-inhibitory effects. Without mutation, deletion, or downregulation of TGF-β receptors, Smad proteins, or other downstream signaling molecules, a considerable portion of prostate tumors become TGFβ-resistant. Not much is known about the physiological and molecular processes that lead to resistance to TGF-β effects on cell proliferation when TGF-β signaling is otherwise normal. It is known that the expression of TGF-β ligands and receptors is changed in prostate cancer compared to normal prostate cells, and this change is further accelerated in aggressive androgen-refractory prostate cancer cells, along with the transition of TGF-β from a growth-inhibitory signal to a growth-promoting signal [163, 164]. Reducing proliferation in the murine High-Grade Prostatic Intraepithelial Neoplasia (HGPIN) model by inhibiting TGF-β receptors implies that TGF-β acts as a tumor promoter rather than a tumor suppressor in these cells [165]. Researchers have looked at the TGF-β signaling pathway as a possible target for treating prostate cancer. Inhibitors of the TGF-β receptor have been tested in both in vivo models used for preclinical research and in clinical trials with patients diagnosed with prostate cancer [166]. Nevertheless, at various points in the disease progression, TGF-β acts as both a tumor suppressor and a tumor promoter, making it difficult to achieve a therapeutic effect by blocking its signaling [166].

Interleukin-4 (IL-4) and Interleukin-13 (IL-13) In human peri-urethral prostate tissues from males with LUTS, IL-4Rα, IL-13Rα1, and collagen are all up-regulated at the same time. Both IL-4 and IL-13 stimulate the expression of their respective cognate receptors, IL-4Rα and IL-13Rα1, in addition to their own expression. As cytokines, IL-4 and IL-13 at low doses encourage prostate fibroblast proliferation, whereas, at high quantities (>40 ng/ml), they inhibit cellular proliferation. Prostate stromal fibroblasts' collagen transcript and protein expression is strongly and selectively enhanced by IL-4 and IL-13, with this enhancement being JAK/STAT dependent. In addition, the activation of the IL-4Rα receptor is related to the JAK/STAT signaling that is mediated by IL-4 and IL-13 [167].

Peroxisome Proliferation-Activated Receptor Gamma (PPARy) The discovery of PPARγ occurred in 1994, and the Thiazolidinediones (TZDs) rosiglitazone and pioglitazone were commercialized for the treatment of type 2 diabetes in 1999 [168–170]. Our understanding of PPARγ has been enhanced during the past 20 years of scientific research, and ongoing studies keep pointing to its involvement in prostate cancer. Although PPARγ1 was previously believed to be specific to adipocytes, PPARγ2 has now been identified as a distinct "tumor suppressor" in contrast to its more carcinogenic counterpart. But it's still not apparent how these two variations interacted with one another or what part they played in PC's evolution and development; the details depend on the environment. Moreover, medical evidence shows that PPARγ levels increase during PC progression, and PC has the potential to rely on PPARγ for lipogenesis and mitochondrial biogenesis, especially when it comes to in vivo processes. This could indicate that blocking PPARγ could be a good way to prevent the development of PC. Researchers have created and tested PPARγ antagonists such as betulinic acid in mouse models to see if they can treat diabetes without the negative effects of PPARγ antagonism [171]. On the other hand, small molecule inhibitors might be even safer. In vitro experiments with the PC cell lines Lipid Composition Profile (LCP) and PC3 revealed that the use of a single small chemical, T0070907, inhibited cell proliferation [172]. After administering T0070907 to xenografts containing LCP cells, four out of seven tumors disappeared, demonstrating full regression. It was demonstrated that the growth suppression occurred by traditional PPARγ signaling, which led to the downregulation of the fatty acid synthesis genes Fatty Acid Synthase (FASN) and Acetyl-CoA Carboxylase Alpha (ACACA). Additionally, AR-dependent pathways were implicated, indicating that the PPARγ-AR connections may be targeted [172]. Research has illustrated that this tiny molecular inhibitor was found to hinder MAPK signaling and PPARγ-dependent pathways, which in turn inhibited the proliferation of breast cancer cell lines [173]. Further evidence of the effectiveness of the PPARγ antagonist GW9662 in inhibiting PC development has been presented by researchers [174]. Not only did GW9662 hinder growth and colony formation in vitro, but it also hindered the metastasis of a PC3 orthograft. Subsequent research confirmed that GW9662 inhibited PC3-M xenograft development as well [175]. Due to its systemic effects on PPARγ, which result in a decrease of visceral fat throughout the body, GW9662 might not be an appropriate medication for therapeutic use, suggesting that it could impact adipogenesis [176]. Based on these findings, PPARγ antagonism could be a potential treatment target for PC, especially in its latter phases when its activity is becoming more and more dependent. Therapeutics that target various isoforms of PPARγ may also have a significant impact on PC, as these variants appear to play distinct roles in the disease. This would enable the control of cancer-causing PPARγ1 signaling without compromising PPARGγ2's ability to decrease tumors. Investigating PPARγ antagonists and their interactions further will shed light on how to capitalize on PC reliance on PPARγ.

In the Reduction by Dutasteride of Prostate Cancer Events (REDUCE) trial, which included men with negative baseline biopsies, the use of aspirin or NSAIDs was associated with a lower risk of total and high-grade prostate cancer [177, 178]. A number of large-scale studies have also looked at how aspirin and other NSAIDs affect the course of prostate cancer [179, 180]. A study of localized prostate cancer patients treated with radical prostatectomy or radiation therapy found that aspirin use was related to a significantly decreased disease-specific mortality rate, with the trend toward this association being driven mostly by individuals at high risk of death [179]. Moreover, the cohort of newly diagnosed prostate cancer did not show any evidence of a protective link between disease-specific mortality and pre-diagnosis use of low-dose aspirin [180]. There was a weak but statistically significant link between using aspirin before a diagnosis and a lower risk of disease-specific death (hazard ratio = 0.88, 95% confidence interval 0.67–1.15; one cohort demonstrated larger effects with higher doses of aspirin) [181]. A subgroup study of a single cohort found that high-risk prostate cancer patients who took aspirin after their diagnosis had a much decreased disease-specific mortality rate [182]. Celecoxib did not show any effect in the STAMPEDE trial, which was a randomized control study of hormone treatment and celecoxib (a selective COX-2) in men with prostate cancer that had progressed to a local or distant stage [183]. It is possible that NSAIDs have an effect on platelets since a meta-analysis found that men with prostate cancer who took them before or after a diagnosis had a much lower probability of distant metastasis [184].

Celecoxib decreased tumor growth, local MDSCs infiltration, M2 polarization of tumor-infiltrating macrophages, and IL6 secretion by tumor-infiltrating macrophages in a Pten-deficient mouse model under high-fat diet (HFD), but not under a normal diet, according to a report [87]. The dosage of celecoxib was found to be equivalent to that used in human clinical practice. The model did not show any changes in COX-2 (Ptgs2) mRNA expression after HFD and celecoxib administration. Celecoxib may have therapeutic benefits in certain subgroups of prostate malignancies, like those affecting obese people, according to these results. However, local expression of COX-2 may not be a reliable biomarker for celecoxib response in prostate cancer. The lack of information on obesity and COX-2 local expression in the STAMPEDE study necessitates additional research. Although nonsteroidal anti-inflammatory medicines (NSAIDs) may help certain prostate cancer patients, their exact indications are still up for debate. Patients with prostate cancer who are receiving radiation treatment may benefit clinically from nonsteroidal anti-inflammatory drugs (NSAIDs), according to research by Mascan B and colleagues [185]. Possible biomarkers for the antitumor effects of NSAIDs include low levels of PD-L1, a specific single-nucleotide polymorphism, or a somatic PIK3CA mutation [4, 21]. Based on the US "Guidelines for the Use of Preventive Drugs," it is explicitly stated that taking 75–100 mg of aspirin daily—also known as a "low-dose"—has anticancer benefits. Careful consideration is required for the long-term use of aspirin or NSAIDs due to the potential side effects, such as gastrointestinal damage and worsening of pulmonary disease [186].

It is noteworthy that metformin slows the advancement of prostate cancer in multiple ways, many of which have to do with inflammation. One important step in metformin's stimulation of AMP-Activated Protein Kinase (AMPK) and inhibition of mTOR is the suppression of the NF-κB pathway [187]. Metformin can inhibit epithelial-mesenchymal transition by decreasing COX-2, PGE2, and phosphorylated STAT-3 expression, according to Tong et al. [188]. By reducing macrophage recruitment et and downregulating COX-2 and PGE2 in tumor cells, metformin slows the growth of prostate cancer in the Transgenic Adenocarcinoma of the Mouse Prostate (TRAMP) animal model [189]. Through regulating various signaling pathways, metformin significantly slows the formation of prostate cancer in xenograft mice when subjected to high-fat diets (HFD) [190]. Metformin reduces local MDSCs and suppresses prostate cancer growth in Pten-deficient model mice when they are on a high-fat diet (HFD), but it has no effect when they are on a regular diet [191]. Metformin may have therapeutic advantages for prostate cancer, according to these results, in part as it reduces inflammatory infiltration. Metformin has been found to inhibit tumor growth in several different mice models of cancer, specifically in macrophages [192, 193], MDSCs [192], and CD8+ T cells [194].

On top of that several studies that used histological examination found that statins could have an effect on reducing local inflammation. A decreased incidence of inflammation within prostate tumors was associated with individuals undergoing radical prostatectomy who used statins before the surgery [195]. Men who use statins and have a negative prostate biopsy are less likely to have inflammation in their prostates than men who do not take statins [196]. The outcomes of a randomized clinical trial utilizing atorvastatin for a median of 27 days prior to radical prostatectomy were reported by Murtola et al. [197]. The atorvastatin group had a time-dependent reduction in the Ki-67 index, but the placebo group had no change in prostate inflammation.

It has been shown that statins impact inflammation through multiple methods. Crystals of cholesterol in the blood cause the body to produce IL1β and IL6, which are inflammatory cytokines, leading to the creation of C-reactive protein (CRP) [198]. By reducing cholesterol, statins obstruct this mechanism. Also, statins lower CRP levels without affecting cholesterol levels [199]. Additionally, statins may be linked to a lower level of the macrophage and MDSC surface marker CD11b adhesion molecule [200] and a decrease in MCP-1 production [201]. Through stimulating the transcription factor, forkhead box P3, statins are known to raise the quantity of CD4+CD25+ regulatory T cells. These cells regulate immunological responses and ward against immunoinflammatory disorders [202, 203]. In addition to decreasing T cell activation [204] and PPAR activation [205], statins can decrease inducible Major Histocompatibility Complex (MHC) class II expression in antigen-presenting cells, which in turn inhibits inflammation. Figure 3.1 shows the function of inflammation in prostate cancer.

3.5 Conclusion and Perspectives

Inflammation determines whether a tumor grows, advances, or reacts to therapy. Moreover, inflammation and cancer have been better understood in the last 10 years, and the time is right to use what we know to create new cancer treatments based on this core knowledge. To make any progress in the fight against these diseases that are now incurable, we must address every aspect of cancer biology. The tumor microenvironment can be targeted with more targeted and selective tumoricidal medications using a mix of anti-inflammatory techniques. Future therapies should also consider the impact of natural genetic diversity on inflammation and immunity. When developing novel preventive strategies for cancer risk reduction, such factors must be carefully considered. Tumors seize pathways that originally served to mediate immunity to infections and promote tissue homeostasis, according to research on the mechanisms of pro-tumorigenic inflammatory pathways in cancer. Different carcinogenesis phases may be associated with different times of inflammation induction in the tumor microenvironment (TME), which can occur before, during, or after tumorigenesis begins. This timing means that tumor-promoting inflammation can either come out in the early stages of some cancer models, tumor types, or individual tumors, or it can stay silent until late stages of metastasis or drug resistance. Crucially, inflammation in tumors can be induced by a number of different things. Important targets for cancer prevention could include carcinogenic microbes, environmental pollutants (particles, smoke), low-grade inflammation linked to obesity, and commensal microorganisms associated with the deterioration of the epithelial barrier. This would allow for a reduction of tumor-initiating inflammation by eliminating or neutralizing the original stimulus. Vaccinations, dietary changes, more education about antibiotics, and stricter environmental regulations can all help accomplish this goal. Events related to hypoxia, cell death, or genetic and/or epigenetic regulation of tumor suppressors and oncogenes are examples of additional stimuli that are highly relevant to cancer biology but likely can only be targeted within the context of cancer treatment.

Conflict of Interest The authors declare no conflict of interest.

References

1. Singh N, et al. Inflammation and cancer. Ann Afr Med. 2019;18(3):121–6.
2. Greten FR, Grivennikov SI. Inflammation and cancer: triggers, mechanisms, and consequences. Immunity. 2019;51(1):27–41.
3. Medzhitov R. Origin and physiological roles of inflammation. Nature. 2008;454(7203):428–35.
4. Koebel CM, et al. Adaptive immunity maintains occult cancer in an equilibrium state. Nature. 2007;450(7171):903–7.
5. McGranahan N, Swanton C. Cancer evolution constrained by the immune microenvironment. Cell. 2017;170(5):825–7.
6. Rosenthal R, et al. Neoantigen-directed immune escape in lung cancer evolution. Nature. 2019;567(7749):479–85.
7. Schreiber RD, Old LJ, Smyth MJ. Cancer immunoediting: integrating immunity's roles in cancer suppression and promotion. Science. 2011;331(6024):1565–70.
8. Zilionis R, et al. Single-cell transcriptomics of human and mouse lung cancers reveals conserved myeloid populations across individuals and species. Immunity. 2019;50(5):1317–34.
9. Bindea G, et al. Spatiotemporal dynamics of intratumoral immune cells reveal the immune landscape in human cancer. Immunity. 2013;39(4):782–95.
10. Jerby-Arnon L, et al. A cancer cell program promotes T cell exclusion and resistance to checkpoint blockade. Cell. 2018;175(4):984–97.
11. Riaz N, et al. Tumor and microenvironment evolution during immunotherapy with nivolumab. Cell. 2017;171(4):934–49.
12. Spranger S, Gajewski TF. A new paradigm for tumor immune escape: β-catenin-driven immune exclusion. J Immunother Cancer. 2015;3:43.
13. Sweis RF, et al. Molecular drivers of the non-T-cell-inflamed tumor microenvironment in urothelial bladder cancer. Cancer Immunol Res. 2016;4(7):563–8.
14. Binnewies M, et al. Understanding the tumor immune microenvironment (TIME) for effective therapy. Nat Med. 2018;24(5):541–50.
15. Rothwell PM, et al. Effect of daily aspirin on long-term risk of death due to cancer: analysis of individual patient data from randomised trials. Lancet. 2011;377(9759):31–41.
16. Rothwell PM, et al. Effect of daily aspirin on risk of cancer metastasis: a study of incident cancers during randomised controlled trials. Lancet. 2012;379(9826):1591–601.

17. Ridker PM, et al. Effect of interleukin-1β inhibition with canakinumab on incident lung cancer in patients with atherosclerosis: exploratory results from a randomised, double-blind, placebo-controlled trial. Lancet. 2017;390(10105):1833–42.
18. Grivennikov SI, Greten FR, Karin M. Immunity, inflammation, and cancer. Cell. 2010;140(6):883–99.
19. Mantovani A, et al. Cancer-related inflammation. Nature. 2008;454(7203):436–44.
20. Trinchieri G. Cancer and inflammation: an old intuition with rapidly evolving new concepts. Annu Rev Immunol. 2012;30:677–706.
21. Kadariya Y, et al. Inflammation-related IL1β/IL1R signaling promotes the development of asbestos-induced malignant mesothelioma. Cancer Prev Res. 2016;9(5):406–14.
22. Takahashi H, et al. Tobacco smoke promotes lung tumorigenesis by triggering IKKbeta- and JNK1-dependent inflammation. Cancer Cell. 2010;17(1):89–97.
23. Quail DF, Dannenberg AJ. The obese adipose tissue microenvironment in cancer development and progression. Nat Rev Endocrinol. 2019;15(3):139–54.
24. Quail DF, et al. Obesity alters the lung myeloid cell landscape to enhance breast cancer metastasis through IL5 and GM-CSF. Nat Cell Biol. 2017;19(8):974–87.
25. Albrengues J, et al. Neutrophil extracellular traps produced during inflammation awaken dormant cancer cells in mice. Science. 2018;361:6409.
26. Cordon-Cardo C, Prives C. At the crossroads of inflammation and tumorigenesis. J Exp Med. 1999;190(10):1367–70.
27. Karin M. Nuclear factor-kappaB in cancer development and progression. Nature. 2006;441(7092):431–6.
28. Wu S, et al. A human colonic commensal promotes colon tumorigenesis via activation of T helper type 17 T cell responses. Nat Med. 2009;15(9):1016–22.
29. Rakoff-Nahoum S, Medzhitov R. Toll-like receptors and cancer. Nat Rev Cancer. 2009;9(1):57–63.
30. Waldner MJ, Neurath MF. Colitis-associated cancer: the role of T cells in tumor development. Semin Immunopathol. 2009;31(2):249–56.
31. Nickoloff BJ, Ben-Neriah Y, Pikarsky E. Inflammation and cancer: is the link as simple as we think? J Invest Dermatol. 2005;124(6):10–4.
32. Punturieri A, et al. Lung cancer and chronic obstructive pulmonary disease: needs and opportunities for integrated research. J Natl Cancer Inst. 2009;101(8):554–9.
33. Dostert C, et al. Innate immune activation through Nalp3 inflammasome sensing of asbestos and silica. Science. 2008;320(5876):674–7.
34. Calle EE. Obesity and cancer. BMJ. 2007;335(7630):1107–8.
35. Rodier F, et al. Persistent DNA damage signalling triggers senescence-associated inflammatory cytokine secretion. Nat Cell Biol. 2009;11(8):973–9.
36. Zheng L, et al. Fen1 mutations result in autoimmunity, chronic inflammation and cancers. Nat Med. 2007;13(7):812–9.
37. Sparmann A, Bar-Sagi D. Ras-induced interleukin-8 expression plays a critical role in tumor growth and angiogenesis. Cancer Cell. 2004;6(5):447–58.
38. Soucek L, et al. Mast cells are required for angiogenesis and macroscopic expansion of Myc-induced pancreatic islet tumors. Nat Med. 2007;13(10):1211–8.
39. Vakkila J, Lotze MT. Inflammation and necrosis promote tumour growth. Nat Rev Immunol. 2004;4(8):641–8.
40. Kim S, et al. Carcinoma-produced factors activate myeloid cells through TLR2 to stimulate metastasis. Nature. 2009;457(7225):102–6.
41. Dvorak HF. Tumors: wounds that do not heal. Similarities between tumor stroma generation and wound healing. N Engl J Med. 1986;315(26):1650–9.
42. Guerra C, et al. Chronic pancreatitis is essential for induction of pancreatic ductal adenocarcinoma by K-Ras oncogenes in adult mice. Cancer Cell. 2007;11(3):291–302.
43. Sieweke MH, et al. Mediation of wound-related Rous sarcoma virus tumorigenesis by TGF-beta. Science. 1990;248(4963):1656–60.

44. Zong WX, Thompson CB. Necrotic death as a cell fate. Genes Dev. 2006;20(1):1–15.
45. Ammirante M, et al. B-cell-derived lymphotoxin promotes castration-resistant prostate cancer. Nature. 2010;464(7286):302–5.
46. Zitvogel L, et al. Immunological aspects of cancer chemotherapy. Nat Rev Immunol. 2008;8(1):59–73.
47. Ullman TA, Itzkowitz SH. Intestinal inflammation and cancer. Gastroenterology. 2011;140(6):1807–16.
48. Puram SV, et al. Single-cell transcriptomic analysis of primary and metastatic tumor ecosystems in head and neck cancer. Cell. 2017;171(7):1611–24.
49. Mlecnik B, et al. Integrative analyses of colorectal cancer show immunoscore is a stronger predictor of patient survival than microsatellite instability. Immunity. 2016;44(3):698–711.
50. Tosolini M, et al. Clinical impact of different classes of infiltrating T cytotoxic and helper cells (Th1, th2, treg, th17) in patients with colorectal cancer. Cancer Res. 2011;71(4):1263–71.
51. Grivennikov SI, et al. Adenoma-linked barrier defects and microbial products drive IL-23/IL-17-mediated tumour growth. Nature. 2012;491(7423):254–8.
52. Hanahan D, Coussens LM. Accessories to the crime: functions of cells recruited to the tumor microenvironment. Cancer Cell. 2012;21(3):309–22.
53. Mantovani A, et al. Innate immunity, inflammation and tumour progression: double-edged swords. J Intern Med. 2019;285(5):524–32.
54. Sharma P, Allison JP. The future of immune checkpoint therapy. Science. 2015;348(6230):56–61.
55. Ghiringhelli F, et al. Activation of the NLRP3 inflammasome in dendritic cells induces IL-1beta-dependent adaptive immunity against tumors. Nat Med. 2009;15(10):1170–8.
56. Ciampricotti M, et al. Chemotherapy response of spontaneous mammary tumors is independent of the adaptive immune system. Nat Med. 2012;18(3):344–6.
57. Galluzzi L, et al. Molecular mechanisms of cell death: recommendations of the Nomenclature Committee on Cell Death 2018. Cell Death Differ. 2018;25(3):486–541.
58. Weinlich R, et al. Necroptosis in development, inflammation and disease. Nat Rev Mol Cell Biol. 2017;18(2):127–36.
59. Hou J, Greten TF, Xia Q. Immunosuppressive cell death in cancer. Nat Rev Immunol. 2017;17(6):401.
60. Halbrook CJ, et al. Macrophage-released pyrimidines inhibit gemcitabine therapy in pancreatic cancer. Cell Metab. 2019;29(6):1390–9.
61. Jinushi M, et al. Tumor-associated macrophages regulate tumorigenicity and anticancer drug responses of cancer stem/initiating cells. Proc Natl Acad Sci USA. 2011;108(30):12425–30.
62. Malesci A, et al. Tumor-associated macrophages and response to 5-fluorouracil adjuvant therapy in stage III colorectal cancer. Onco Targets Ther. 2017;6(12):e1342918.
63. Wang K, et al. Interleukin-17 receptor a signaling in transformed enterocytes promotes early colorectal tumorigenesis. Immunity. 2014;41(6):1052–63.
64. Meisel M, et al. Microbial signals drive pre-leukaemic myeloproliferation in a Tet2-deficient host. Nature. 2018;557(7706):580–4.
65. Luo JL, et al. Inhibition of NF-kappaB in cancer cells converts inflammation- induced tumor growth mediated by TNFalpha to TRAIL-mediated tumor regression. Cancer Cell. 2004;6(3):297–305.
66. Fearon ER, Vogelstein B. A genetic model for colorectal tumorigenesis. Cell. 1990;61(5):759–67.
67. Hanahan D, Weinberg RA. The hallmarks of cancer. Cell. 2000;100(1):57–70.
68. Hussain SP, Hofseth LJ, Harris CC. Radical causes of cancer. Nat Rev Cancer. 2003;3(4):276–85.
69. Kraus S, Arber N. Inflammation and colorectal cancer. Curr Opin Pharmacol. 2009;9(4):405–10.
70. Meira LB, et al. DNA damage induced by chronic inflammation contributes to colon carcinogenesis in mice. J Clin Invest. 2008;118(7):2516–25.

71. Okayasu I, et al. Promotion of colorectal neoplasia in experimental murine ulcerative colitis. Gut. 1996;39(1):87–92.
72. Hatano K, Fujita K, Nonomura N. Application of anti-inflammatory agents in prostate cancer. J Clin Med. 2020;9(8):2680.
73. Coussens LM, Zitvogel L, Palucka AK. Neutralizing tumor-promoting chronic inflammation: a magic bullet? Science. 2013;339(6117):286–91.
74. Petty AJ, Yang Y. Tumor-associated macrophages: implications in cancer immunotherapy. Immunotherapy. 2017;9(3):289–302.
75. Cassetta L, Pollard JW. Targeting macrophages: therapeutic approaches in cancer. Nat Rev Drug Discov. 2018;17(12):887–904.
76. Pathria P, Louis TL, Varner JA. Targeting tumor-associated macrophages in cancer. Trends Immunol. 2019;40(4):310–27.
77. Gabrilovich DI, Ostrand-Rosenberg S, Bronte V. Coordinated regulation of myeloid cells by tumours. Nat Rev Immunol. 2012;12(4):253–68.
78. Law AMK, Valdes-Mora F, Gallego-Ortega D. Myeloid-derived suppressor cells as a therapeutic target for cancer. Cells. 2020;9(3):561.
79. Liu Y, et al. Targeting myeloid-derived suppressor cells for cancer immunotherapy. Cancer Immunol Immunother. 2018;67(8):1181–95.
80. Nguyen DP, Li J, Tewari AK. Inflammation and prostate cancer: the role of interleukin 6 (IL-6). BJU Int. 2014;113(6):986–92.
81. George DJ, et al. The prognostic significance of plasma interleukin-6 levels in patients with metastatic hormone-refractory prostate cancer: results from cancer and leukemia group B 9480. Clin Cancer Res. 2005;11(5):1815–20.
82. Wu CT, et al. Significance of IL-6 in the transition of hormone-resistant prostate cancer and the induction of myeloid-derived suppressor cells. J Mol Med. 2012;90(11):1343–55.
83. Kitamura H, et al. Interleukin-6/STAT3 signaling as a promising target to improve the efficacy of cancer immunotherapy. Cancer Sci. 2017;108(10):1947–52.
84. Kortylewski M, et al. Inhibiting Stat3 signaling in the hematopoietic system elicits multicomponent antitumor immunity. Nat Med. 2005;11(12):1314–21.
85. Yu H, Pardoll D, Jove R. STATs in cancer inflammation and immunity: a leading role for STAT3. Nat Rev Cancer. 2009;9(11):798–809.
86. Hellsten R, et al. The STAT3 inhibitor galiellalactone inhibits the generation of MDSC-like monocytes by prostate cancer cells and decreases immunosuppressive and tumorigenic factors. Prostate. 2019;79(14):1611–21.
87. Hayashi T, et al. High-fat diet-induced inflammation accelerates prostate cancer growth via IL6 signaling. Clin Cancer Res. 2018;24(17):4309–18.
88. van Rhee F, et al. Siltuximab for multicentric Castleman's disease: a randomised, double-blind, placebo-controlled trial. Lancet Oncol. 2014;15(9):966–74.
89. Wallner L, et al. Inhibition of interleukin-6 with CNTO328, an anti-interleukin-6 monoclonal antibody, inhibits conversion of androgen-dependent prostate cancer to an androgen-independent phenotype in orchiectomized mice. Cancer Res. 2006;66(6):3087–95.
90. Dorff TB, et al. Clinical and correlative results of SWOG S0354: a phase II trial of CNTO328 (siltuximab), a monoclonal antibody against interleukin-6, in chemotherapy-pretreated patients with castration-resistant prostate cancer. Clin Cancer Res. 2010;16(11):3028–34.
91. Fizazi K, et al. Randomised phase II study of siltuximab (CNTO 328), an anti-IL-6 monoclonal antibody, in combination with mitoxantrone/prednisone versus mitoxantrone/prednisone alone in metastatic castration-resistant prostate cancer. Eur J Cancer. 2012;48(1):85–93.
92. Karkera J, et al. The anti-interleukin-6 antibody siltuximab down-regulates genes implicated in tumorigenesis in prostate cancer patients from a phase I study. Prostate. 2011;71(13):1455–65.
93. Chen W, et al. Niclosamide: beyond an antihelminthic drug. Cell Signal. 2018;41:89–96.
94. Sekulovski N, et al. Niclosamide suppresses macrophage-induced inflammation in endometriosis. Biol Reprod. 2020;102(5):1011–9.

95. Liu C, et al. Niclosamide inhibits androgen receptor variants expression and overcomes enzalutamide resistance in castration-resistant prostate cancer. Clin Cancer Res. 2014;20(12):3198–210.
96. Moreira D, et al. STAT3 inhibition combined with CpG immunostimulation activates antitumor immunity to eradicate genetically distinct castration-resistant prostate cancers. Clin Cancer Res. 2018;24(23):5948–62.
97. Ferrer FA, et al. Vascular endothelial growth factor (VEGF) expression in human prostate cancer: in situ and in vitro expression of VEGF by human prostate cancer cells. J Urol. 1997;157(6):2329–33.
98. Tong Y, et al. Role of interleukin-1 family in bone metastasis of prostate cancer. Front Oncol. 2022;12:951167.
99. Thomas-Jardin SE, et al. Identification of an IL-1-induced gene expression pattern in AR(+) PCa cells that mimics the molecular phenotype of AR(-) PCa cells. Prostate. 2018;78(8):595–606.
100. Jemaa AB, et al. Cytokine profiling identifies an interaction of IL-6 and IL-1α to drive PSMA-PSA prostate clones. Immunobiology. 2016;221(12):1424–31.
101. Longoni N, et al. ETS transcription factor ESE1/ELF3 orchestrates a positive feedback loop that constitutively activates NF-κB and drives prostate cancer progression. Cancer Res. 2013;73(14):4533–47.
102. Le Brun G, et al. Upregulation of endothelin 1 and its precursor by IL-1beta, TNF-alpha, and TGF-beta in the PC3 human prostate cancer cell line. Cytokine. 1999;11(2):157–62.
103. Klein RD, et al. Interleukin-1beta secreted from monocytic cells induces the expression of matrilysin in the prostatic cell line LNCaP. J Biol Chem. 1997;272(22):14188–92.
104. Ricote M, et al. Interleukin-1 (IL-1alpha and IL-1beta) and its receptors (IL-1RI, IL-1RII, and IL-1Ra) in prostate carcinoma. Cancer. 2004;100(7):1388–96.
105. Ben-Baruch A. The inflammatory milieu of tumors: cytokines and chemokines that affect tumor growth and metastasis. Potomac: Bentham Science Publishers; 2012.
106. Ries CH, et al. Targeting tumor-associated macrophages with anti-CSF-1R antibody reveals a strategy for cancer therapy. Cancer Cell. 2014;25(6):846–59.
107. Xu J, et al. CSF1R signaling blockade stanches tumor-infiltrating myeloid cells and improves the efficacy of radiotherapy in prostate cancer. Cancer Res. 2013;73(9):2782–94.
108. Escamilla J, et al. CSF1 receptor targeting in prostate cancer reverses macrophage-mediated resistance to androgen blockade therapy. Cancer Res. 2015;75(6):950–62.
109. Tap WD, et al. Pexidartinib versus placebo for advanced tenosynovial giant cell tumour (ENLIVEN): a randomised phase 3 trial. Lancet. 2019;394(10197):478–87.
110. Guan W, et al. Inhibition of TAMs improves the response to docetaxel in castration-resistant prostate cancer. Endocr Relat Cancer. 2019;26(1):131–40.
111. Raymond E, et al. Mechanisms of action of tasquinimod on the tumour microenvironment. Cancer Chemother Pharmacol. 2014;73(1):1–8.
112. Gupta N, et al. Mechanism of action and clinical activity of tasquinimod in castrate-resistant prostate cancer. Onco Targets Ther. 2014;7:223–34.
113. Sternberg C, et al. Randomized, double-blind, placebo-controlled phase III study of tasquinimod in men with metastatic castration-resistant prostate cancer. J Clin Oncol. 2016;34(22):2636–43.
114. Gunderson AJ, et al. Bruton tyrosine kinase-dependent immune cell cross-talk drives pancreas cancer. Cancer Discov. 2016;6(3):270–85.
115. Molina-Cerrillo J, et al. Bruton's tyrosine kinase (BTK) as a promising target in solid tumors. Cancer Treat Rev. 2017;58:41–50.
116. O'Neill LA, Kishton RJ, Rathmell J. A guide to immunometabolism for immunologists. Nat Rev Immunol. 2016;16(9):553–65.
117. Uyttenhove C, et al. Evidence for a tumoral immune resistance mechanism based on tryptophan degradation by indoleamine 2,3-dioxygenase. Nat Med. 2003;9(10):1269–74.

118. Godin-Ethier J, et al. Indoleamine 2,3-dioxygenase expression in human cancers: clinical and immunologic perspectives. Clin Cancer Res. 2011;17(22):6985–91.
119. Prendergast GC, et al. Indoleamine 2,3-dioxygenase pathways of pathogenic inflammation and immune escape in cancer. Cancer Immunol Immunother. 2014;63(7):721–35.
120. Prendergast GC, et al. Discovery of IDO1 inhibitors: from bench to bedside. Cancer Res. 2017;77(24):6795–811.
121. Fox E, et al. Indoximod: an immunometabolic adjuvant that empowers T cell activity in cancer. Front Oncol. 2018;8:370.
122. Yoshimura T. The production of monocyte chemoattractant protein-1 (MCP-1)/CCL2 in tumor microenvironments. Cytokine. 2017;98:71–8.
123. Yoshimura T. The chemokine MCP-1 (CCL2) in the host interaction with cancer: a foe or ally? Cell Mol Immunol. 2018;15(4):335–45.
124. Lu Y, et al. Monocyte chemotactic protein-1 (MCP-1) acts as a paracrine and autocrine factor for prostate cancer growth and invasion. Prostate. 2006;66(12):1311–8.
125. Loberg RD, et al. CCL2 is a potent regulator of prostate cancer cell migration and proliferation. Neoplasia. 2006;8(7):578–86.
126. Loberg RD, et al. CCL2 as an important mediator of prostate cancer growth in vivo through the regulation of macrophage infiltration. Neoplasia. 2007;9(7):556–62.
127. Loberg RD, et al. Targeting CCL2 with systemic delivery of neutralizing antibodies induces prostate cancer tumor regression in vivo. Cancer Res. 2007;67(19):9417–24.
128. Pienta KJ, et al. Phase 2 study of carlumab (CNTO 888), a human monoclonal antibody against CC-chemokine ligand 2 (CCL2), in metastatic castration-resistant prostate cancer. Investig New Drugs. 2013;31(3):760–8.
129. Hughes R, et al. Perivascular M2 macrophages stimulate tumor relapse after chemotherapy. Cancer Res. 2015;75(17):3479–91.
130. Deng Y, et al. Hepatic carcinoma-associated fibroblasts enhance immune suppression by facilitating the generation of myeloid-derived suppressor cells. Oncogene. 2017;36(8):1090–101.
131. Teicher BA, Fricker SP. CXCL12 (SDF-1)/CXCR4 pathway in cancer. Clin Cancer Res. 2010;16(11):2927–31.
132. Chen Q, Zhong T. The association of CXCR4 expression with clinicopathological significance and potential drug target in prostate cancer: a meta-analysis and literature review. Drug Des Devel Ther. 2015;9:5115–22.
133. Hatano K, et al. Residual prostate cancer cells after docetaxel therapy increase the tumorigenic potential via constitutive signaling of CXCR4, ERK1/2 and c-Myc. Mol Cancer Res. 2013;11(9):1088–100.
134. Gravina GL, et al. CXCR4 pharmacogical inhibition reduces bone and soft tissue metastatic burden by affecting tumor growth and tumorigenic potential in prostate cancer preclinical models. Prostate. 2015;75(12):1227–46.
135. Saha A, et al. Proinflammatory CXCL12-CXCR4/CXCR7 signaling axis drives myc-induced prostate cancer in obese mice. Cancer Res. 2017;77(18):5158–68.
136. Domanska UM, et al. CXCR4 inhibition with AMD3100 sensitizes prostate cancer to docetaxel chemotherapy. Neoplasia. 2012;14(8):709–18.
137. De Clercq E. Mozobil® (Plerixafor, AMD3100), 10 years after its approval by the US Food and Drug Administration. Antivir Chem Chemother. 2019;27:2040206619829382.
138. Dennis KL, et al. Current status of interleukin-10 and regulatory T-cells in cancer. Curr Opin Oncol. 2013;25(6):637–45.
139. Samiea A, et al. Interleukin-10 induces expression of neuroendocrine markers and PDL1 in prostate cancer cells. Prostate Cancer. 2020;2020:5305306.
140. Hutchins AP, Diez D, Miranda-Saavedra D. The IL-10/STAT3-mediated anti-inflammatory response: recent developments and future challenges. Brief Funct Genomics. 2013;12(6):489–98.
141. Ouyang W, O'Garra A. IL-10 family cytokines IL-10 and IL-22: from basic science to clinical translation. Immunity. 2019;50(4):871–91.

142. Ugge H, et al. Circulating inflammation markers and prostate cancer. Prostate. 2019;79(11):1338–46.
143. Dwivedi S, et al. Diagnostic and prognostic significance of prostate specific antigen and serum interleukin 18 and 10 in patients with locally advanced prostate cancer: a prospective study. Asian Pac J Cancer Prev. 2011;12(7):1843–8.
144. Chen Q, et al. Production of IL-10 by melanoma cells: examination of its role in immunosuppression mediated by melanoma. Int J Cancer. 1994;56(5):755–60.
145. Gastl GA, et al. Interleukin-10 production by human carcinoma cell lines and its relationship to interleukin-6 expression. Int J Cancer. 1993;55(1):96–101.
146. Hao NB, et al. Macrophages in tumor microenvironments and the progression of tumors. Clin Dev Immunol. 2012;2012:948098.
147. Chen Y, et al. Tumor-associated macrophages: an accomplice in solid tumor progression. J Biomed Sci. 2019;26(1):78.
148. Taube JM, et al. Differential expression of immune-regulatory genes associated with PD-L1 display in melanoma: implications for PD-1 pathway blockade. Clin Cancer Res. 2015;21(17):3969–76.
149. Butte MJ, et al. Programmed death-1 ligand 1 interacts specifically with the B7-1 costimulatory molecule to inhibit T cell responses. Immunity. 2007;27(1):111–22.
150. Brown JA, et al. Blockade of programmed death-1 ligands on dendritic cells enhances T cell activation and cytokine production. J Immunol. 2003;170(3):1257–66.
151. Stearns ME, Hu Y, Wang M. IL-10 signaling via IL-10E1 is dependent on tyrosine phosphorylation in the IL-10R alpha chain in human primary prostate cancer cell lines. Oncogene. 2003;22(24):3781–91.
152. Wang M, Hu Y, Stearns ME. A novel IL-10 signalling mechanism regulates TIMP-1 expression in human prostate tumour cells. Br J Cancer. 2003;88(10):1605–14.
153. Stearns ME, et al. Interleukin 10 blocks matrix metalloproteinase-2 and membrane type 1-matrix metalloproteinase synthesis in primary human prostate tumor lines. Clin Cancer Res. 2003;9(3):1191–9.
154. Escaff S, et al. Study of matrix metalloproteinases and their inhibitors in prostate cancer. Br J Cancer. 2010;102(5):922–9.
155. Bishop JL, et al. PD-L1 is highly expressed in Enzalutamide resistant prostate cancer. Oncotarget. 2015;6(1):234–42.
156. Tavassoli P, et al. Rapid, non-destructive, cell-based screening assays for agents that modulate growth, death, and androgen receptor activation in prostate cancer cells. Prostate. 2007;67(4):416–26.
157. Ware JL. Growth factors and their receptors as determinants in the proliferation and metastasis of human prostate cancer. Cancer Metastasis Rev. 1993;12(3-4):287–301.
158. Lee C, et al. Transforming growth factor-beta in benign and malignant prostate. Prostate. 1999;39(4):285–90.
159. Thompson-Elliott B, Johnson R, Khan SA. Alterations in TGFβ signaling during prostate cancer progression. Am J Clin Exp Urol. 2021;9(4):318–28.
160. Kaminska B, Wesolowska A, Danilkiewicz M. TGF beta signalling and its role in tumour pathogenesis. Acta Biochim Pol. 2005;52(2):329–37.
161. Bhowmick NA, et al. TGF-beta signaling in fibroblasts modulates the oncogenic potential of adjacent epithelia. Science. 2004;303(5659):848–51.
162. Robson CN, et al. Transforming growth factor-beta1 up-regulates p15, p21 and p27 and blocks cell cycling in G1 in human prostate epithelium. J Endocrinol. 1999;160(2):257–66.
163. Williams RH, et al. Reduced levels of transforming growth factor beta receptor type II in human prostate cancer: an immunohistochemical study. Clin Cancer Res. 1996;2(4):635–40.
164. Wikström P, et al. Alterations of transforming growth factor beta1 (TGF-beta1) and TGFbeta receptor expressions with progression in Dunning rat prostatic adenocarcinoma sublines. Urol Res. 1999;27(3):185–93.

165. Qin T, et al. A novel highly potent trivalent TGF-β receptor trap inhibits early-stage tumorigenesis and tumor cell invasion in murine Pten-deficient prostate glands. Oncotarget. 2016;7(52):86087–102.
166. Massagué J. TGF-β signaling in development and disease. FEBS Lett. 2012;586(14):1833.
167. D'Arcy Q, et al. The IL-4/IL-13 signaling axis promotes prostatic fibrosis. PLoS One. 2022;17(10):e0275064.
168. Kliewer SA, et al. Differential expression and activation of a family of murine peroxisome proliferator-activated receptors. Proc Natl Acad Sci USA. 1994;91(15):7355–9.
169. Rosen CJ. The rosiglitazone story–lessons from an FDA Advisory Committee meeting. N Engl J Med. 2007;357(9):844–6.
170. Hartley A, Ahmad I. The role of PPARγ in prostate cancer development and progression. Br J Cancer. 2023;128(6):940–5.
171. Brusotti G, et al. Betulinic acid is a PPARγ antagonist that improves glucose uptake, promotes osteogenesis and inhibits adipogenesis. Sci Rep. 2017;7(1):5777.
172. Elix CC, et al. Peroxisome proliferator-activated receptor gamma controls prostate cancer cell growth through AR-dependent and independent mechanisms. Prostate. 2020;80(2):162–72.
173. Zaytseva YY, et al. The PPARgamma antagonist T0070907 suppresses breast cancer cell proliferation and motility via both PPARgamma-dependent and -independent mechanisms. Anticancer Res. 2011;31(3):813–23.
174. Ahmad I, et al. Sleeping Beauty screen reveals Pparg activation in metastatic prostate cancer. Proc Natl Acad Sci USA. 2016;113(29):8290–5.
175. Al-Jameel W, et al. Inhibitor SBFI26 suppresses the malignant progression of castration-resistant PC3-M cells by competitively binding to oncogenic FABP5. Oncotarget. 2017;8(19):31041–56.
176. Nakano R, et al. Antagonism of peroxisome proliferator-activated receptor gamma prevents high-fat diet-induced obesity in vivo. Biochem Pharmacol. 2006;72(1):42–52.
177. Hayashi T, et al. Main inflammatory cells and potentials of anti-inflammatory agents in prostate cancer. Cancer. 2019;11(8):1153.
178. Vidal AC, et al. Aspirin, NSAIDs, and risk of prostate cancer: results from the REDUCE study. Clin Cancer Res. 2015;21(4):756–62.
179. Choe KS, et al. Aspirin use and the risk of prostate cancer mortality in men treated with prostatectomy or radiotherapy. J Clin Oncol. 2012;30(28):3540–4.
180. Cardwell CR, et al. Low-dose aspirin and survival in men with prostate cancer: a study using the UK Clinical Practice Research Datalink. Cancer Causes Control. 2014;25(1):33–43.
181. Flahavan EM, et al. A cohort study investigating aspirin use and survival in men with prostate cancer. Ann Oncol. 2014;25(1):154–9.
182. Jacobs EJ, et al. Daily aspirin use and prostate cancer-specific mortality in a large cohort of men with nonmetastatic prostate cancer. J Clin Oncol. 2014;32(33):3716–22.
183. James ND, et al. Celecoxib plus hormone therapy versus hormone therapy alone for hormone-sensitive prostate cancer: first results from the STAMPEDE multiarm, multistage, randomised controlled trial. Lancet Oncol. 2012;13(5):549–58.
184. Zhao X, Xu Z, Li H. NSAIDs use and reduced metastasis in cancer patients: results from a meta-analysis. Sci Rep. 2017;7(1):1875.
185. Mascan B, Marignol L. Aspirin in the management of patients with prostate cancer undergoing radiotherapy: friend or foe? Anticancer Res. 2018;38(4):1897–902.
186. Hua H, et al. Complex roles of the old drug aspirin in cancer chemoprevention and therapy. Med Res Rev. 2019;39(1):114–45.
187. Kim HG, et al. Metformin inhibits P-glycoprotein expression via the NF-κB pathway and CRE transcriptional activity through AMPK activation. Br J Pharmacol. 2011;162(5):1096–108.
188. Tong D, et al. Metformin inhibits castration-induced EMT in prostate cancer by repressing COX2/PGE2/STAT3 axis. Cancer Lett. 2017;389:23–32.
189. Liu Q, et al. Metformin inhibits prostate cancer progression by targeting tumor-associated inflammatory infiltration. Clin Cancer Res. 2018;24(22):5622–34.

190. Sarmento-Cabral A, et al. Metformin reduces prostate tumor growth, in a diet-dependent manner, by modulating multiple signaling pathways. Mol Cancer Res. 2017;15(7):862–74.
191. Hayashi T, et al. Metformin inhibits prostate cancer growth induced by a high-fat diet in Pten-deficient model mice. Int J Urol. 2019;26(2):307–9.
192. Uehara T, et al. Metformin induces CD11b+-cell-mediated growth inhibition of an osteosarcoma: implications for metabolic reprogramming of myeloid cells and anti-tumor effects. Int Immunol. 2019;31(4):187–98.
193. Incio J, et al. PlGF/VEGFR-1 signaling promotes macrophage polarization and accelerated tumor progression in obesity. Clin Cancer Res. 2016;22(12):2993–3004.
194. Eikawa S, et al. Immune-mediated antitumor effect by type 2 diabetes drug, metformin. Proc Natl Acad Sci USA. 2015;112(6):1809–14.
195. Bañez LL, et al. Association between statins and prostate tumor inflammatory infiltrate in men undergoing radical prostatectomy. Cancer Epidemiol Biomarkers Prev. 2010;19(3):722–8.
196. Allott EH, et al. Statin use, serum lipids, and prostate inflammation in men with a negative prostate biopsy: results from the REDUCE trial. Cancer Prev Res. 2017;10(6):319–26.
197. Murtola TJ, et al. Atorvastatin versus placebo for prostate cancer before radical prostatectomy-a randomized, double-blind, placebo-controlled clinical trial. Eur Urol. 2018;74(6):697–701.
198. Ridker PM. From C-reactive protein to interleukin-6 to interleukin-1: moving upstream to identify novel targets for atheroprotection. Circ Res. 2016;118(1):145–56.
199. Sugiyama M, et al. Effects of atorvastatin on inflammation and oxidative stress. Heart Vessel. 2005;20(4):133–6.
200. Weber C, et al. HMG-CoA reductase inhibitors decrease CD11b expression and CD11b-dependent adhesion of monocytes to endothelium and reduce increased adhesiveness of monocytes isolated from patients with hypercholesterolemia. J Am Coll Cardiol. 1997;30(5):1212–7.
201. Romano M, et al. Inhibition of monocyte chemotactic protein-1 synthesis by statins. Lab Investig. 2000;80(7):1095–100.
202. Mallat Z, Ait-Oufella H, Tedgui A. Regulatory T cell responses: potential role in the control of atherosclerosis. Curr Opin Lipidol. 2005;16(5):518–24.
203. Mausner-Fainberg K, et al. The effect of HMG-CoA reductase inhibitors on naturally occurring CD4+CD25+ T cells. Atherosclerosis. 2008;197(2):829–39.
204. Kwak B, et al. Statins as a newly recognized type of immunomodulator. Nat Med. 2000;6(12):1399–402.
205. Paumelle R, Staels B. Peroxisome proliferator-activated receptors mediate pleiotropic actions of statins. Circ Res. 2007;100(10):1394–5.

Chapter 4
Prostate Cancer, Apoptosis, Autophagy and Ferroptosis: Cell Death Mechanisms and Their Cross-talk

Mehrdad Hashemi, Atena Sadat Hosseini, Sajad Monjezi, Saina Hasany, Sara Binaei, Mobina Nejat, Hadis Melyani, Nader Bashandeh, Arash Matinahmadi, Zoofa Zayani, Sima Orouei, Seyed Hesamoddin Bidooki, Rasoul Raesi, Najma Farahani, and Maliheh Entezari

Abstract A crucial mechanism for maintaining organismic homeostasis is cell death, which is the last cellular choice taken after intricate communications. When cells stop performing their essential life duties, it is called cell death. Typically, cell death is categorized as either controlled cell death (RCD) or accidental cell death (ACD). The irreversible end of life occurs at cell death. Involved in embryonic

M. Hashemi · M. Entezari
Farhikhtegan Medical Convergence Sciences Research Center, Farhikhtegan Hospital Tehran Medical Sciences, Islamic Azad University, Tehran, Iran

Faculty of Advanced Science and Technology, Department of Genetics, Tehran Medical Sciences, Islamic Azad University, Tehran, Iran

A. S. Hosseini · S. Hasany
Farhikhtegan Medical Convergence Sciences Research Center, Farhikhtegan Hospital Tehran Medical Sciences, Islamic Azad University, Tehran, Iran

S. Monjezi
Department of Clinical Biochemistry, School of Medicine, Ahvaz Jundishapur University Medical Sciences, Ahvaz, Iran

S. Binaei
Endocrinology and Metabolism Research Center, Hormozgan University of Medical Sciences, Bandar Abbas, Iran

M. Nejat
Faculty of Advanced Science and Technology, Tehran Medical Sciences, Islamic Azad University, Tehran, Iran

H. Melyani
Biology Teaching Groupe, Farhangian University, Ahvaz, Iran

N. Bashandeh
Biology Science Groupe, University of Sistan and Baluchestan, Zahedan, Iran

G. Sethi et al. (eds.), *Prostate Cancer: Molecular Events and Therapeutic Modalities*, https://doi.org/10.1007/978-981-97-4612-5_4

development, organ maintenance, and autoimmunity, it is also the fundamental physiological mechanism of all living things. Apoptosis, necroptosis, autophagy, and pyroptosis are all forms of "programmed cell death" that have been better understood in recent years, and we have also identified several important genes involved in these processes. However, the use of these various cell death processes in illnesses and their conversion is underexplored in these earlier studies. Overall, the area of cell death has made several important discoveries in the past few years, but there are still a lot of unanswered questions. The facts show that cell death is a complicated game, with a number of key players that can upset the cell environment's delicate balance, switching it from anti-inflammatory to pro-inflammatory, and from survival to death. There will undoubtedly be thrilling new research in this area in the coming years, thanks to the exhaustive investigation of the intricate regulatory mechanism of cell death.

Keywords Prostate cancer · Cell death · Apoptosis · Ferroptosis · Cancer

4.1 Introduction

While massive damage can cause cell death, the vast majority of cell deaths in animals are initiated by specific signaling events [1]. The outward appearance of the dying cell is a key indicator of the kind of cell death that has occurred: apoptosis, autophagic cell death, and necrosis [2]. Cellulose degradation, blebbing of the cell membrane, and chromatin condensation (pyknosis) are hallmarks of cell death, as

A. Matinahmadi
Department of Cellular and Molecular Biology, Nicolaus Copernicus University, Torun, Poland

Z. Zayani
Centre for Modern Interdisciplinary Technologies, Nicolaus Copernicus University, Torun, Poland

S. Orouei
Department of Biology, Science and Research Branch, Islamic Azad University, Tehran, Iran

S. H. Bidooki
Faculty of Veterinary Medicine, Department of Biochemistry and Molecular and Cellular Biology, Health Research Institute of Aragon-University of Zaragoza, Zaragoza, Spain

R. Raesi
Department of Nursing, Torbat Jam Faculty of Medical Sciences, Torbat Jam, Iran

Department of Health Services Management, Mashhad University of Medical Sciences, Mashhad, Iran

N. Farahani (✉)
Farhikhtegan Medical Convergence Sciences Research Center, Farhikhtegan Hospital Tehran Medical Sciences, Islamic Azad University, Tehran, Iran

described by Kerr and colleagues in 1972 [3]. Moreover, the activation of caspase proteases is a hallmark of this form of cell death [4]. The death receptor route and the mitochondrial pathway are the two main signaling mechanisms that initiate apoptotic cell death. The second type of contact contains the traditional ligand-cell-surface-receptor triangle. One member of the tumor necrosis factor receptor (TNFR) family, cytotoxic lymphocytes (CTLs), expresses ligands for death receptors (DRs), which allow them to kill altered or contaminated cells. Assuming the target cells have these DRs, these ligands cause them to undergo apoptotic cell death. Immune system homeostasis and function depend on DR-induced cell death in general. The mitochondrial apoptotic pathway, on the other hand, is typically begun by the cell itself. When cells are irreparably damaged, apoptosis is actively engaged by the majority of cellular stressors, including DNA damage (caused by genotoxic chemicals or DNA repair errors) and endoplasmic reticulum (ER) stress (caused by the buildup of unfolded proteins). Furthermore, cell death can occur in the absence of a signal, such as those activated by growth factors (such as cytokines and neurotrophic factors). The procedure is predicted to kill half of the neurons created, although it is crucial for vertebrates' nervous system development [5]. A lack of neurotrophic factor stimulation, which occurs when some neuronal progenitors do not migrate or innervate their targets correctly, contributes to this cell death. In the same way, the rapid reduction of the lymphocyte number following pathogen clearance is caused by cytokine deprivation in conjunction with the DR pathway during an immunological response. Another type of cell death caused by "loss-of-signal" is anoikis, which happens when cells in the cell membrane (epithelial or endothelial cells) separate from the Extracellular Matrix (ECM). Here, apoptosis results from the loss of pro-survival signaling pathways induced by unligated integrin family ECM receptors. This process stops cells that have shed from their initial site from spreading to other areas, which is a hallmark of cancer cells that have metastasized. As a last line of defense against cancer, oncogenes (like Myc) can trigger cell death. When oncogene overexpression or mutation triggers abnormal mitogenic signals, a p53-dependent apoptotic pathway is activated and helps to regulate this process. Thus, it is frequently necessary to avoid apoptotic cell death in order to maintain oncogene transformation [6].

The presence of large intracellular vesicles and activation of the autophagy machinery are hallmarks of autophagic cell death. It is worth noting that autophagy, which involves engulfing sections of the cytoplasm and catabolic breakdown, is a well-defined process. However, its role as a mechanism for active cell death is still highly debated. To remove damaged organelles (such as mitochondria with low membrane potential) and protein aggregates, or in reaction to a metabolic crisis (such as low ATP levels or food and amino acid deprivation), autophagy is primarily activated. Moreover, Shen and collaborators revealed that autophagy is more often seen as a stress response that fails to drive cell death but rather occurs in tandem with it. But there are also cases where cell death cannot occur without the autophagy process [7]. The steroid hormone ecdysone triggers extensive autophagic cell death during Drosophila metamorphosis, allowing obsolete larval organs including the midgut and salivary glands to retreat. On top of that, the cell death program is affected when genes involved in the autophagic signaling pathway are lacking [8]. One potential defense mechanism against oncogenic transformation is autophagic cell death, which has been observed in response to dysregulated H-Ras activity [9]. The hallmarks of necrosis include the enlargement of cells, rupture of their plasma membranes, and the disappearance of organellar structure in the absence of chromatin condensation. There is at least one functioning necrosis route, even though necrosis can happen due to irreparable cell damage. The activation of receptor-interacting protein kinase 3 (RIP3) is the final step in this cascade of events that leads to cell death, which is also known as necroptosis. RIP3 becomes active when it is recruited to macromolecular complexes by distinct cell-surface receptors, such as DRs, TLRs, and the T-Cell Receptor (TCR). Furthermore, RIP3-activation platform creation can be directly induced by DNA damage, apart from cell-surface receptor ligation. Lastly, after a virus infection and the presence of double-stranded viral DNA in the cytosol, the cytosolic DNA sensor and the DNA-dependent activator of interferon (DAI) regulatory factors promote RIP3-dependent necrosis.

4.2 Autophagy Flux

The regulatory control of cellular mass, the correct distribution of organelles, and the elimination of toxic and detrimental components are all aided by autophagy, a well-conserved homeostatic process [10]. The intricate process of autophagy interacts with various biological activities, including the development and differentiation of tissues, the regulation of the immune system, and the removal of cancer cells [11, 12]. Combinatorial actions of the ATG1/ULK1 (Unc-51 such as autophagy activating kinase-1) complex and the PI3K-III complex initiate autophagy in response to cellular energy demands. The next stage in phagophore nucleation is the formation of autophagosomes, which are double-membrane structures, by phagocytizing intracellular cargos. When these autophagosomes combine with lysosomes, they create autolysosomes. The contents of these autolysosomes are then broken down to liberate amino acids and other substances involved in metabolism [13]. There are many different physiological processes in cells, and they all play an important part in keeping things in check and stopping disease from progressing [14–16]. When electron microscopy was originally developed in the 1950s, it was used to discover autophagy, a physiological process [17, 18]. An integral part of this process is the formation of autophagosomes and the mediation of their fusion with lysosomes, which leads to the degradation and recycling of cargo [19]. In autophagy, microautophagy, macroautophagy, and chaperone-mediated autophagy (CMA) are the three main varieties. When it comes to lysosome-limiting membrane sequestration pathways, the least well-studied is microautophagy, which is a catch-all word for a non-selective mechanism that involves membrane invagination [20]. Specifically, CMA identifies proteins for lysosomal breakdown, making it a selective autophagy mechanism [21]. When cells undergo autophagy, the most common type is macroautophagy, which involves the production of temporary double-membrane compartments called phagophores to ingest payloads, which are then contained within autophagosomes and eventually degraded when they fuse with lysosomes. For cellular homeostasis to be maintained, this form of autophagy is of significant importance [22].

In order to effectively design future studies and create innovative therapeutic treatments, it is crucial to understand the molecular mechanism of autophagy, regardless of its form [23, 24]. There are a total of six stages to autophagy: induction, growth, maturation, fusion, breakdown, and recycling [25]. Autophagy activation is facilitated by the ULK1 complex, which also includes ATG13, ATG101, and RB1CC1. Specifically, ULK1 is a serine/threonine kinase that promotes phagophore formation at the endoplasmic reticulum (ER) and participates in the phosphorylation of phosphatidylinositol 3-kinase complex I components, such as BECN1 and PIK3C3/VPS34 [26]. During the expansion step, the phagophore membrane is targeted by the formation of the ATG12-ATG5 complex by means of the ATG7 and ATG10 enzymes. Following translation into precursor forms, ATG4 cleaves two subfamilies of proteins called Atg8-family proteins because of their homology with yeast Atg8, and MAP1LC3/LC3 (microtubule-associated protein 1 light chain 3) and GABARAP proteins. Proteins undergo proteolytic processing before being covalently linked to phosphatidylethanolamine at the phagophore membrane. This mechanism, similar to that which generates the ATG12-ATG5 conjugate, is dependent on ATG3 and ATG7. Mature autophagosome development follows phagophore expansion for cargo engulfment. In order to finish maturation and allow fusion with either lysosomes or endosomes directly, LC3-II is removed from the autophagosome surface at this stage [27–29]. Molecular components such as soluble *N*-ethylmaleimide-sensitive factor-activating membrane fusion proteins (SNAREs) and tethering factors like RAB7 facilitate fusion [30]. At last, lysosomal enzymes break down the contents upon fusion with a lysosome, and the cytosol receives the breakdown products for reuse. This is the overarching process for initiating and finishing autophagy. Additional biochemical pathways and signaling networks involved in autophagy have been uncovered by other research. An example of an autophagy inhibitor is MTOR (mechanistic target of rapamycin kinase). An increase in Adenosine Monophosphate (AMP) levels triggers the activation of AMP-activated protein kinase (AMPK) when AMP-sensitive kinase (MTOR) is active. AMP-activated protein kinase (AMPK) inhibits mTOR, which leads to autophagy and an increase in cellular energy. Autophagy is essential for cellular survival and homeostasis, and its proper functioning is ensured by interconnected, intricate signaling networks. Figure 4.1 shows the autophagy mechanism.

Moreover, the role of autophagy in cancer is controversial, and researchers disagree on the precise ways in which it aids in cancer development and prevention. It is worth considering autophagy as a potential therapeutic target to decrease cancer-related mortality and morbidity. Autophagy, on the other side, can have opposite effects on cancer progression. An investigation into autophagy's role in cancer has recently revealed that its function is context-dependent [27]. Many studies have focused on autophagy in an effort to learn more about its dual regulatory roles in cancer and how to inhibit or activate it. Two main pathways in cancer cells'

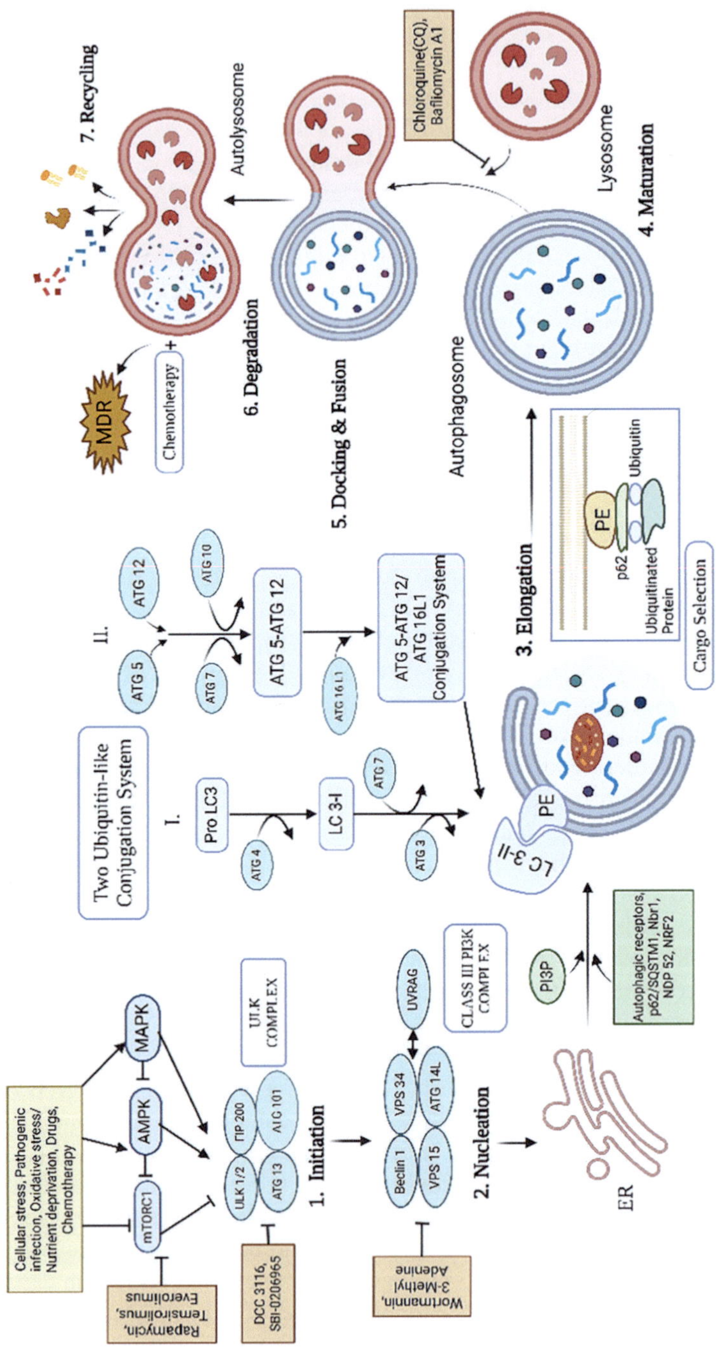

Fig. 4.1 The autophagy profile in cells (Biorender.com)

programmed cell death (PCD) are autophagy and apoptosis. Sustaining autophagy promotes cancer cell survival by reducing apoptosis, which allows cancer to develop [31]. On the other hand, inducing autophagy and apoptosis can lead to cancer suppression when autophagy functions as a tumor suppressor. One example is the finding that pancreatic cancer cells can have their MTOR inhibition by AMPK boosted by autophagy, which in turn increases the likelihood of cell death [32]. Cancer treatment can be advanced with the discovery of molecular mechanisms that regulate autophagy. The activation of pro-survival autophagy by hypoxic conditions is enhanced by phosphorylation of ATG5, which is caused by PAK1 (p21 (RAC1) activated kinase 1) [33]. All of these investigations point to autophagy as a key player in cancer metastasis [34]. Whether or if autophagy is associated with cancer spread is the next natural inquiry. Autophagy can increase or decrease cancer migration and invasion in different settings, hence the answer is favorable from an experimental standpoint [35]. Through inducing transitions from epithelial to mesenchymal cells, autophagy can greatly facilitate the spread of cancer. Levels of mesenchymal markers, including VIM (vimentin) and CDH2/N-cadherin, are downregulated during autophagy suppression, providing further evidence that autophagy is involved in cancer spread [36]. There is mounting evidence that autophagy regulates immune system function [37, 38], in addition to proliferation and migration. Autophagy ensures tumor growth by limiting anti-tumor T cell immunity against pancreatic cancer cells and preventing major histocompatibility complex class I (MHCI) expression [39]. Lastly, autophagy can control how cancer cells react to chemotherapy. A new study found that inhibiting autophagy makes stomach cancer cells more sensitive to chemotherapy [40].

While the core machinery appears to be controlled at numerous cytoplasmic sites in mammals, it has only been found at one site in yeast cells [41]. Protein Beclin-1, encoded by the BECN1 gene, is one of the primary regulators of autophagy. The vesicle-trafficking mechanisms are mediated by the phosphatidylinositol-3-kinase (PI3K) complex, which this protein is a component of [42]. A lack of Beclin-1 has been associated with the growth of solid tumors. Indeed, an increased risk of cancer in humans has been linked to its elimination. In addition, malignancies can arise on their own in BECN1 heterozygous mice [43, 44]. As a regulator of cellular metabolism, mammalian target of rapamycin complex 1 (mTORC1) is an important player. Phosphorylation of ULK1 and ATG13 by the mTORC1 complex initiates the metabolic behavior switch into anabolism in response to energy abundance. Autophagic activity is suppressed by the phosphorylated ULK1 complex [45]. In addition, autophagy regulates mitochondrial activity in response to stress. The activation of PTEN-induced putative kinase 1 (PINK1) occurs when mitochondria that are not functioning properly lose their membrane potential. PINK1 triggers the E3 ligase parkin (PARK2), which ubiquitylates proteins on the outer membrane of mitochondria and sends recognition signals to the autophagy machinery to break them down. An approach to reducing metabolic stress and reactive oxygen species (ROS) production while maintaining high mitochondrial quality involves the selective removal of damaged mitochondria [46, 47]. CaMKK2 is a member of the family of protein kinases that are selective for serine and threonine. Many metabolic pathways rely on

CaMMKs to control inflammation, food intake, adipogenesis, and glucose metabolism. In addition, its role in carcinogenesis has been established. Since androgen-receptor hyperactivity contributes to prostate cancer, CaMKK2 is also overexpressed in this disease [48]. New evidence suggests that CAMKK2 knockdown causes vesicle-trafficking disruption disturbances. Because CAMKK2 influences organelle integrity and membrane transport, it sustains cell proliferation, which is compatible with the role of autophagy in cancer development [49].

The connection between autophagy and cancer progression is complicated, though, and there may be some inconsistencies to consider. Disrupting Beclin-1 may enhance autophagic activity, which in turn increases lifespan and quality of life in mice [50, 51]. This could be feasible since Beclin-1 promotes cell survival by inhibiting B-cell lymphoma 2 (Bcl2). Nonetheless, these results are in line with the fact that cells have a higher chance of becoming cancers when apoptotic control is inaccurate. Autophagy has emerged as a mechanism that can regulate the response of tumor cells to chemotherapy. The dysregulation of autophagy can cause drug resistance in various human cancers [52, 53]. Moreover, autophagy has been specifically connected to the progression of a number of cancers such as pancreatic cancer in which the aberrant activation or inhibition of autophagy can change proliferation, metastasis and therapy response of tumor cells [54].

4.3 Autophagy in Prostate Cancer

Autophagy has several impacts, one of which is to increase the survival and multiplication of prostate cancer cells [14]. This is complex and the product of multiple molecular pathways interacting with one another. By activating autophagy, AR signaling contributes to the advancement of prostate cancer, for instance [55, 56]. Transcription Factor EB (TFEB) plays a prominent role in controlling the formation and operation of lysosomes. Autophagy induction is promoted by AR-stimulated TFEB expression. Additionally, AR regulates additional autophagy upstream mediators, such as ATG4B, ATG4D, ULK1, and ULK2, which contribute to the advancement of prostate cancer. Additional research has linked AR-mediated autophagy induction to a bad prognosis and has shown that it is critical for the proliferation and viability of prostate cancer cells [57]. The function of AR signaling in controlling autophagy in prostate cancer cells is demonstrated in a different experiment. As an autophagy modulator, androgens direct transcriptional regulation of GABARAPL1 (GABA type A receptor associated protein like 1), and blocking autophagy slows the growth of prostate cancer cells. Androgen deprivation enhances prostate cancer cell survival and proliferation by downregulating GABARAPL1, which in turn induces autophagy (GABARAPL1 is autophagy repressive in this situation) [58]. The function of androgen restriction treatment in autophagy-related prostate cancer needs further exploration.

One characteristic of tumor microenvironments is hypoxia, which can promote cancer growth [59]. One study found that oxygen deprivation promotes cancer growth by influencing DNA replication, metastasis, and angiogenesis [60, 61]. The activation of hypoxia inducible factor 1 subunit alpha, which is known as HIF1A/HIF-1α, occurs in hypoxic conditions and improves the proliferation and survival of prostate cancer cells [62, 63]. Results show that HIF1A has a dual function in cancer regulation of autophagy [64]. By influencing autophagy, HIF1A promotes tumor growth in prostate cancer. Autophagy induction occurs at the transcriptional level, where HIF1A binds to the Atg5 promoter and increases Atg5 expression. For tumor formation in nude mice, the HIF1A-ATG5-autophagy axis is crucial [65]. For upstream mediators involved in autophagy induction and the enhancement of prostate cancer progression, ATG5 could be a target [66]. Fibroblast growth factors (FGFs) are thought to have a wide variety of biological roles, such as regulating metabolism, development, angiogenesis, differentiation, and growth [67]. Metabolic homeostasis is linked to FGF21, which is released by the liver [68]. Reduced proliferation and survival rates are associated with downregulating FGF21, which may indicate an anti-tumor effect. Curiously, FGF21 slows the growth of prostate cancer by inducing autophagy and blocking the PI3K-AKT-MTOR axis [69]. Furthermore, there has been recent research on how an autophagic genetic signature affects prostate cancer susceptibility and prognosis. Using the Prostate adenocarcinoma (PRAD) dataset from The Cancer Genome Atlas (TCGA), Cheng and colleagues have discovered Differentially Expressed Autophagy-Related Genes (DEARGs), or differentially expressed autophagy-related genes. They found 16 DEARGs, 7 of which were linked to OS in prostate cancer patients. Furthermore, three prognostic genes (NPC1, BNIP3, and TP53) were linked to clinical features: increased levels of Niemann-Pick C1 protein (NPC1) and BCL2 interacting protein 3 (BNIP3) were strongly linked to advanced pathological T stages, and overexpression of NPC1 was substantially associated with higher International Society of Urological Pathology (ISUP) grades [70]. More than 20 Autophagy-Related Genes (ARGs) influencing disease-free survival (DFS) associated with T status, N status, and Gleason score were also demonstrated in a study by Hu and colleagues [71]. The Human Autophagy Database retrieved the data; they compared the ARGs that were found to be differently expressed with over 230 ARGs that were collected from the Cancer Genome Atlas (TCGA) database. The results corroborate earlier findings from studies using biopsy samples. Indeed, studies have looked into how the expression of the four main autophagy proteins—LC3A, LC3B, Beclin 1, p62, and lactate dehydrogenase 5-LDH5—relates to the aggressiveness of cancer. When LDH5 levels were high and the Gleason score was high, it was because LC3A, LC3B, and p62 were highly expressed in the cytoplasm of the tumor cells (more than 50% of the cells in each region). In addition, there was a strong correlation between substantial Beclin-1 overexpression and extraprostatic invasion [72]; these results suggest that ARGs and phenotypical autophagy expression could be useful prognostic indicators.

In both cancer progression and autophagy regulation, mTORC plays an essential role. It is possible that carcinogenesis is involved in reduced autophagy caused by impaired mTORC1 activity. As a matter of fact, hepatocellular cancer develops in mice lacking either the liver-specific phosphatase and tensin homolog (PTEN) or tuberous sclerosis complex 1 (TSC1) gene, which is responsible for autophagy [73].

Once a tumor mass has formed, autophagy activation is critical for cancer cell survival, despite the fact that it suppresses tumors in non-tumor cells and during early tumor cell formation. In order to achieve their higher energy rate and building block use, cancer cells exhibit an elevated metabolic demand. Adapting to metabolic deprivation, they increase autophagic flux and rely on energy supply [74]. As prostate cancer develops from normal to malignant tissue, research has revealed that STK11/LKB1 expression declines. Prostate carcinogenesis is defined histologically by a gradual progression from normal epithelium to invasive prostate cancer, as shown in high-grade prostate intraepithelial neoplasia (PIN). When using immunohistochemistry, only normal or atrophic cells will display staining for STK11/LKB1 [75]. Dysplastic cells will not stain. Furthermore, it was demonstrated that stak11/LKB1 expression influenced the effect of p38MAPK inhibition on prostate cancer cell survival. Particularly, a treatment strategy based on p38MAPK inhibitors in conjunction with ADT may be beneficial for prostate cancer patients lacking STK11/LKB1 expression. Patients with prostate cancer that express a lot of STK11/LKB1 could benefit from treatments that target the autophagic machinery or dual kinase inhibition, which targets both p38MAPK and AMPK.

A process largely associated with autophagic regulation mediates the effects of the androgen receptor (AR) on the progression of prostate cancer. Autophagy, energy utilization, and cell replication are the downstream targets of AR's effects. The results demonstrate that CaMKK2 is an AR target gene in prostate cancer. In line with the pro-survival function of CaMKK2-mediated autophagy, it has been noted that tumors with CaMKK2 knockdown showed elevated necrosis, particularly in regions deficient in energy nutrients. Since CAMKK2 allows cells to survive in a tumor microenvironment that is nutritionally poor, our results may imply that it is essential for prostate cancer growth in vivo [76].

Restoring sensitivity to docetaxel or ADT has been the goal of multiple research that have attempted to combat autophagy. Considering that anticancer treatment leads to increased cell death when autophagy is inhibited, the results in preclinical models are encouraging. To validate the findings of preclinical studies in patients with refractory cancers, the focus of current research has switched to clinical trials [77]. Also, small interfering RNAs (siRNAs) and 3-methyladenine (3-MA) have been shown to block autophagy in vitro. Unfortunately, siRNAs are not yet used in clinical practice and are only used in preclinical investigations as a confirmatory technique. Chloroquine and its derivative hydroxychloroquine, on the other hand, may be more practically useful autophagy inhibitors [78]. Chloroquine may be useful in improving clinical outcomes; a study is under underway to determine whether or not this is possible (NCT04011410, NCT00726596). The effectiveness of chloroquine in conjunction with metal-based chemotherapy medications, including palladium, has recently been studied by Erkisa and collaborators [79]. Palladium complexes enhance prostate cancer cell death, as demonstrated by their research. It is true that chloroquine pre-treatment increased apoptosis through a mitochondria-mediated route and reduced PI3K/AKT/mTOR-related protein expressions.

Researchers have also looked at other inhibitors, such as metabolic modulators like fenofibrate or metformin. Currently, people with type II diabetes use metformin, an oral biguanide. Its autophagy-inhibiting effects are well-documented, and its method of action involves blocking mTOR through AMPK activation. This trigger is supposed to increase autophagic activity, however it instead blocks Beclin-1 and suppresses autophagy even after activating AMPK [80]. Nevertheless, metformin inhibits autophagy activity in a way that is reliant on environmental factors. To that end, Chen and colleagues found that metformin may improve autophagy in prostate cancer cells in their most recent study. It has been demonstrated that metformin reduces cell proliferation by activating the AMPK system, which is linked to an increase in apoptotic activity and a larger autophagic flux [81]. Autophagy has multiple effects that determine cell viability, and these results are in line with those effects.

One further use for fenofibrate is in the treatment of docetaxel-resistant prostate cancer cells via regulating autophagy. Actually, a new study found that prostate cancer cells become more sensitive to taxanes and undergo autophagy when fenofibrate and docetaxel are combined [82]. An energy-depleted environment results when fibrates disrupt the cell's metabolic balance. Based on these results, autophagic induction may be an effort to speed up cell death or restore energy balance [82].

However, these medications' clinical efficacy and their practical use remain very questionable. One of the medications that has been considered for use as an adjuvant in chemotherapy is pantoprazole. Indeed, it was shown that several solid tumors might be effectively treated with large doses of pantoprazole to suppress autophagy and avoid taxanes resistance [83]. To demonstrate that pantoprazole improves docetaxel's efficacy in metastatic CRPCa, a phase II trial known as Pantoprazole Affecting Docetaxel Resistance Pathways via Autophagy (PANDORA) was undertaken. Despite the treatment's good safety profile in the group, the resulting clinical activity fell short of the stated target, necessitating more testing [84].

Reducing the proliferation and survival rate of prostate cancer cells can be achieved by activating autophagy, which is a double edged sword when it comes to biological activities in cells. Additionally, metabolic reprogramming has the potential to impact the proliferation and development of cancer cells. A key player in this scenario are mitochondria. Under the control of DNM1L/DRP1 (dynamin 1 like) [85, 86], prostate cancer cells can have their mitochondria changed in form, connectivity, and subcellular distribution to speed up the disease. Downregulation of DNM1L induces autophagy and proliferation suppression, whereas overexpression of DNM1L via AR signaling impacts metabolism and carcinogenesis, according to a recent study [87]. Serine/threonine kinase Aurora Kinase A (AURKA), which stands for aurora kinase A, may regulate spindle assembly, centrosome separation, and chromosomal segregation, all of which have the potential to contribute to genetic stability [88, 89]. In prostate cancer, AURKA overexpression plays a critical role in carcinogenesis and may help tumor cells avoid treatment [90, 91]. Through its suppression of Protein Kinase B (AKT) phosphorylation, AURKA suppresses autophagy's tumor suppressor component [92]. This means that reducing AURKA expression can inhibit prostate cancer cell proliferation by inducing autophagy. Despite oxidative stress's prominence in the apoptotic process, it has been postulated that it can mediate autophagic cell death in prostate cancer cells when activated [93]. Other molecular pathways that contribute to the progression of prostate cancer are also associated with autophagy's anti-tumor effects [94]. An example of this would be the finding that overexpression of the hydroxysteroid 17-beta dehydrogenase 4 gene enhances the growth and cancerous behavior of prostate cancer cells. Reduced prostate cancer progression is the result of HSD17B4 being acetylated, which increases its breakdown by CMA [95]. Although autophagy is not involved in cell death in this scenario, it does lead to the degradation of a component that promotes the growth of prostate cancer.

The cells that have spread from the prostate show signs of autophagy induction. Therefore, autophagy is crucial for migration and metastases. There are many different types of cells in a tumor microenvironment (TME), including inflammatory cells, fibroblasts associated with malignancy, and vascular cells [96]. based on reports, endothelial cells are one of the components of the tumor microenvironment (TME) that significantly contributes to the spread of prostate cancer. Prostatic microvasculature undergoes apoptosis during androgen-deprivation therapy (ADT), while endothelial cells regenerate instantly [97]. Metastasis of prostate cancer is linked to an increase in microvascular infiltration, which is mediated by AR signaling [98, 99]. Both in vivo and in vitro studies linked autophagy to the spread of prostate cancer. This happens because endothelial cells offer autophagy induction by inhibiting AR signaling. As a result of focal adhesion protein disintegration, autophagy activation increases migration and invasion of prostate cancer cells [100].

Regarding the twofold function of autophagy, it is also possible to inhibit the spread of prostate cancer cells. Histone deacetylase 6 (HADC6) is closely related to cell autophagy. Cancer suppression is induced by the maturation of autophagy by HDAC6 [101]. In addition, deacetylation of TUBA/α-tubulin can be used by HDAC6 to suppress autophagy [101]. Microtubule acetylation inhibits migration and invasion in prostate cancer cells via inducing autophagosome formation and autophagy flux. Nevertheless, SQSTM1/p62 promotes tumor growth by secreting HDAC6 to inhibit microtubule acetylation-mediated autophagy, which in turn causes prostate cancer to spread [102]. This work highlights the significance of autophagy in reducing prostate cancer metastasis and initiating autophagy flux.

4.4 Apoptosis Mechanism

There is an intricate chain reaction of molecular events taking place during apoptosis, and it is dependent on energy [103]. Moreover, the two primary apoptotic mechanisms that have been identified thus far in the field are the intrinsic or mitochondrial pathway and the extrinsic or death receptor pathway. In addition, new data suggests a connection between the two routes, with chemicals acting on one pathway potentially influencing the other [104]. The second route completely relies on perforin-granzyme-dependent cell death and T-cell mediated cytotoxicity. One of two granzymes, B or A, can trigger cell death in the perforin/granzyme pathway. One terminal, or execution pathway, is shared by the extrinsic, intrinsic, and granzyme B pathways. Breakdown of cytoskeletal and nuclear proteins, DNA fragmentation, cross-linking of proteins, creation of apoptotic bodies, production of ligands for phagocytic cell receptors, and absorption by phagocytic cells are all steps in this process that begins with caspase-3 cleavage. A parallel cell death process that does not rely on caspases is activated by the granzyme A pathway through damage to single-stranded DNA [105]. Figure 4.2 shows the molecular profile of apoptosis.

Furthermore, the unique structural pathology mentioned earlier is the consequence of a number of biochemical variations that apoptotic cells exhibit, including protein cleavage, protein cross-linking, DNA disintegration, and phagocytic recognition [106]. The majority of cells express caspases in their inactive proenzyme form; when activated, these caspases can initiate a protease cascade by activating other procaspases. It is also possible for some procaspases to cluster and autoactivate. By provoking additional caspases, this proteolytic cascade speeds up the apoptotic signaling pathway, which in turn causes cells to die off quickly.

On top of that caspases are proteolytic enzymes that may cleave proteins at aspartic acid residues; however, their specificities in recognizing adjacent amino acids vary among caspases. It appears that there is an irrevocable commitment toward cell death once caspases are initially activated. From what researchers can tell, there are ten main caspases: those that initiate the cascade (caspase-2, -8, -9, -10), those that carry out the cascade (caspase-3, -6, -7) and those that cause

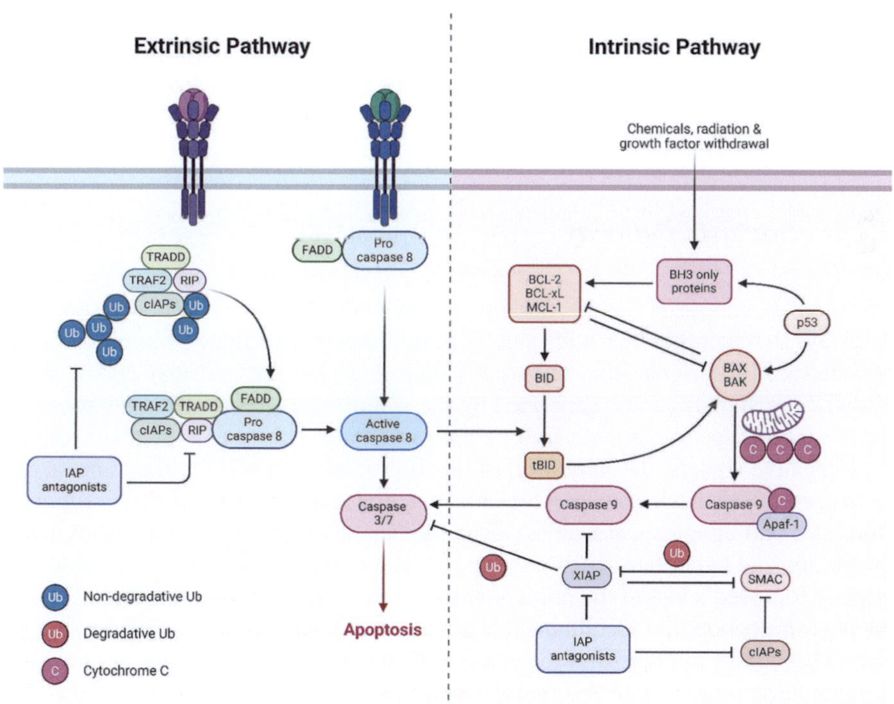

Fig. 4.2 The molecular profile of apoptosis (Biorender.com)

inflammation (caspase-1, -4, -5) [107, 108]. Not to mention, caspase-11 is known to control cytokine maturation and apoptosis in septic shock, caspase-12 is involved in endoplasmic-specific apoptosis and cytotoxicity caused by amyloid-β, caspase-13 is thought to be a gene specific to cattle, and caspase-14 is abundant in embryonic tissues but not in adult tissues [109–112]. Apoptotic cells also express and activate tissue transglutaminase, leading to extensive protein cross-linking [113]. Moreoevr, fragments of 180–200 bp of DNA are also produced by endonucleases that are reliant on Ca^{2+} and Mg^{2+} [114]. Due to the ethidium bromide stain and ultraviolet light used in agarose gel electrophoresis, a distinctive "DNA ladder" may be seen. One such biochemical characteristic is the production of cell surface signals, which allow neighboring cells to quickly phagocytose apoptotic cells with little damage to the surrounding tissue. To do this, the normally inward-facing phosphatidylserine of the cell's lipid bilayer is transferred to the outer layers of the plasma membrane for expression [115]. While phosphatidylserine externalization is a well-known phagocyte recognition ligand, newer research has demonstrated that additional proteins may also be exposed on the surface of apoptotic cells during clearance. Two examples are calreticulin and annexin I.

One tool for detecting apoptosis is annexin V, a recombinant phosphatidylserine-binding protein [116]. It interacts firmly and selectively with phosphatidylserine residues. There is evidence that calcreticulin, in conjunction with phosphatidylserine, acts as a recognition signal by binding to an engulfing cell protein that is linked to Low-Density Lipoprotein (LDL) receptors [117]. On the surface of active microvascular endothelial cells, you may find the sticky glycoprotein thrombospondin-1. This protein, along with CD36 and other proteins like caspase-3-like proteases, can trigger receptor-mediated death [118].

4.4.1 Intrinsic Pathway

Initiation of apoptosis occurs through mitochondrial-initiated intrinsic signaling pathways that incorporate a wide variety of non-receptor-mediated stimuli that generate intracellular signals that act directly on cell targets. Both positive and negative intracellular signals can be generated by the stimuli that start the intrinsic route. In the absence of specific growth factors, hormones, and cytokines, which are considered negative signals, the inhibition of death processes can fail, and apoptosis can be triggered. Taken together, these events include factor removal, apoptotic suppression loss, and apoptosis activation. Free radicals, hypoxia, radiation, toxins, viral infections, and hyperthermia are among the many stimuli that can have a beneficial effect. Moreover, a loss of the mitochondrial transmembrane potential, alterations to the inner mitochondrial membrane that allow the mitochondrial permeability transition (MPT) pore to open, and the release of two classes of normally intracellular pro-apoptotic proteins into the cytosol are all outcomes of these stimuli [119]. This first set includes cytochrome *c*, Smac/DIABLO (Direct IAP-Binding Protein with Low PI), and the HtrA2/Omi serine protease [120]. A mechanism involving mitochondria that is dependent on caspase is activated by these proteins. Forming a "apoptosome," cytochrome *c* binds to and activates procaspase-9 and Apaf-1 [121, 122].

When procaspase-9 clumps together in this way, caspase-9 gets activated. It has been found that Smac/DIABLO and HtrA2/Omi can enhance apoptosis by blocking the activity of inhibitors of apoptosis proteins (IAP) [123, 124]. Several other mitochondrial proteins have been found to bind to IAP and inhibit its activity; however, results from gene knockout studies raise doubts about whether or not this is sufficient proof to classify a mitochondrial protein as "pro-apoptotic" [125]. Although Apoptosis-Inducing Factor (AIF), endonuclease G, and Caspase-Activated DNase (CAD) are the second set of pro-apoptotic proteins produced from mitochondria during apoptosis, this process happens after the cell has already decided to die. When AIF moves into the nucleus, it causes the DNA to be broken up into around 50–300 kb pairs and the nuclear chromatin surrounding the nucleus to condense [126]. The term for this initial step of nuclear condensation is "stage I condensation" [127]. Furthermore, endonuclease G gets into the nucleus and splits nuclear chromatin into oligonucleosomal DNA pieces [128]. There is no caspase requirement for the activity of AIF or endonuclease G. Further release from mitochondria causes CAD to translocate to the nucleus, where it causes oligonucleosomal DNA breakage and progressive chromatin condensation after caspase-3 cleavage [129]. What happens later on is known as "stage II" condensation, and it is much more noticeable than stage I condensation [127].

These apoptotic mitochondrial processes are regulated and controlled by proteins belonging to the Bcl-2 family [130]. Despite the importance of the tumor suppressor protein p53 in regulating the Bcl-2 family of proteins, the precise processes by which it does this remain unclear [131]. The Bcl-2 family of proteins governs mitochondrial membrane permeability and can be either pro-apoptotic or anti-apoptotic. It is noteworthy that a total of 25 genes have been identified in the Bcl-2 family. Some of the anti-apoptotic proteins include Bcl-2, Bcl-x, Bcl-XL, Bcl-XS, Bcl-w, BAG, and some of the pro-apoptotic proteins include Bcl-10, BCL2-Associated X Protein (Bax), Bak, Bid, Bad, Bim, Bik, and Blk. These proteins have special significance since they can determine if the cell commits to apoptosis or aborts the process. It is thought that the main mechanism of action of the Bcl-2 family of proteins is the regulation of cytochrome *c* release from the mitochondria via alteration of mitochondrial membrane permeability.

A few possible mechanisms have been studied but none have been proven definitively. Mitochondrial damage in the Fas pathway of apoptosis is mediated by the caspase-8 cleavage of Bid [132, 133]. This is one example of the "cross-talk" between the death receptor (extrinsic) pathway and the mitochondrial (intrinsic) pathway [104]. Serine phosphorylation of Bad is associated with 14-3-3, a member of a family of multifunctional phosphoserine binding molecules. When Bad is phosphorylated, it is trapped by 14-3-3 and sequestered in the cytosol but once Bad is unphosphorylated, it will translocate to the mitochondria to release cytochrome *c* [134].

Bad can also heterodimerize with Bcl-Xl or Bcl-2, neutralizing their protective effect and promoting cell death [135]. The process by which Bcl-2 and Bcl-Xl, when Bad is not present, prevent mitochondrial cytochrome *c* release is unclear.

More research has demonstrated that Bcl-2 and Bcl-XL mainly regulate caspase protease activation to prevent apoptotic death [20]. An additional protein designated "Aven" appears to bind both Bcl-Xl and Apaf-1, thereby preventing activation of procaspase-9 [20]. There is evidence that overexpression of either Bcl-2 or Bcl-Xl will down-regulate the other, indicating a reciprocal regulation between these two proteins.

The Bcl2 family includes the pro-apoptotic proteins Puma and Noxa. In p53-mediated apoptosis, Puma is a key player. In vitro studies demonstrated that Puma overexpression is associated with BAX overexpression, BAX conformational change, mitochondrial translocation, cytochrome *c* release, and decreased mitochondrial membrane potential [136]. Noxa is also a candidate mediator of p53-induced apoptosis. Studies show that this protein can localize to the mitochondria and interact with anti-apoptotic Bcl-2 family members, resulting in the activation of caspase-9 [137]. Since both Puma and Noxa are induced by p53, they might mediate the apoptosis that is elicited by geno-toxic damage or oncogene activation. The Myc oncoprotein has also been reported to potentiate apoptosis through both p53-dependent and -independent mechanisms [138].

4.4.2 Extrinsic Pathway

Apoptosis initiation pathways involving extrinsic signaling entail connections mediated by transmembrane receptors. Part of the tumor necrosis factor (TNF) receptor gene superfamily, these include death receptors [139]. In addition to having cyteine-rich extracellular domains, TNF receptors also share a "death domain" in their cytoplasm that is around 80 amino acids long [140]. An absolutely essential function of this death domain is to relay the death signal from the surface of the cell to the signaling pathways within the cell. The most well-studied ligands and death receptors so far are FasL/FasR, TNF-α/TNFR1, Apo3L/DR3, Apo2L/DR4, and Apo2L/DR5 [140–143].

To fully understand the extrinsic phase of apoptosis, one should use the FasL/FasR and TNF-α/TNFR1 models. Receptor clustering and binding to homologous trimeric ligands are features of these models. To connect with receptors, ligands trigger the recruitment of cytoplasmic adapter proteins, which include death domains. Adherence of Fas ligand to Fas receptor initiates the binding of the adapter protein Fas-Associated Death Domain Protein (FADD) [144, 145]. Similarly, when TNF ligand binds to TNF receptor, the binding of the adapter protein TNF Receptor-Associated Death Domain (TRADD) with recruitment of FADD and RIP follows. Dimerization of the death effector domain is the next step for FADD to bind with procaspase-8. A death-inducing signaling complex (DISC) is created at this moment, which causes procaspase-8 to be auto-catalytically activated [146]. Moreover, activation of caspase-8 initiates the final stage of cell death. By attaching to FADD and caspase-8, a protein known as c-FLIP can suppress death receptor-mediated apoptosis [147, 148]. An additional possible regulator of cell death is a protein named

Toso. This protein has been demonstrated to prevent T cell death caused by Fas by inhibiting caspase-8 processing [149].

4.4.3 Perforin/Granzyme Pathway

In T-cell mediated cytotoxicity, antigen-bearing cells are killed by sensitized CD8+ cells, a kind of type IV hypersensitivity. Through the FasL/FasR connection, cytotoxic T lymphocytes (CTLs) trigger apoptosis, which allows them to destroy target cells via the extrinsic pathway [150]. On the other hand, there is a new way for them to kill tumor cells and cells infected with viruses. This involves secreting the molecule perforin, which forms transmembrane pores, and then exophytically releasing cytoplasmic granules into the cell of interest [151]. Granzyme A and granzyme B, two serine proteases, are the granules' most crucial components.

It should be mentioned that granzyme B can activate procaspase-10 and cleave factors like ICAD (Inhibitor of Caspase Activated DNAse) by cleaving proteins at aspartate residues [152]. There have been reports indicating that granzyme B can enhance the death signal through the mitochondrial route, namely by cleaving Bid and inducing the release of cytochrome *c* [153, 154]. On the other hand, granzyme B can activate caspase-3 directly. This initiates the execution phase of apoptosis directly, skipping the upstream signaling cascades.

Granzyme B-induced death is thought to rely on the mitochondrial pathway as well as the direct activation of caspase-3 [155]. In order to regulate the proliferation of type 2 helper T (Th2) cells, new research shows that this granzyme B cytotoxicity technique is essential [156]. Furthermore, since inhibiting the ligands of death receptors and caspases does not affect apoptosis, the results show that these pathways are unrelated to the T cell receptor-induced death of activated Th2 cells. Contrarily, granzyme B does not influence apoptosis or the regulation of cytotoxic type 1 helper cells; nonetheless, Fas-Fas ligand interaction, adaptor proteins with death domains, and caspases are all involved.

Granzyme A activates caspase-independent pathways and plays a crucial role in cytotoxic T cell mediated apoptosis. When granzyme A reaches a cell, it triggers DNA nicking through the tumor suppressor gene product DNAse NM23-H1 [23]. By inducing tumor cell death, this DNAse plays a crucial function in immunological surveillance for cancer prevention. The NM23-H1 gene is generally inhibited by the nucleosome assembly protein SET. Protease granzyme A breaks down the SET complex, which releases NM23-H1 inhibition and causes DNA to be degraded in an apoptotic manner. Not only does the SET complex suppress NM23-H1, but it also plays a crucial role in DNA repair and chromatin shape. It appears that the proteins SET, Ape1, pp32, and HMG2 collaborate to safeguard DNA and chromatin structure (23). Hence, granzyme A's inactivation of this complex likely adds to apoptosis by preventing the integrity of DNA and chromatin structure from being maintained.

4.5 Apoptosis in Prostate Cancer

When it comes to cancer-related deaths among American men, prostate cancer is second only due to lung cancer [157, 158]. More importantly, it is also the most often diagnosed cancer in this demographic. Androgen ablation therapy is effective in reducing the size of most prostate cancers since it removes the hormone that the tumor cells use to grow [159]. Regrettably, hormone ablation causes prostate cancer to develop to androgen-independent illness, which is resistant to hormone ablation and other systemic chemotherapies [160]. Radiosensitivity in prostate cancer is influenced by apoptosis, which seems to be the main mechanism by which tumor cells die off in response to androgen ablation and chemotherapeutic drugs [159, 160]. The development of treatment resistance in advanced prostate cancer is caused by the acquisition of anti-apoptotic signal transduction.

Prostate cancer, like other cancers, is thought to progress by the interplay of cell growth, proliferation, and apoptotic components. Interactions like these, issues with apoptosis regulation, cause prostate cancer cells to differentiate, avoid apoptosis, and proliferate indefinitely [161]. Research including a large number of clinical factors and biochemical markers is necessary to determine the effective apoptotic mechanisms in the advancement of prostate cancer [162, 163].

With regard to prostate cancer, there are two mechanisms for apoptosis: the intrinsic and the extrinsic. The extrinsic pathway is activated by death receptors and involves caspase-8, which in turn activates caspase-3 to produce apoptosis. Bcl family anti-apoptotic regulators can block the intrinsic pathway's cytochrome *c* release, which activates caspase-9. Apoptosis is triggered by the activation of caspase-3, the last step. Important dietary regulators in this apoptotic pathway include bioactive chemicals like flavones [163].

Moreover, malignant prostate cancer results from a mutated gene. Some examples of these alterations include changes in biosynthesis and amplification, such as point mutations in the ligand-binding domain (LBD) of AR or AR overexpression [164]. Furthermore, the apoptotic pathway of prostate cancer is inhibited by mutations in the RNase L gene, which is an inherited allele of prostate cancer type 1 (HPC1) [165].

In reaction to various cellular stressors, including DNA or free radical damage, the tumor suppressor gene p53, which is most often linked with cell death, controls cell-cycle progression and cell death. P53 can trigger apoptosis by mitochondrial overexpression of BAX; however, this mutation of P53 prevents apoptosis, allowing cancer cells to multiply endlessly [158, 166]. As metastatic illness or hormone-independent tumors advance, p53 mutations in prostate cancer become increasingly common, although they are rare in the early, well-differentiated stage [167].

In addition, proteins belonging to the Bcl-2 family impact mitochondrial activity; these proteins include both pro- and anti-apoptotic molecules [168]. The outer mitochondrial membrane is a stable anchor for several members of the Bcl-2 family due to a hydrophobic region of amino acids close to their carboxyl-terminus. Bid, Bim, and Bad are members of the Bcl-2 family that target mitochondria but do not have these membrane anchoring domains. Members that prevent cell death, such as Bcl-2 and Bcl-xL, prevent mitochondrial apoptosis by blocking the release of cytochrome *c*. Bax, Bad, and Bid are proapototic Bcl-2 family members that inhibit their activity, which in turn triggers the release of cytochrome *c* from mitochondria and the activation of caspase cascades [168]. Tumor cell survival is regulated by the relative abundance of pro- and anti-apoptotic family members.

Research has shown that aggressive prostate cancer morphologies are characterized by a large upregulation of Bcl-2 and other members of its family, which inhibit cell death [169, 170]. More research has represented that prostate cancer and other cancers can develop resistance to radiation and chemotherapy when Bcl-2 and Bcl-xL are overexpressed. In addition, the androgen-signaling axis in prostate cancer cells relies on the Bcl-2 family [170]. Moreover, Coffey and colleagues demonstrated that androgens suppress the expression of pro-apoptotic Bcl-2 family members such as Bax in cells that are susceptible to androgens in prostate cancer [171]. More investigations, in this field, has revealed that there is evidence that prostate cancer cells can survive in androgen-free environments due to increased Bcl-2 and Bcl-xL expression [169, 172]. This suggests that Bcl-2/Bcl-xL overexpression is important for both the function and prediction of androgen-independent recurrences in prolonged androgen ablation therapy [170]. While it is true that Bcl-2 family expression alterations can lead to treatment resistance, it is equally important to recognize and explain the dynamic cross-talk between this "powerful" family and other anti-apoptotic pathways affected by external ligand-receptor communication.

Furthermore, an extremely conserved tumor suppressor gene, Phosphatase and tensin homolog deleted on chromosome 10 (PTEN) regulates the P13K/AKT signal transduction pathway, leading to cellular death. The activation and targeting of AKT's numerous downstream effectors are dependent on its phosphorylation, which PTEN blocks [173]. Apoptotic resistance and constitutive activation of the P13K/AKT pathway are outcomes of PTEN loss, which is prevalent in treatment resistant and poorly differentiated prostate tumors [174]. By restoring PTEN activity in PTEN deficient prostate cancer cell lines, researchers were able to enhance their susceptibility to caspase-8-mediated apoptosis and facilitate BH3 Interacting Domain Death Agonist (BIDD) breakage, which led to the release of cytochrome *c* and mitochondrial-driven apoptosis [175]. Second messengers activate AKTs through phosphatidylinositol 3′-kinases (P13Ks). On the other hand, PTEN phosphatases work to counteract this phosphorylation [176]. Plasmid negativity in prostate cancer can lead to constitutive AKT phosphorylation, whereas tumors positive for PTEN can experience autocrine and paracrine cell membrane receptor-ligand interactions that stimulate and upregulate AKT [177]. Phosphorylated AKT appears to suppress cellular apoptosis in prostate cancer due to the strong interaction between this effector and various other anti-apoptotic pathways. It has been demonstrated that activated AKT activates MDM2, which in turn causes p53 proteolysis and the suppression of p53 mediated apoptosis, while simultaneously stimulating cell-cycle progression [176, 178]. In addition to releasing Bcl-2 and inhibiting mitochondrial apoptosis, activated AKT inactivates Bad and caspase-9 [173, 176, 179]. In addition, phosphorylation of IκB occurs as a result of upregulated P13K/AKT activity, which in turn permits the nuclear translocation of NF-κB and the consequent inhibition of apoptosis caused by NF-κB [173, 176]. Inhibition of androgen-deprivation-induced apoptosis can result from phosphorylated AKT inducing AR phosphorylation and upregulating AR expression [179, 180].

The hallmarks of aggressive prostate cancer include both PTEN inactivation and AKT phosphorylation, according to a growing body of recent findings. On the other hand, xenograft models produced from metastatic prostate cancer cell lines show a loss of PTEN in 60% of cases, while only 10–15% of original prostate malignancies had PTEN inactivation [173, 177]. In addition, a Gleason score more than 6 and aggressive local disease (T3b-T4 tumors) have been linked to PTEN depletion [181]. Independent prognostic indicators and markers for aggressive illness include AKT phosphorylation. Only benign tissues, not prostate cancer, are linked to high levels of AKT phosphorylation [182]. In poorly differentiated tumors (Gleason 8–10), nearly 90% of tissues tested exhibit a substantial level of phosphorylated AKT [183], and AKT phosphorylation correlates with Gleason score [184]. Recurrence was indicated by higher AKT phosphorylation in prostate cancer specimens with Gleason scores of 5–6, a group of patients whose prognosis is notoriously difficult to predict [184]. Furthermore, it was recently determined that AKT phosphorylation, rather than mitotic index or Gleason score, was a better predictive indication of recurrence [185]. The advancement of resistant prostate cancer following long-term androgen ablation therapy has been linked to the loss of PTEN and phosphorylation of AKT, which is not surprising given their associations with chemotherapy resistance [175, 179]. Experimental evidence suggests that new targeting techniques that restore PTEN activity or suppress AKT phosphorylation might induce significant cell death and make cancer cells more sensitive to chemotherapy, both in laboratory settings and using xenograft models [175, 179].

One emerging class of medications that may make prostate cancer treatment more challenging is apoptosis inhibitors. The IAPs are a kind of caspase inhibitors that decrease cell death by directly inhibiting caspases 3, 7, and 9 [123]. As of this writing, eight human IAPs have been the subject of substantial research: survivin, X-linked inhibitor of apoptosis protein (XIAP), IAP1, and IAP2 [186]. It has been suggested in reference that there might be a positive feedback loop involving the two pathways, even if they can all decrease effector caspases, since IAP1 and IAP2 can upregulate NF-κB expression [187]. Evidence from animal studies and patient specimens taken after prostatectomy suggests that these four IAPs are overexpressed during the early stages of prostate cancer [186]. Numerous tumor models have demonstrated that IAPs can suppress apoptosis in response to various chemotherapeutic drugs [188], but the role of IAPs in treatment resistance in prostate cancer is a topic of "active" research that has only just begun to emerge. It has been found that inhibiting XIAP increases chemotherapy sensitivity in prostate cancer cell lines that are normally resistant to the treatment [189]. It has been suggested that IAPs may play a role in androgen independence, according to another small research of 23 patients who underwent neoadjuvant androgen ablation, wherein the expression of IAP1 and IAP2 was significantly increased [187]. More and more evidence is pointing to IAPs as a cause of treatment resistance in prostate cancer. By manipulating IAP pathways, we may be able to bypass the apoptotic resistance in intracellular apoptotic escape mechanisms like AKT and Bcl-2.

Moreover, Survivin, XIAP, c-IAP1, and c-IAP2 levels were decreased in PC-3 and DU145 prostate cancer cells treated with apigenin. The apoptotic cascades involved an increase in cytochrome *c* (5, 10, 20, 40 μM), a decrease in Bcl-xL and Bcl-2, and a peak in BAX [190]. In addition, at doses of 1, 5, 10, and 20 μM, LNCaP cells showed an increase in the expression of the cancer suppressor protein p21 [191]. At 2.5, 5, 10, and 20 μM concentrations, it was observed that IκB Kinase α (IKK α) was inhibited in PC-3 and 22Rv1 cells, and that p65 activation was suppressed as well [192]. The activation of NF-κB by IKK α regulates inflammation and the advancement of cancer. Additionally, research has demonstrated that apigenin can cause extrinsic apoptosis in PC-3 cells and prostate cancer stem cell (CSC) (CD44+) isolated from there at a concentration of 25 μM by increasing the production of caspase-8, -3, and TNF-a [193].

Twenty weeks of oral administration of apigenin at doses of 20 or 50 μg/mouse/day (wt/vol) was carried out on male Transgenic Adenocarcinoma of the Mouse Prostate (TRAMP) mice that were 8 weeks old. Hence, the PI3K/AKT/FOXO pathway was able to suppress the growth of prostate cancer without causing any harm or weight loss [194]. Doses like these are consistent with what humans have been shown to consume on a regular basis in flavonoid studies [195]. After injecting PC-3 and 22Rv1 cells subcutaneously into the flanks of mice, researchers found that giving the same dose of apigenin orally slowed tumor growth, reduced tumor growth via blocking IKK phosphorylation, and induced cell death. Using two different amounts of apigenin did not seem to have any negative consequences in this mouse model [192].

With a molecular weight of 284.26 g/mol and a chemical formula of $C_{16}H_{12}O_5$, acetin is a 5,7-dihydroxy-4′-methoxyflavone [196]. Plants belonging to the Asteraceae family, as well as safflower and propolis, are the primary sources of acctin [197]. Levels of phospho-AKT and phospho-GSK-3β were decreased in DU145 prostate cancer cells treated with acacetin, whereas levels of the cancer suppressor p53 were increased (12.5 and 5 μM, respectively). In addition, apoptosis was caused by a decrease in XIAP and Bcl-2 levels, and the activation of phospho-IκB and NFκB was hindered [196].

By lowering STAT3 phosphorylation in DU145 cells, acacetin (20, 30, and 50 μM) reduces cancer cell proliferation and growth. It then induces apoptosis by inhibiting the expression of STAT3 target proteins, including Bcl-2, Bcl-xL, Mcl-1, cyclin D1, with survivin among them. Direct binding by interacting with the SH-2 domain of numerous signaling proteins, including the Src (steroid receptor coactivator) tumor protein of STAT3, was another mechanism by which acetin demonstrated anticancer action [198].

In LNCaP and DU145 cells, Acacetin (25, 50, 100 μM) inhibited cell growth and caused a cell-cycle arrest in the G1 or G2-M phase as a result of an increase in Ciap/p21 and a decrease in CDK2, CDK4, and CDK6. G2-M phase arrest was more pronounced in LNCaP cells compared to DU145 cells because Cdc25C, Cdc2/p34, and cyclin B1 were reduced to greater extents in the former. Closure of poly-(ADP-ribose) polymerase (PARP) also contributed to cell death [199]. The possibility of toxicity due to cytochrome P450 inhibition was documented by Zhou et al. in their study of rats given 50 mg/kg of acacetin intraperitoneally. Nevertheless, the particular toxicity has not been reported as of yet. Therefore, additional studies are necessary [200].

4.6 Ferroptosis Machinery

In order for cells to produce glutathione, System X_c^-, an antiporter that does not rely on sodium, exports internal glutamate and imports extracellular cystine across the membrane in a ratio of 1:1 [201, 202]. The two components that make it up are SLC7A11 and SLC3A2. The conserved site cys158 of SLC7A11 and cys109 of SLC3A2 form a disulfide link that connects the two proteins [203]. Another subtype of CD44, CD44v, interacts with and stabilizes SLC7A11 on cancer cell surfaces [204]. SLC7A11 is an integral part of system X_c^- and is a multichannel transmembrane protein. The molecular chaperone responsible for ensuring the stability and correct localization of the SLC7A11 protein is SLC3A2, a single transmembrane protein [203]. To enhance ferroptosis, new small compounds like erastin and sorafenib have been discovered as inhibitors of system X_c^- [205, 206]. One of the many environmental pollutants is the poisonous metal cadmium, or Cd. Consumption of tainted food and drink, along with inhalation and smoking, are the main routes of Cd exposure. Some epidemiological studies, like those conducted by the International Cancer Society, have linked Cd to an increased risk of prostate cancer [207]. Moreover, Zhang and colleagues have illustrated that prolonged exposure to cadmium impeded ferroptosis and enhanced prostate cancer cell proliferation. Cd-induced prostate cancer metastasized, and RNA sequencing showed that lncRNA OIP5-AS1 was upregulated in a considerable way. Through the miR-128-3p/SLC7A11 axis, OIP5-AS1 suppresses ferroptosis [208]. Inhibiting tumor growth is one of the key functions of the tumor suppressor gene p53 [209]. Inhibiting cystine uptake by reducing SLC7A11 expression and making cells more susceptible to ferroptosis, p53 is involved in ferroptosis, according to recent studies [210] To stop castration-resistant prostate cancer (CRPC) from spreading, flubendazole promotes ferroptosis, downregulates glutathione peroxidase 4 (GPX4), and inhibits SLC7A11 expression through p53 induction. Furthermore, when it came to treating colorectal cancer, flubendazole and 5-fluorouracil (5-FU) worked together in a synergistic fashion. It enhances the pharmacological efficacy and induces ferroptosis by reducing SLC7A11 expression after concurrent use [211].

Protecting cells and membranes from peroxidation, the antioxidant enzyme GPX4 employs glutathione as a cofactor to ward against lipid peroxidation. By alternating between its reduced (GSH) and oxidized (GSSG) forms, glutathione is able to take part in redox biological reactions [212]. In order to make prostate cancer cells more sensitive to docetaxel, ChaC1, an enzyme that is specific for glutathione, can reduce the amount of GSH within the cells. When GPX4 is not functioning properly, it can cause lipid peroxidation and the buildup of reactive oxygen species (ROS), which can then lead to ferroptosis [213]. On top of that, GPX4 can convert harmful lipid peroxides (like R-OOH) into their corresponding alcohols (like R-OH). To render GPX4 inactive, RSL3 binds to selenocysteine in the enzyme's active site [214]. One of the main inhibitors of ferroptosis is GPX4. Researchers and cancer patients alike have found serum miRNA to be an exciting new target in the fight against the disease. Alterations to regulatory components in cellular physiological processes are brought about by microRNAs, which primarily interact with the '3'-UTR of target mRNAs and either cause their destruction or block their translation. Prostate cancer patients exhibited a decrease in miR-15a expression. Negative regulation of GPX4 expression can occur when miR-15a interacts with the 3′-untranslated region (UTR) of GPX4 messenger RNA. One way to increase cell death in prostate cancer is to utilize a miR-15a mimic or siGPX4 [215]. Cells from more advanced prostate cancers express SLC7A11 and GPX4 at high levels. One way to enhance cancer cell death is by inducing ferroptosis with the ferroptosis activator erastin or RSL3. When ferroptosis activator is used alongside second-generation anti-androgen medications such enzalutamide or abiraterone, the conventional treatment for advanced prostate cancer can further suppress tumor development [216]. Figure 4.3 highlights the ferroptosis mechanism.

Typically, reactive oxygen species (ROS) include free radicals, peroxides, and superoxide [217]. They are normal metabolites made in live cells; as unstable compounds, they are important for signal transduction and tissue homeostasis [218]. Metabolism, inflammation, neurogenesis, and carcinogenesis are just a few of the physiological and pathological processes that ROS are engaged in [219, 220]. Damage to DNA, lipids, and proteins occurs as a result of oxidative stress, which in turn causes cells to release dangerous levels of reactive oxygen species (ROS) [221]. The most notable aspect of ferroptosis is the high levels of polyunsaturated fatty acids (PUFA) in the cell membrane, which makes it extremely susceptible to damage from reactive oxygen species (ROS). Cancer cells are more susceptible to ferroptosis and ROS buildup than normal ones. An anticancer medication that is commonly used is cisplatin. Cisplatin resistance is a major problem for prostate cancer patients undergoing chemotherapy. By increasing ROS production, exacerbating cell-cycle arrest, and cisplatin-induced apoptosis, the ferroptosis activator RSL3 makes prostate cancer cells more sensitive to the drug [222]. As allicin breaks down, one of its primary active components is diallyl trisulfide, or Dopamine Transporter (DAT). According to research, DAT has many biological functions, including anti-tumor, bacteriostasis, oxidative stress, and involvement in inflammatory response modulation. It suppresses cancer cell proliferation in prostate cancer by increasing reactive oxygen species, which in turn induces ferritin breakdown and, ultimately, ferroptosis [223]. It was in 1971 when Tu youyou initially isolated artemisinin from Artemisia annua [224]. An antimalarial action is imparted by this semiterpene lactone. Research in recent years has shown that it induces ferroptosis and has anticancer effects. There was no discernible impact of artemisinin on PC3 and LNCaP cell lines, while it was found to cause ferroptosis in prostate cancer cell DU145 [225]. One of artemisinin's active metabolites is dihydroartemisinin, or

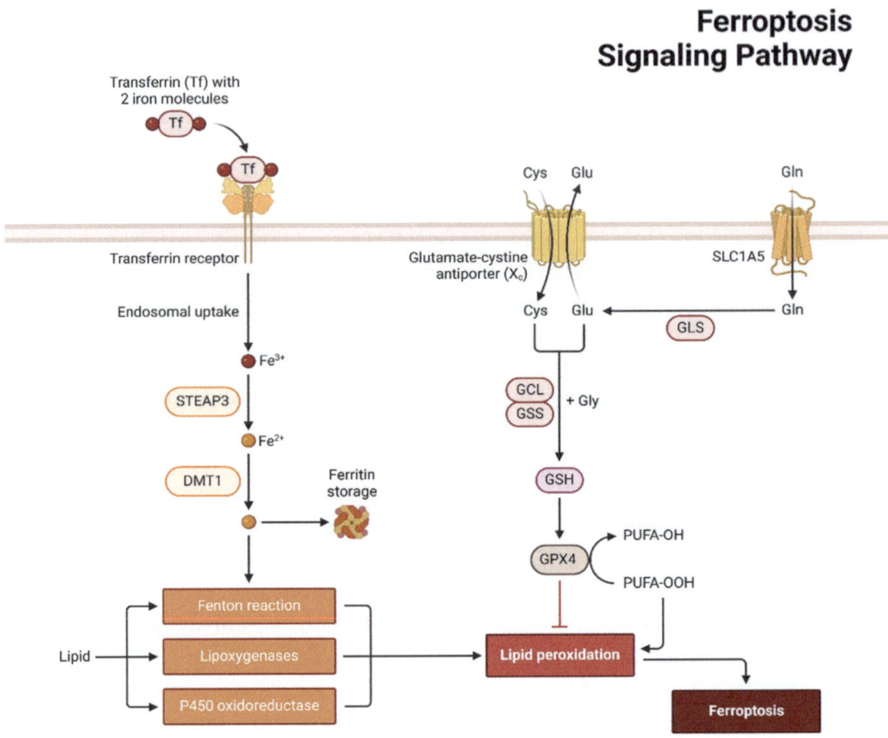

Fig. 4.3 The mechanism of ferroptosis (Biorender.com)

Docosahexaenoic Acid (DHA). Several cancer cells, including those in the lung and brain, have been found to be cytotoxic to DHA, according to a plethora of studies [226, 227]. It has the ability to decrease cancer cell proliferation, activate autophagy and ferroptosis in cancer cells. Current study does not establish its involvement in prostate cancer ferroptosis; nonetheless, this could be an area for future investigation. The active ingredients in traditional Chinese medicine often work in tandem with one another or in addition to one another. By controlling ADAMTS18, ROS, Nrf2, GPX4, and other molecules to regulate ferroptosis, traditional Chinese medicine (TCM) has the properties of many targets and can regulate a range of signal pathways, in contrast to specific medications. Research into inducing ferroptosis in prostate cancer cells using traditional Chinese medicine could be a promising avenue for future investigation.

Several biological processes rely on iron as a cofactor [228]. Iron excess causes lipid peroxidation and deadly reactive oxygen species (ROS) generation [229]. The transmembrane glycoprotein known as transferrin receptor 1 (TFR1) is in charge of importing iron, which is stored and delivered as an iron-protein complex, primarily ferritin [230]. An enzyme titled iron oxide reductase steam3 (STEAP3) converts ferric ions from Fe^{3+} to Fe^{2+} [231]. At last, the endosome, which is mediated by divalent metal transporter 1 (DMT1), releases Fe^{2+} into the cytoplasm's unstable iron pool [232]. Iron acts as a crucial component in the production of reactive oxygen species (ROS) through enzymatic and non-enzymatic processes, which in turn makes cells more susceptible to ferroptosis. In a specific investigation, Bordini and colleagues exhibited that oxidative damage can be used by high-dose iron to suppress the proliferation of prostate cancer cells. Iron had a synergistic impact with bicalutamide in cells that were resistant to the drug [233]. A great deal of research in the last several years has concentrated on ferroptosis inducers and how they work.

4.7 Ferroptosis in Prostate Cancer

Numerous human disorders have been linked to ferroptosis, including neurodegeneration, ischemia-reperfusion injury, and malignancies (including prostate cancer) [201, 234–236]. When compared to normal cells, tumor cells rely on iron more for their rapid growth. Iron addiction is the name given to this condition [231]. A new light on the origins and progression of tumor disorders has been shed by the revelation of ferroptosis. Ferroptosis inhibits tumor growth, according to mounting data. An anticancer method that involves the use of inducers to induce ferroptosis or alter genes associated to ferroptosis is being considered. Consequently, learning about ferroptosis and how it works in prostate cancer research is crucial.

New research has identified the phosphatase and tensin homolog (PTEN) gene as a tumor suppressor located on chromosome 10. Its final product, the PTEN protein, can phosphorylate both lipids and proteins. By inhibiting the PI3K/AKT signaling pathway, PTEN primarily blocks the anti-tumor impact of PI3K by acting on its downstream target molecule, PIP3 [237]. Encoding numerous genes for important enzymes in the adipogenesis pathway (including SCD, FASN, and ACLY), sterol regulatory element-binding protein 1 (SREBP1) is a critical transcription factor that controls lipid metabolism. Researchers discovered that the PI3K/AKT/mTOR pathway, which inhibits ferroptosis, is activated when the PTEN gene is defective or when PI3K is activated, promoting SREBP1/SCD mediated adipogenesis. An emerging strategy for prostate cancer treatment could involve blocking mTOR [238].

In vivo and in vitro research shown that knocking down these two genes enhances ferroptosis [239]. The genes AIFM2 and NFSI were identified in a prostate cancer gene risk model as being involved in ferroptosis. Additionally, prostate cancer is associated with elevated levels of pannexin2 (PANX2). By preventing the proliferation of prostate cancer cells, this gene knockout enhances ferroptosis [240]. It is intriguing to note that ferroptosis-related genes have emerged as possible therapeutic targets and prognostic indicators in prostate cancer patients, thanks to the discovery of database mining. The androgen receptor (AR) and its splice variants continue to be the primary drivers of castration-resistant prostate cancer (CRPC) progression, which is dependent on the ongoing activation of androgens for cell growth in prostate cancer. As a traditional ferroptosis inducer, erastin has the ability to block the AR and its splice variants' transcriptional activity both in test tubes and living organisms. Furthermore, it was discovered that the growth inhibitory impact of docetaxel was improved when administered in combination with erastin to treat CRPC. With minimal toxicity and adverse effects, erastin can further increase the anticancer effect of docetaxel in in vivo tests, and it causes no visible damage to numerous organs of mice [241]. Additionally, Li et al. discovered that ferroptosis activator RSL3 in conjunction with anti-androgens slowed the proliferation of prostate cancer cells in xenografts from mice [216]. In the future, additional clinical trials can be carried out to establish the significance of ferroptosis in the management of prostate cancer. Gene analysis for AR inhibitor resistance led to the discovery of 2,4-Dienoyl-CoA reductase (DECR1). One gene that AR negatively regulates is DECR1. Ferroptosis is enhanced in CRPC cells when this gene is deleted [242]. Recent research has shown that antagonists of AR that contain isothiocyanate (ITC) can reduce AR and its spliceosome levels. Lipid peroxidation and ferroptosis are enhanced in prostate cancer cells when BSO, a GSH inhibitor, is combined with it [243]. Based on the research conducted by Kumar et al., which shown that supraphysiological testosterone can hinder tumor proliferation through the production of lipid peroxides, one potential therapeutic approach could involve targeting the lipid metabolism associated with prostate cancer cells in order to halt their growth [244].

In another investigation Fu and collaborators revealed that in prostate cancer cells, luteolin promotes TFEB nuclear translocation and increases ferritinophagy, leading to ferroptosis [245]. Following treatment with 60 μM luteolin, RWPE-1 did not alter significantly at 12, 24, and 48 h. Nevertheless, DU145 and PC-3 cells were found to be significantly different. Luteolin promoted the demise of PCa cells. Lutein administration resulted in an increase of AnV-PI-positive dead cells and a decrease of cell viability and Ki67 expression. Fer-1, Nec-1, 3-MA, and Z-VAD-FMK were able to counteract the effects of luteolin on the viability, proliferation, and AnV-PI-positive dead cells of DU145 and PC-3 cells. The two most effective were Fer-1 and 3-MA. Autophagy and ferroptosis were enhanced in DU145 and PC-3 cells when exposed to luteolin. Additionally, DU145 and PC-3 cells experienced enhanced autophagy due to luteolin, which facilitated ferroptosis. Nevertheless, luteolin's capacity to stimulate ferritin lysosome degradation was reversed upon TFEB knockdown. Luteinolytic induction by luteolin also enhanced PCa ferroptosis in vivo.

A key component of ferroptosis is the endoplasmic reticulum stress response, as has been shown in recent research. Cancer cells can decrease ferroptosis and contribute to drug resistance generation by activating the endoplasmic reticulum stress pathway, on the one hand. Endoplasmic reticulum stress, in contrast, may play a role in the co-regulation of ferroptosis and apoptosis and can enhance cell ferroptosis [246]. Research has also demonstrated that ferroptosis inducers can activate the ERK-eIF2 pathway through the ATFα-ATF4-CHOP stress cascade in the endoplasmic reticulum, even though they do not cause apoptosis. The expression of ATF6 is greater in LNCaP-AI cells compared to LNCap-A cells. The tolerance to ferroptosis is mediated by the highly expressed ATF6 through the transcriptional activation of PLA2G4A, and the effect of enzalutamide on CRPC xenograft growth is enhanced when Ceapin-A7 inhibits ATF6α signaling [247]. It is crucial to comprehend the connection between ferroptosis and ER stress, apoptosis, and autophagy in order to conquer cancer cells' resistance to drugs. However, this subfield of prostate cancer has received surprisingly little attention from researchers. Additional investigation on the possibility of such reciprocal control in prostate cancer is warranted.

Moreover, Zou and colleagues demonstrated that Polyphyllin I activates the ERK/DNMT1/ACSL4 axis, leading to ferroptosis in castration-resistant prostate cancer cells [248]. PPI slowed the growth of CRPC cells, decreased GSH and GPX4 levels, and increased Malondialdehyde (MDA), Fe^{2+}, and ROS levels; however, an Extracellular Signal-Regulated Kinase (ERK) inhibitor undid PPI's effect on ferroptosis. Inhibiting DNMT1 was the mechanism by which PPI reduced the ACSL4 promoter methylation level. DNMT1 downregulation enhanced CRPC cell ferroptosis through regulation of ACSL4. In naked mice, PPI inhibited the development of CRPC and caused ferroptosis. One potential novel approach to treating CRPC is the use of PPI, which can trigger ferroptosis in CRPC cells through the ERK/DNMT1/ACSL4 axis.

4.8 Conclusion and Remarks

In multicellular creatures, homeostasis and the selective death of dangerous or diseased cells are both maintained by active or programmed cell death. Thus, catastrophic diseases like cancer and autoimmune disorders (too little cell death) and degenerative diseases (too much cell death) can occur when the signaling pathways that cause cell death are not properly regulated. Therefore, it is reasonable to assume that the development of multicellular creatures is the rationale behind the presence of effective and well-regulated methods to cause cell death. It may seem paradoxical, though, that there must be so many distinct mechanisms for death signaling. When seen as a whole, cell death induction is best understood as a straightforward signaling pathway leading to a single effect: cell death. Nonetheless, nearby cells and, at occasion, the entire organism are affected by the manner in which a cell dies. The inflammatory characteristics and immunological responses elicited by apoptotic and necrotic cells, for instance, are distinct. Furthermore, specific death programs involve the secretion of signals that stimulate the growth of adjacent tissues in order to compensate for the loss of their own. The signals may vary depending on the kind of cell death. Lastly, there is a definite interconnection between the routes that indicate death.

Conflict of Interest The authors declare no conflict of interest.

References

1. Green DR, Llambi F. Cell death signaling. Cold Spring Harb Perspect Biol. 2015;7(12):a006080.
2. Galluzzi L, et al. Cell death modalities: classification and pathophysiological implications. Cell Death Differ. 2007;14(7):1237–43.
3. Kerr JF, Wyllie AH, Currie AR. Apoptosis: a basic biological phenomenon with wide-ranging implications in tissue kinetics. Br J Cancer. 1972;26(4):239–57.
4. Galluzzi L, et al. Molecular definitions of cell death subroutines: recommendations of the Nomenclature Committee on Cell Death 2012. Cell Death Differ. 2012;19(1):107–20.
5. Buss RR, Sun W, Oppenheim RW. Adaptive roles of programmed cell death during nervous system development. Annu Rev Neurosci. 2006;29:1–35.
6. Sever R, Brugge JS. Signal transduction in cancer. Cold Spring Harb Perspect Med. 2015;5(4):a006098.
7. Shen S, Kepp O, Kroemer G. The end of autophagic cell death? Autophagy. 2012;8(1):1–3.
8. Berry DL, Baehrecke EH. Growth arrest and autophagy are required for salivary gland cell degradation in Drosophila. Cell. 2007;131(6):1137–48.
9. Elgendy M, et al. Oncogenic Ras-induced expression of Noxa and Beclin-1 promotes autophagic cell death and limits clonogenic survival. Mol Cell. 2011;42(1):23–35.
10. Loizzo D, et al. Novel insights into autophagy and prostate cancer: a comprehensive review. Int J Mol Sci. 2022;23(7):3826.
11. Jiang GM, et al. The relationship between autophagy and the immune system and its applications for tumor immunotherapy. Mol Cancer. 2019;18(1):17.
12. Kuballa P, et al. Autophagy and the immune system. Annu Rev Immunol. 2012;30:611–46.
13. Bento CF, et al. Mammalian autophagy: how does it work? Annu Rev Biochem. 2016;85:685–713.
14. Ashrafizadeh M, et al. Targeting autophagy in prostate cancer: preclinical and clinical evidence for therapeutic response. J Exp Clin Cancer Res. 2022;41(1):105.
15. Ichimiya T, et al. Autophagy and autophagy-related diseases: a review. Int J Mol Sci. 2020;21(23):8974.
16. Bhardwaj M, et al. Regulation of autophagy by canonical and non-canonical ER stress responses. Semin Cancer Biol. 2020;66:116–28.
17. Singh SS, et al. Dual role of autophagy in hallmarks of cancer. Oncogene. 2018;37(9):1142–58.
18. Deng S, et al. Targeting autophagy using natural compounds for cancer prevention and therapy. Cancer. 2019;125(8):1228–46.
19. De Duve C, et al. Tissue fractionation studies. 6. Intracellular distribution patterns of enzymes in rat-liver tissue. Biochem J. 1955;60(4):604–17.
20. Li WW, Li J, Bao JK. Microautophagy: lesser-known self-eating. Cell Mol Life Sci. 2012;69(7):1125–36.
21. Tasset I, Cuervo AM. Role of chaperone-mediated autophagy in metabolism. FEBS J. 2016;283(13):2403–13.
22. Mizushima N, Ohsumi Y, Yoshimori T. Autophagosome formation in mammalian cells. Cell Struct Funct. 2002;27(6):421–9.
23. Tavakol S, et al. Autophagy modulators: mechanistic aspects and drug delivery systems. Biomol Ther. 2019;9(10):530.
24. Bordoloi D, et al. TIPE family of proteins and its implications in different chronic diseases. Int J Mol Sci. 2018;19(10):2974.
25. Acevo-Rodríguez PS, et al. Autophagy regulation by the translation machinery and its implications in cancer. Front Oncol. 2020;10:322.
26. Dikic I, Elazar Z. Mechanism and medical implications of mammalian autophagy. Nat Rev Mol Cell Biol. 2018;19(6):349–64.
27. Wen X, Klionsky DJ. At a glance: a history of autophagy and cancer. Semin Cancer Biol. 2020;66:3–11.

28. Yu L, Chen Y, Tooze SA. Autophagy pathway: cellular and molecular mechanisms. Autophagy. 2018;14(2):207–15.
29. Yin Z, et al. The roles of ubiquitin in mediating autophagy. Cells. 2020;9(9):2025.
30. Benvenuto M, et al. Polyphenol-mediated autophagy in cancer: evidence of in vitro and in vivo studies. Int J Mol Sci. 2020;21(18):6635.
31. Zhang HM, et al. MKL1/miR-5100/CAAP1 loop regulates autophagy and apoptosis in gastric cancer cells. Neoplasia. 2020;22(5):220–30.
32. Kong F, et al. Downregulation of METTL14 increases apoptosis and autophagy induced by cisplatin in pancreatic cancer cells. Int J Biochem Cell Biol. 2020;122:105731.
33. Feng X, et al. Hypoxia-induced acetylation of PAK1 enhances autophagy and promotes brain tumorigenesis via phosphorylating ATG5. Autophagy. 2021;17(3):723–42.
34. Li JP, et al. miR-133a-3p/FOXP3 axis regulates cell proliferation and autophagy in gastric cancer. J Cell Biochem. 2020;121(5–6):3392–405.
35. Babaei G, Aziz SG, Jaghi NZZ. EMT, cancer stem cells and autophagy; the three main axes of metastasis. Biomed Pharmacother. 2021;133:110909.
36. Alizadeh J, et al. Autophagy modulates transforming growth factor beta 1 induced epithelial to mesenchymal transition in non-small cell lung cancer cells. Biochim Biophys Acta Mol Cell Res. 2018;1865(5):749–68.
37. de Souza ASC, et al. The role of autophagy in tumor immunology-complex mechanisms that may be explored therapeutically. Front Oncol. 2020;10:603661.
38. Chavez-Dominguez R, et al. The double-edge sword of autophagy in cancer: from tumor suppression to pro-tumor activity. Front Oncol. 2020;10:578418.
39. Yamamoto K, et al. Selective autophagy of MHC-I promotes immune evasion of pancreatic cancer. Autophagy. 2020;16(8):1524–5.
40. Hou G, et al. Inhibition of autophagy improves resistance and enhances sensitivity of gastric cancer cells to cisplatin. Can J Physiol Pharmacol. 2020;98(7):449–58.
41. Mizushima N. The role of the Atg1/ULK1 complex in autophagy regulation. Curr Opin Cell Biol. 2010;22(2):132–9.
42. Menon MB, Dhamija S. Beclin 1 phosphorylation—at the center of autophagy regulation. Front Cell Dev Biol. 2018;6:137.
43. Qu X, et al. Promotion of tumorigenesis by heterozygous disruption of the beclin 1 autophagy gene. J Clin Invest. 2003;112(12):1809–20.
44. Mizushima N, et al. Autophagy fights disease through cellular self-digestion. Nature. 2008;451(7182):1069–75.
45. Rabanal-Ruiz Y, Otten EG, Korolchuk VI. mTORC1 as the main gateway to autophagy. Essays Biochem. 2017;61(6):565–84.
46. Padman BS, et al. The protonophore CCCP interferes with lysosomal degradation of autophagic cargo in yeast and mammalian cells. Autophagy. 2013;9(11):1862–75.
47. White E. Deconvoluting the context-dependent role for autophagy in cancer. Nat Rev Cancer. 2012;12(6):401–10.
48. Massie CE, et al. The androgen receptor fuels prostate cancer by regulating central metabolism and biosynthesis. EMBO J. 2011;30(13):2719–33.
49. Stewart LM, et al. CaMKK2 facilitates Golgi-associated vesicle trafficking to sustain cancer cell proliferation. Cell Death Dis. 2021;12(11):1040.
50. Fernández ÁF, et al. Disruption of the beclin 1-BCL2 autophagy regulatory complex promotes longevity in mice. Nature. 2018;558(7708):136–40.
51. Wong RSY. Apoptosis in cancer: from pathogenesis to treatment. J Exp Clin Cancer Res. 2011;30(1):87.
52. Yang Y, et al. Autophagy-driven regulation of cisplatin response in human cancers: exploring molecular and cell death dynamics. Cancer Lett. 2024;587:216659.
53. Qin Y, et al. Autophagy and cancer drug resistance in dialogue: pre-clinical and clinical evidence. Cancer Lett. 2023;570:216307.

54. Ashrafizadeh M, et al. A bioinformatics analysis, pre-clinical and clinical conception of autophagy in pancreatic cancer: complexity and simplicity in crosstalk. Pharmacol Res. 2023;194:106822.
55. Ding M, et al. SIRT7 depletion inhibits cell proliferation and androgen-induced autophagy by suppressing the AR signaling in prostate cancer. J Exp Clin Cancer Res. 2020;39(1):28.
56. Wadosky KM, et al. Riluzole induces AR degradation via endoplasmic reticulum stress pathway in androgen-dependent and castration-resistant prostate cancer cells. Prostate. 2019;79(2):140–50.
57. Blessing AM, et al. Transcriptional regulation of core autophagy and lysosomal genes by the androgen receptor promotes prostate cancer progression. Autophagy. 2017;13(3):506–21.
58. Xie CW, et al. Gabarapl1 mediates androgen-regulated autophagy in prostate cancer. Tumour Biol. 2015;36(11):8727–33.
59. Bertout JA, Patel SA, Simon MC. The impact of O2 availability on human cancer. Nat Rev Cancer. 2008;8(12):967–75.
60. Young SD, Marshall RS, Hill RP. Hypoxia induces DNA overreplication and enhances metastatic potential of murine tumor cells. Proc Natl Acad Sci U S A. 1988;85(24):9533–7.
61. Young SD, Hill RP. Effects of reoxygenation on cells from hypoxic regions of solid tumors: analysis of transplanted murine tumors for evidence of DNA overreplication. Cancer Res. 1990;50(16):5031–8.
62. Xia L, et al. PRKAR2B-HIF-1α loop promotes aerobic glycolysis and tumour growth in prostate cancer. Cell Prolif. 2020;53(11):e12918.
63. Shanmugam MK, et al. Potential role of natural compounds as anti-angiogenic agents in cancer. Curr Vasc Pharmacol. 2017;15(6):503–19.
64. Deng M, et al. HIF-1a regulates hypoxia-induced autophagy via translocation of ANKRD37 in colon cancer. Exp Cell Res. 2020;395(1):112175.
65. Yu K, et al. HIF1α promotes prostate cancer progression by increasing ATG5 expression. Anim Cells Syst (Seoul). 2019;23(5):326–34.
66. Zhang N, et al. PAX5-induced upregulation of IDH1-AS1 promotes tumor growth in prostate cancer by regulating ATG5-mediated autophagy. Cell Death Dis. 2019;10(10):734.
67. Beenken A, Mohammadi M. The FGF family: biology, pathophysiology and therapy. Nat Rev Drug Discov. 2009;8(3):235–53.
68. Potthoff MJ, Kliewer SA, Mangelsdorf DJ. Endocrine fibroblast growth factors 15/19 and 21: from feast to famine. Genes Dev. 2012;26(4):312–24.
69. Dai H, et al. FGF21 facilitates autophagy in prostate cancer cells by inhibiting the PI3K-Akt-mTOR signaling pathway. Cell Death Dis. 2021;12(4):303.
70. Cheng Y, et al. Autophagy-related genes are potential diagnostic and prognostic biomarkers in prostate cancer. Transl Androl Urol. 2020;9(6):2616–28.
71. Hu D, et al. Development of an autophagy-related gene expression signature for prognosis prediction in prostate cancer patients. J Transl Med. 2020;18(1):160.
72. Giatromanolaki A, et al. Autophagy proteins in prostate cancer: relation with anaerobic metabolism and Gleason score. Urol Oncol. 2014;32(1):39.e11–8.
73. Menon S, et al. Chronic activation of mTOR complex 1 is sufficient to cause hepatocellular carcinoma in mice. Sci Signal. 2012;5(217):ra24.
74. Guo JY, White E. Autophagy, metabolism, and cancer. Cold Spring Harb Symp Quant Biol. 2016;81:73–8.
75. Grossi V, et al. Loss of STK11 expression is an early event in prostate carcinogenesis and predicts therapeutic response to targeted therapy against MAPK/p38. Autophagy. 2015;11(11):2102–13.
76. Lin C, et al. Inhibition of CAMKK2 impairs autophagy and castration-resistant prostate cancer via suppression of AMPK-ULK1 signaling. Oncogene. 2021;40(9):1690–705.
77. Farrow JM, Yang JC, Evans CP. Autophagy as a modulator and target in prostate cancer. Nat Rev Urol. 2014;11(9):508–16.

78. Yang ZJ, et al. The role of autophagy in cancer: therapeutic implications. Mol Cancer Ther. 2011;10(9):1533–41.
79. Erkisa M, et al. A promising therapeutic combination for metastatic prostate cancer: chloroquine as autophagy inhibitor and palladium(II) barbiturate complex. Biochimie. 2020;175:159–72.
80. Ben Sahra I, et al. Targeting cancer cell metabolism: the combination of metformin and 2-deoxyglucose induces p53-dependent apoptosis in prostate cancer cells. Cancer Res. 2010;70(6):2465–75.
81. Chen C, et al. Metformin exerts anti-AR-negative prostate cancer activity via AMPK/autophagy signaling pathway. Cancer Cell Int. 2021;21(1):404.
82. Luty M, et al. Fenofibrate augments the sensitivity of drug-resistant prostate cancer cells to docetaxel. Cancers (Basel). 2019;11(1):77.
83. Tan Q, et al. Up-regulation of autophagy is a mechanism of resistance to chemotherapy and can be inhibited by pantoprazole to increase drug sensitivity. Cancer Chemother Pharmacol. 2017;79(5):959–69.
84. Hansen AR, et al. Pantoprazole affecting docetaxel resistance pathways via autophagy (PANDORA): phase II trial of high dose pantoprazole (autophagy inhibitor) with docetaxel in metastatic castration-resistant prostate cancer (mCRPC). Oncologist. 2019;24(9):1188–94.
85. Mishra P, Chan DC. Metabolic regulation of mitochondrial dynamics. J Cell Biol. 2016;212(4):379–87.
86. Senft D, Ronai ZA. Regulators of mitochondrial dynamics in cancer. Curr Opin Cell Biol. 2016;39:43–52.
87. Lee YG, et al. Androgen-induced expression of DRP1 regulates mitochondrial metabolic reprogramming in prostate cancer. Cancer Lett. 2020;471:72–87.
88. Glover DM, et al. Mutations in aurora prevent centrosome separation leading to the formation of monopolar spindles. Cell. 1995;81(1):95–105.
89. Zhou H, et al. Tumour amplified kinase STK15/BTAK induces centrosome amplification, aneuploidy and transformation. Nat Genet. 1998;20(2):189–93.
90. Jones D, et al. Aurora A regulates expression of AR-V7 in models of castrate resistant prostate cancer. Sci Rep. 2017;7:40957.
91. Buschhorn HM, et al. Aurora-A over-expression in high-grade PIN lesions and prostate cancer. Prostate. 2005;64(4):341–6.
92. Zhang S, et al. Aurora-A regulates autophagy through the Akt pathway in human prostate cancer. Cancer Biomark. 2017;19(1):27–34.
93. You D, et al. KML001 induces apoptosis and autophagic cell death in prostate cancer cells via oxidative stress pathway. PLoS One. 2015;10(9):e0137589.
94. Chopra P, et al. Polo-like kinase inhibitors: an emerging opportunity for cancer therapeutics. Expert Opin Investig Drugs. 2010;19(1):27–43.
95. Huang H, et al. Acetylation-mediated degradation of HSD17B4 regulates the progression of prostate cancer. Aging (Albany NY). 2020;12(14):14699–717.
96. Balkwill FR, Capasso M, Hagemann T. The tumor microenvironment at a glance. J Cell Sci. 2012;125(Pt 23):5591–6.
97. Godoy A, et al. Androgen deprivation induces rapid involution and recovery of human prostate vasculature. Am J Physiol Endocrinol Metab. 2011;300(2):E263–75.
98. Wang X, et al. Endothelial cells enhance prostate cancer metastasis via IL-6→androgen receptor→TGF-β→MMP-9 signals. Mol Cancer Ther. 2013;12(6):1026–37.
99. Tomić TT, et al. Castration resistant prostate cancer is associated with increased blood vessel stabilization and elevated levels of VEGF and Ang-2. Prostate. 2012;72(7):705–12.
100. Zhao R, et al. Endothelial cells promote metastasis of prostate cancer by enhancing autophagy. J Exp Clin Cancer Res. 2018;37(1):221.
101. Liang T, et al. HDAC6-mediated α-tubulin deacetylation suppresses autophagy and enhances motility of podocytes in diabetic nephropathy. J Cell Mol Med. 2020;24(19):11558–72.

102. Jiang X, et al. Metastatic prostate cancer-associated P62 inhibits autophagy flux and promotes epithelial to mesenchymal transition by sustaining the level of HDAC6. Prostate. 2018;78(6):426–34.
103. Elmore S. Apoptosis: a review of programmed cell death. Toxicol Pathol. 2007;35(4):495–516.
104. Igney FH, Krammer PH. Death and anti-death: tumour resistance to apoptosis. Nat Rev Cancer. 2002;2(4):277–88.
105. Martinvalet D, Zhu P, Lieberman J. Granzyme A induces caspase-independent mitochondrial damage, a required first step for apoptosis. Immunity. 2005;22(3):355–70.
106. Hengartner MO. The biochemistry of apoptosis. Nature. 2000;407(6805):770–6.
107. Cohen GM. Caspases: the executioners of apoptosis. Biochem J. 1997;326(Pt 1):1–16.
108. Rai NK, et al. Apoptosis: a basic physiologic process in wound healing. Int J Low Extrem Wounds. 2005;4(3):138–44.
109. Hu S, et al. Caspase-14 is a novel developmentally regulated protease. J Biol Chem. 1998;273(45):29648–53.
110. Nakagawa T, et al. Caspase-12 mediates endoplasmic-reticulum-specific apoptosis and cytotoxicity by amyloid-beta. Nature. 2000;403(6765):98–103.
111. Koenig U, Eckhart L, Tschachler E. Evidence that caspase-13 is not a human but a bovine gene. Biochem Biophys Res Commun. 2001;285(5):1150–4.
112. Kang SJ, et al. Distinct downstream pathways of caspase-11 in regulating apoptosis and cytokine maturation during septic shock response. Cell Death Differ. 2002;9(10):1115–25.
113. Nemes Z Jr, et al. Expression and activation of tissue transglutaminase in apoptotic cells of involuting rodent mammary tissue. Eur J Cell Biol. 1996;70(2):125–33.
114. Bortner CD, Oldenburg NB, Cidlowski JA. The role of DNA fragmentation in apoptosis. Trends Cell Biol. 1995;5(1):21–6.
115. Bratton DL, et al. Appearance of phosphatidylserine on apoptotic cells requires calcium-mediated nonspecific flip-flop and is enhanced by loss of the aminophospholipid translocase. J Biol Chem. 1997;272(42):26159–65.
116. Arur S, et al. Annexin I is an endogenous ligand that mediates apoptotic cell engulfment. Dev Cell. 2003;4(4):587–98.
117. Gardai SJ, et al. Cell-surface calreticulin initiates clearance of viable or apoptotic cells through trans-activation of LRP on the phagocyte. Cell. 2005;123(2):321–34.
118. Jiménez B, et al. Signals leading to apoptosis-dependent inhibition of neovascularization by thrombospondin-1. Nat Med. 2000;6(1):41–8.
119. Saelens X, et al. Toxic proteins released from mitochondria in cell death. Oncogene. 2004;23(16):2861–74.
120. Du C, et al. Smac, a mitochondrial protein that promotes cytochrome c-dependent caspase activation by eliminating IAP inhibition. Cell. 2000;102(1):33–42.
121. Chinnaiyan AM. The apoptosome: heart and soul of the cell death machine. Neoplasia. 1999;1(1):5–15.
122. Hill MM, et al. Analysis of the composition, assembly kinetics and activity of native Apaf-1 apoptosomes. EMBO J. 2004;23(10):2134–45.
123. Schimmer AD. Inhibitor of apoptosis proteins: translating basic knowledge into clinical practice. Cancer Res. 2004;64(20):7183–90.
124. van Loo G, et al. The serine protease Omi/HtrA2 is released from mitochondria during apoptosis. Omi interacts with caspase-inhibitor XIAP and induces enhanced caspase activity. Cell Death Differ. 2002;9(1):20–6.
125. Ekert PG, Vaux DL. The mitochondrial death squad: hardened killers or innocent bystanders? Curr Opin Cell Biol. 2005;17(6):626–30.
126. Joza N, et al. Essential role of the mitochondrial apoptosis-inducing factor in programmed cell death. Nature. 2001;410(6828):549–54.
127. Susin SA, et al. Two distinct pathways leading to nuclear apoptosis. J Exp Med. 2000;192(4):571–80.

128. Li LY, Luo X, Wang X. Endonuclease G is an apoptotic DNase when released from mitochondria. Nature. 2001;412(6842):95–9.
129. Enari M, et al. A caspase-activated DNase that degrades DNA during apoptosis, and its inhibitor ICAD. Nature. 1998;391(6662):43–50.
130. Cory S, Adams JM. The Bcl2 family: regulators of the cellular life-or-death switch. Nat Rev Cancer. 2002;2(9):647–56.
131. Schuler M, Green DR. Mechanisms of p53-dependent apoptosis. Biochem Soc Trans. 2001;29(Pt 6):684–8.
132. Li H, et al. Cleavage of BID by caspase 8 mediates the mitochondrial damage in the Fas pathway of apoptosis. Cell. 1998;94(4):491–501.
133. Esposti MD. The roles of bid. Apoptosis. 2002;7(5):433–40.
134. Zha J, et al. Serine phosphorylation of death agonist BAD in response to survival factor results in binding to 14-3-3 not BCL-X(L). Cell. 1996;87(4):619–28.
135. Yang E, et al. Bad, a heterodimeric partner for Bcl-XL and Bcl-2, displaces Bax and promotes cell death. Cell. 1995;80(2):285–91.
136. Liu FT, Newland AC, Jia L. Bax conformational change is a crucial step for PUMA-mediated apoptosis in human leukemia. Biochem Biophys Res Commun. 2003;310(3):956–62.
137. Oda E, et al. Noxa, a BH3-only member of the Bcl-2 family and candidate mediator of p53-induced apoptosis. Science. 2000;288(5468):1053–8.
138. Meyer N, Kim SS, Penn LZ. The Oscar-worthy role of Myc in apoptosis. Semin Cancer Biol. 2006;16(4):275–87.
139. Locksley RM, Killeen N, Lenardo MJ. The TNF and TNF receptor superfamilies: integrating mammalian biology. Cell. 2001;104(4):487–501.
140. Ashkenazi A, Dixit VM. Death receptors: signaling and modulation. Science. 1998;281(5381):1305–8.
141. Chicheportiche Y, et al. TWEAK, a new secreted ligand in the tumor necrosis factor family that weakly induces apoptosis. J Biol Chem. 1997;272(51):32401–10.
142. Rubio-Moscardo F, et al. Characterization of 8p21.3 chromosomal deletions in B-cell lymphoma: TRAIL-R1 and TRAIL-R2 as candidate dosage-dependent tumor suppressor genes. Blood. 2005;106(9):3214–22.
143. Suliman A, et al. Intracellular mechanisms of TRAIL: apoptosis through mitochondrial-dependent and -independent pathways. Oncogene. 2001;20(17):2122–33.
144. Wajant H. The Fas signaling pathway: more than a paradigm. Science. 2002;296(5573):1635–6.
145. Hsu H, Xiong J, Goeddel DV. The TNF receptor 1-associated protein TRADD signals cell death and NF-kappa B activation. Cell. 1995;81(4):495–504.
146. Kischkel FC, et al. Cytotoxicity-dependent APO-1 (Fas/CD95)-associated proteins form a death-inducing signaling complex (DISC) with the receptor. EMBO J. 1995;14(22):5579–88.
147. Kataoka T, et al. FLIP prevents apoptosis induced by death receptors but not by perforin/granzyme B, chemotherapeutic drugs, and gamma irradiation. J Immunol. 1998;161(8):3936–42.
148. Scaffidi C, et al. The role of c-FLIP in modulation of CD95-induced apoptosis. J Biol Chem. 1999;274(3):1541–8.
149. Hitoshi Y, et al. Toso, a cell surface, specific regulator of Fas-induced apoptosis in T cells. Immunity. 1998;8(4):461–71.
150. Brunner T, et al. Fas (CD95/Apo-1) ligand regulation in T cell homeostasis, cell-mediated cytotoxicity and immune pathology. Semin Immunol. 2003;15(3):167–76.
151. Trapani JA, Smyth MJ. Functional significance of the perforin/granzyme cell death pathway. Nat Rev Immunol. 2002;2(10):735–47.
152. Sakahira H, Enari M, Nagata S. Cleavage of CAD inhibitor in CAD activation and DNA degradation during apoptosis. Nature. 1998;391(6662):96–9.
153. Russell JH, Ley TJ. Lymphocyte-mediated cytotoxicity. Annu Rev Immunol. 2002;20:323–70.
154. Barry M, Bleackley RC. Cytotoxic T lymphocytes: all roads lead to death. Nat Rev Immunol. 2002;2(6):401–9.

155. Goping IS, et al. Granzyme B-induced apoptosis requires both direct caspase activation and relief of caspase inhibition. Immunity. 2003;18(3):355–65.
156. Devadas S, et al. Granzyme B is critical for T cell receptor-induced cell death of type 2 helper T cells. Immunity. 2006;25(2):237–47.
157. Jemal A, et al. Cancer statistics, 2005. CA Cancer J Clin. 2005;55(1):10–30.
158. McKenzie S, Kyprianou N. Apoptosis evasion: the role of survival pathways in prostate cancer progression and therapeutic resistance. J Cell Biochem. 2006;97(1):18–32.
159. Arnold JT, Isaacs JT. Mechanisms involved in the progression of androgen-independent prostate cancers: it is not only the cancer cell's fault. Endocr Relat Cancer. 2002;9(1):61–73.
160. Debes JD, Tindall DJ. Mechanisms of androgen-refractory prostate cancer. N Engl J Med. 2004;351(15):1488–90.
161. Jeong SH, et al. Flavones: the apoptosis in prostate cancer of three flavones selected as therapeutic candidate models. Int J Mol Sci. 2023;24(11):9240.
162. Khan N, Adhami VM, Mukhtar H. Apoptosis by dietary agents for prevention and treatment of prostate cancer. Endocr Relat Cancer. 2010;17(1):R39–52.
163. Xiang Y, et al. Effects of RNase L mutations associated with prostate cancer on apoptosis induced by 2′,5′-oligoadenylates. Cancer Res. 2003;63(20):6795–801.
164. Fujita K, Nonomura N. Role of androgen receptor in prostate cancer: a review. World J Mens Health. 2019;37(3):288–95.
165. Hernandez I, et al. Prostate-specific expression of p53R172L differentially regulates p21, Bax, and mdm2 to inhibit prostate cancer progression and prolong survival. Mol Cancer Res. 2003;1(14):1036–47.
166. Gurova KV, et al. Cooperation of two mutant p53 alleles contributes to Fas resistance of prostate carcinoma cells. Cancer Res. 2003;63(11):2905–12.
167. Zhou Y, et al. Natural polyphenols for prevention and treatment of cancer. Nutrients. 2016;8(8):515.
168. DiPaola RS, Patel J, Rafi MM. Targeting apoptosis in prostate cancer. Hematol Oncol Clin North Am. 2001;15(3):509–24.
169. Kajiwara T, et al. Effect of Bcl-2 overexpression in human prostate cancer cells in vitro and in vivo. Int J Urol. 1999;6(10):520–5.
170. McCarty MF. Targeting multiple signaling pathways as a strategy for managing prostate cancer: multifocal signal modulation therapy. Integr Cancer Ther. 2004;3(4):349–80.
171. Coffey RN, et al. Androgen-mediated resistance to apoptosis. Prostate. 2002;53(4):300–9.
172. Furuya Y, et al. Expression of bcl-2 and the progression of human and rodent prostatic cancers. Clin Cancer Res. 1996;2(2):389–98.
173. Wang S, et al. Prostate-specific deletion of the murine Pten tumor suppressor gene leads to metastatic prostate cancer. Cancer Cell. 2003;4(3):209–21.
174. Davies MA, et al. Regulation of Akt/PKB activity, cellular growth, and apoptosis in prostate carcinoma cells by MMAC/PTEN. Cancer Res. 1999;59(11):2551–6.
175. Yuan XJ, Whang YE. PTEN sensitizes prostate cancer cells to death receptor-mediated and drug-induced apoptosis through a FADD-dependent pathway. Oncogene. 2002;21(2):319–27.
176. Stern DF. More than a marker... phosphorylated Akt in prostate carcinoma. Clin Cancer Res. 2004;10(19):6407–10.
177. Pfeil K, et al. Long-term androgen-ablation causes increased resistance to PI3K/Akt pathway inhibition in prostate cancer cells. Prostate. 2004;58(3):259–68.
178. Gao N, et al. Role of PI3K/AKT/mTOR signaling in the cell cycle progression of human prostate cancer. Biochem Biophys Res Commun. 2003;310(4):1124–32.
179. Ghosh PM, et al. Akt in prostate cancer: possible role in androgen-independence. Curr Drug Metab. 2003;4(6):487–96.
180. Lin HK, et al. Akt suppresses androgen-induced apoptosis by phosphorylating and inhibiting androgen receptor. Proc Natl Acad Sci U S A. 2001;98(13):7200–5.
181. McMenamin ME, et al. Loss of PTEN expression in paraffin-embedded primary prostate cancer correlates with high Gleason score and advanced stage. Cancer Res. 1999;59(17):4291–6.

182. Ayala G, et al. High levels of phosphorylated form of Akt-1 in prostate cancer and non-neoplastic prostate tissues are strong predictors of biochemical recurrence. Clin Cancer Res. 2004;10(19):6572–8.
183. Malik SN, et al. Immunohistochemical demonstration of phospho-Akt in high Gleason grade prostate cancer. Clin Cancer Res. 2002;8(4):1168–71.
184. Liao Y, et al. Increase of AKT/PKB expression correlates with Gleason pattern in human prostate cancer. Int J Cancer. 2003;107(4):676–80.
185. Kreisberg JI, et al. Phosphorylation of Akt (Ser473) is an excellent predictor of poor clinical outcome in prostate cancer. Cancer Res. 2004;64(15):5232–6.
186. Krajewska M, et al. Elevated expression of inhibitor of apoptosis proteins in prostate cancer. Clin Cancer Res. 2003;9(13):4914–25.
187. McEleny KR, Watson RW, Fitzpatrick JM. Defining a role for the inhibitors of apoptosis proteins in prostate cancer. Prostate Cancer Prostatic Dis. 2001;4(1):28–32.
188. Debatin KM, Krammer PH. Death receptors in chemotherapy and cancer. Oncogene. 2004;23(16):2950–66.
189. Amantana A, et al. X-linked inhibitor of apoptosis protein inhibition induces apoptosis and enhances chemotherapy sensitivity in human prostate cancer cells. Mol Cancer Ther. 2004;3(6):699–707.
190. Shukla S, Fu P, Gupta S. Apigenin induces apoptosis by targeting inhibitor of apoptosis proteins and Ku70-Bax interaction in prostate cancer. Apoptosis. 2014;19(5):883–94.
191. Shukla S, et al. Apigenin blocks IKKα activation and suppresses prostate cancer progression. Oncotarget. 2015;6(31):31216–32.
192. Erdogan S, et al. The flavonoid apigenin reduces prostate cancer CD44+ stem cell survival and migration through PI3K/Akt/NF-κB signaling. Life Sci. 2016;162:77–86.
193. Shukla S, et al. Apigenin inhibits prostate cancer progression in TRAMP mice via targeting PI3K/Akt/FoxO pathway. Carcinogenesis. 2014;35(2):452–60.
194. Hollman PCH, Katan MB. Dietary flavonoids: intake, health effects and bioavailability. Food Chem Toxicol. 1999;37(9–10):937–42.
195. Singh S, et al. Acacetin, a flavone with diverse therapeutic potential in cancer, inflammation, infections and other metabolic disorders. Food Chem Toxicol. 2020;145:111708.
196. Kim HR, Park CG, Jung JY. Acacetin (5,7-dihydroxy-4′-methoxyflavone) exhibits in vitro and in vivo anticancer activity through the suppression of NF-κB/Akt signaling in prostate cancer cells. Int J Mol Med. 2014;33(2):317–24.
197. Singh RP, et al. Acacetin inhibits cell growth and cell cycle progression, and induces apoptosis in human prostate cancer cells: structure-activity relationship with linarin and linarin acetate. Carcinogenesis. 2005;26(4):845–54.
198. Yun S, et al. Acacetin inhibits the growth of STAT3-activated DU145 prostate cancer cells by directly binding to signal transducer and activator of transcription 3 (STAT3). Molecules. 2021;26(20):6204.
199. Zhou Y, et al. Evaluation of acacetin inhibition potential against cytochrome P450 in vitro and in vivo. Chem Biol Interact. 2020;329:109147.
200. Ko YC, et al. Inhibitory effects of tangeretin, a citrus peel-derived flavonoid, on breast cancer stem cell formation through suppression of Stat3 signaling. Molecules. 2020;25(11):2599.
201. Wang Y, Ma Y, Jiang K. The role of ferroptosis in prostate cancer: a novel therapeutic strategy. Prostate Cancer Prostatic Dis. 2023;26(1):25–9.
202. Bridges RJ, Natale NR, Patel SA. System xc^- cystine/glutamate antiporter: an update on molecular pharmacology and roles within the CNS. Br J Pharmacol. 2012;165(1):20–34.
203. Pfeiffer R, et al. Functional heterodimeric amino acid transporters lacking cysteine residues involved in disulfide bond. FEBS Lett. 1998;439(1–2):157–62.
204. Liu T, et al. The deubiquitylase OTUB1 mediates ferroptosis via stabilization of SLC7A11. Cancer Res. 2019;79(8):1913–24.
205. Dixon SJ, et al. Pharmacological inhibition of cystine-glutamate exchange induces endoplasmic reticulum stress and ferroptosis. elife. 2014;3:e02523.

206. Patel D, et al. Novel analogs of sulfasalazine as system x(c)(−) antiporter inhibitors: insights from the molecular modeling studies. Drug Dev Res. 2019;80(6):758–77.
207. Genchi G, et al. The effects of cadmium toxicity. Int J Environ Res Public Health. 2020;17(11):3782.
208. Zhang Y, et al. LncRNA OIP5-AS1 inhibits ferroptosis in prostate cancer with long-term cadmium exposure through miR-128-3p/SLC7A11 signaling. Ecotoxicol Environ Saf. 2021;220:112376.
209. Liu J, et al. Tumor suppressor p53 and its mutants in cancer metabolism. Cancer Lett. 2015;356(2 Pt A):197–203.
210. Jiang L, et al. Ferroptosis as a p53-mediated activity during tumour suppression. Nature. 2015;520(7545):57–62.
211. Zhou X, et al. Flubendazole, FDA-approved anthelmintic, elicits valid antitumor effects by targeting P53 and promoting ferroptosis in castration-resistant prostate cancer. Pharmacol Res. 2021;164:105305.
212. Su LJ, et al. Reactive oxygen species-induced lipid peroxidation in apoptosis, autophagy, and ferroptosis. Oxidative Med Cell Longev. 2019;2019:5080843.
213. Jelinek A, et al. Mitochondrial rescue prevents glutathione peroxidase-dependent ferroptosis. Free Radic Biol Med. 2018;117:45–57.
214. Yang WS, et al. Regulation of ferroptotic cancer cell death by GPX4. Cell. 2014;156(1–2):317–31.
215. Xu P, et al. MicroRNA-15a promotes prostate cancer cell ferroptosis by inhibiting GPX4 expression. Oncol Lett. 2022;23(2):67.
216. Ghoochani A, et al. Ferroptosis inducers are a novel therapeutic approach for advanced prostate cancer. Cancer Res. 2021;81(6):1583–94.
217. Li R, Jia Z, Trush MA. Defining ROS in biology and medicine. React Oxyg Species (Apex). 2016;1(1):9–21.
218. He L, et al. Antioxidants maintain cellular redox homeostasis by elimination of reactive oxygen species. Cell Physiol Biochem. 2017;44(2):532–53.
219. Zhao M, et al. Mitochondrial ROS promote mitochondrial dysfunction and inflammation in ischemic acute kidney injury by disrupting TFAM-mediated mtDNA maintenance. Theranostics. 2021;11(4):1845–63.
220. Peng X, Gandhi V. ROS-activated anticancer prodrugs: a new strategy for tumor-specific damage. Ther Deliv. 2012;3(7):823–33.
221. Wang S, et al. Verticillium dahliae chromatin remodeling facilitates the DNA damage repair in response to plant ROS stress. PLoS Pathog. 2020;16(4):e1008481.
222. Li M, et al. RSL3 enhances the antitumor effect of cisplatin on prostate cancer cells via causing glycolysis dysfunction. Biochem Pharmacol. 2021;192:114741.
223. Samy A, et al. Can diallyl trisulfide, a dietary garlic-derived compound, activate ferroptosis to overcome therapy resistance in prostate cancer? Nutr Health. 2022;28(2):207–12.
224. Ma N, et al. The birth of artemisinin. Pharmacol Ther. 2020;216:107658.
225. Vakhrusheva O, et al. Artesunate inhibits the growth behavior of docetaxel-resistant prostate cancer cells. Front Oncol. 2022;12:789284.
226. Yuan B, et al. Dihydroartemisinin inhibits the proliferation, colony formation and induces ferroptosis of lung cancer cells by inhibiting PRIM2/SLC7A11 Axis. Onco Targets Ther. 2020;13:10829–40.
227. Chen Y, et al. Dihydroartemisinin-induced unfolded protein response feedback attenuates ferroptosis via PERK/ATF4/HSPA5 pathway in glioma cells. J Exp Clin Cancer Res. 2019;38(1):402.
228. Pantopoulos K, et al. Mechanisms of mammalian iron homeostasis. Biochemistry. 2012;51(29):5705–24.
229. Nakamura T, Naguro I, Ichijo H. Iron homeostasis and iron-regulated ROS in cell death, senescence and human diseases. Biochim Biophys Acta Gen Subj. 2019;1863(9):1398–409.

230. Zhang F, et al. Metalloreductase Steap3 coordinates the regulation of iron homeostasis and inflammatory responses. Haematologica. 2012;97(12):1826–35.
231. Basuli D, et al. Iron addiction: a novel therapeutic target in ovarian cancer. Oncogene. 2017;36(29):4089–99.
232. Xue X, et al. Iron uptake via DMT1 integrates cell cycle with JAK-STAT3 signaling to promote colorectal tumorigenesis. Cell Metab. 2016;24(3):447–61.
233. Bordini J, et al. Iron induces cell death and strengthens the efficacy of antiandrogen therapy in prostate cancer models. Clin Cancer Res. 2020;26(23):6387–98.
234. Hambright WS, et al. Ablation of ferroptosis regulator glutathione peroxidase 4 in forebrain neurons promotes cognitive impairment and neurodegeneration. Redox Biol. 2017;12:8–17.
235. Li Y, et al. Ischemia-induced ACSL4 activation contributes to ferroptosis-mediated tissue injury in intestinal ischemia/reperfusion. Cell Death Differ. 2019;26(11):2284–99.
236. Wang M, et al. Correction to: long noncoding RNA LINC00336 inhibits ferroptosis in lung cancer by functioning as a competing endogenous RNA. Cell Death Differ. 2020;27(4):1447.
237. Chen C-Y, et al. PTEN: tumor suppressor and metabolic regulator. Front Endocrinol. 2018;9:338.
238. Yi J, et al. Oncogenic activation of PI3K-AKT-mTOR signaling suppresses ferroptosis via SREBP-mediated lipogenesis. Proc Natl Acad Sci U S A. 2020;117(49):31189–97.
239. Lv Z, et al. Identifying a ferroptosis-related gene signature for predicting biochemical recurrence of prostate cancer. Front Cell Dev Biol. 2021;9:666025.
240. Liao D, et al. Identification of pannexin 2 as a novel marker correlating with ferroptosis and malignant phenotypes of prostate cancer cells. Onco Targets Ther. 2020;13:4411–21.
241. Yang Y, et al. Ferroptosis inducer erastin downregulates androgen receptor and its splice variants in castration-resistant prostate cancer. Oncol Rep. 2021;45(4):25.
242. Nassar ZD, et al. Human DECR1 is an androgen-repressed survival factor that regulates PUFA oxidation to protect prostate tumor cells from ferroptosis. elife. 2020;9:e54166.
243. Qin Z, et al. Design and synthesis of isothiocyanate-containing hybrid androgen receptor (AR) antagonist to downregulate AR and induce ferroptosis in GSH-deficient prostate cancer cells. Chem Biol Drug Des. 2021;97(5):1059–78.
244. Kumar R, et al. Supraphysiologic testosterone induces ferroptosis and activates immune pathways through nucleophagy in prostate cancer. Cancer Res. 2021;81(23):5948–62.
245. Fu W, et al. Luteolin induces ferroptosis in prostate cancer cells by promoting TFEB nuclear translocation and increasing ferritinophagy. Prostate. 2024;84(3):223–36.
246. Lee YS, et al. Ferroptosis-induced endoplasmic reticulum stress: cross-talk between ferroptosis and apoptosis. Mol Cancer Res. 2018;16(7):1073–6.
247. Zhao R, et al. ATF6α promotes prostate cancer progression by enhancing PLA2G4A-mediated arachidonic acid metabolism and protecting tumor cells against ferroptosis. Prostate. 2022;82(5):617–29.
248. Zou P, et al. Polyphyllin I induces ferroptosis in castration-resistant prostate cancer cells through the ERK/DNMT1/ACSL4 axis. Prostate. 2024;84(1):64–73.

Chapter 5
Prostate Cancer and Metastasis: An Emphasis on EMT Mechanism

Mehrdad Hashemi, Shima Hajimazdarany, Reza Morovatshoar, Abbas Amini, Amirsoheil Karami, Alireza Hajimohammad, Zahra Rahbar Zare, Anis Mashhad Merdasi, Hosein Izadi, Saba Asadi, Sima Orouei, Behdokht Jamali, Rasoul Raesi, Najma Farahani, and Maliheh Entezari

Abstract Metastasis from prostate cancer is still a major problem, affecting patients' mortality rates and quality of life in general. Moreover, the presence of metastases is a direct determinant of the prognosis and clinical outcome of prostate cancer. Furthermore, metastasis thrives in the bone microenvironment. The progression of androgen-sensitive to castration-resistant and metastatic prostate cancer is a major clinical concern in prostate cancer treatment. In their normal state, epithelial cells form a monolayer that is adherently held in place by proteins that inhibit cell movement. Epithelial cells in prostate cancer can change their shape from cuboidal to spindle-shaped as the disease advances; this process is called epithelial-

M. Hashemi · M. Entezari
Farhikhtegan Medical Convergence Sciences Research Center, Farhikhtegan Hospital Tehran Medical Sciences, Islamic Azad University, Tehran, Iran

Faculty of Advanced Science and Technology, Department of Genetics, Tehran Medical Sciences, Islamic Azad University, Tehran, Iran

S. Hajimazdarany · A. Karami · H. Izadi · S. Asadi
Farhikhtegan Medical Convergence Sciences Research Center, Farhikhtegan Hospital Tehran Medical Sciences, Islamic Azad University, Tehran, Iran

R. Morovatshoar
Molecular Medicine Research Center, Hormozgan Health Institute, Hormozgan University of Medical Sciences, Bandar Abbas, Iran

A. Amini
College of Engineering and Energy, Abdullah Al Salem University (AASU), Khaldiya, Kuwait

Centre for Infrastructure Engineering, Western Sydney University, Penrith, NSW, Australia

A. Hajimohammad
Department of Molecular Cell Biology, Tehran Medical Branch, Islamic Azad University, Tehran, Iran

G. Sethi et al. (eds.), *Prostate Cancer: Molecular Events and Therapeutic Modalities*, https://doi.org/10.1007/978-981-97-4612-5_5

mesenchymal transition (EMT). Despite efforts to block the androgen receptor (AR) signaling axis, the exact molecular process by which androgen independence kills is yet unknown. The involvement of cancer stem cells (CSCs) and epithelial-to-mesenchymal transition (EMT) in the progression of prostate cancer to castration-resistant and metastasis are being more and more highlighted by new findings. This EMT procedure may be evolving over time. It is worth noting that metastatic disease development in prostate tumors may trigger the reactivation of a dormant embryonic pathway known as the epithelial-mesenchymal transition (EMT). A mesenchymal phenotype resembling cancer stem cells can be achieved by malignancies by EMT.

Keywords Prostate cancer · Metastasis · EMT · Cancer

5.1 Introduction

Of all the cancers that affect men, the most frequent non-skin cancer is prostate cancer, which also happens to be the biggest killer of men. Different forms of this complex disease manifest in different ways at the genetic, clinical, and molecular levels [1]. From low-grade prostatic intraepithelial neoplasia (PINs) to aggressive adenocarcinoma and castration-resistant prostate cancer (CRPC), there is a multi-stage process culminating in metastatic prostate cancer [2, 3]. To treat prostate cancer, androgen deprivation therapy (ADT) was widely used since testosterone and the androgen receptor (AR) are essential for the normal growth and maintenance of homeostasis in normal prostate tissues. Although radiation and surgery are excellent

Z. R. Zare
Biology Group, Central Branch, Islamic Azad University, Tehran, Iran

A. M. Merdasi
Cell and Molecular Biology Group, Shiraz University, Shiraz, Iran

S. Orouei
Department of Biology, Science and Research Branch, Islamic Azad University, Tehran, Iran

B. Jamali
Department of Microbiology and Genetics, Kherad Institute of Higher Education, Bushehr, Iran

R. Raesi
Department of Nursing, Torbat Jam Faculty of Medical Sciences, Torbat Jam, Iran

Department of Health Services Management, Mashhad University of Medical Sciences, Mashhad, Iran

N. Farahani (✉)
Farhikhtegan Medical Convergence Sciences Research Center, Farhikhtegan Hospital Tehran Medical Sciences, Islamic Azad University, Tehran, Iran

solutions for localized prostate cancer, ADT remains the treatment of choice for metastatic cancer [4, 5]. It has also been demonstrated that AR is involved in AR-dependent and AR-independent prostate cancers in modulating differential gene transcription programming [6]. Metastatic CRPC or primary CRPC can develop as a result of ADT resistance [7]. Nevertheless, newer recommendations suggest enhancing patient survival rates by combining ADT with additional chemotherapeutic medications, such as docetaxel [8, 9]. In addition, multiple studies have demonstrated the ways in which pathways that are androgen-dependent or -independent contribute to the development of prostate tumors [3, 10–12]. Resistance to pharmacological treatments and the development of evasive mechanisms by tumor cells have diminished the impact of these accomplishment breakthroughs in the treatment of prostate cancer. Therefore, this condition continues to be a significant obstacle in healthcare today.

Moreover, metastatic illness is the leading cause of mortality from prostate cancer [7]. Patients reach the last stage of prostate cancer when the tumor has spread. Treatment choices and prognosis are poor at this point in the disease's progression. The overall survival rate for patients with metastatic prostate cancer was anticipated to be fewer than 5 years in 98% of cases [13]. Osteoblastic lesions strewn with osteolytic regions are a common imaging pattern of prostate tumor cells metastasizing to bone [14]. The lymph nodes, liver, lungs, and brain are among the other organs that can be affected by metastasis [15–17]. Metastatic prostate cancer is often classified into two primary groups: ADT-naïve and ADT-resistant prostate cancer [8]. Small cell prostate cancer and neuroendocrine (NE) prostate cancer are two additional recognized phenotypes of prostate cancer. NE and NE are both AR negative and manifest as aggressive disease forms. In addition to AR, other genes such as TP53, PTEN, RB1, ETS, and SPOP may be involved in certain tumor types' aberrant gene alterations and expression [8, 18]. Bone cells, tumor cells, endothelial cells, immune cells, cytokines, chemokines, and a plethora of growth factors are all intricately interdependent in the formation and upkeep of the bone metastatic microenvironment, as detailed by Taichman and colleagues [19]. When tumor cells migrate to a new location, only a small fraction of them are able to re-establish clones and develop into macrometastases. The remaining cells either die off in the bloodstream, do not start growing after extravasation, or can not continue to grow into micrometastases [20].

An enormous variety of research in recent years has linked the progression of prostate cancer to the involvement of cancer stem cells (CSCs) and the epithelial-to-mesenchymal transition (EMT) [21]. Future therapeutic options for metastatic prostate cancer might benefit from a better understanding of the molecular pathways underlying EMT and CSCs. Our present knowledge of EMT and CSCs in CRPC will be summarized in this study, along with any potential links between these two concepts and the particular signaling pathways that play a role in their development.

5.2 The Definition of Metastasis

The last and worst stage of cancer is metastasis, which is the spread of cancer cells to other parts of the body. Most cancer patients do not succumb to primary tumors but rather metastatic illness [22]. Metastasis is a complex biological process that begins with a primary tumor's cells gaining the ability to invade deeper tissues through the mucosa. From there, they can spread through the blood, lymphatics, or direct infiltration of nearby structures. Additionally, they can seed distant organs and eventually resume proliferation at distant sites in order to colonize them [23, 24]. In order to fuel their growth and elude the immune system, tumor cells are able to take on several phenotypic cell states and enlist the help of the stromal and immune cells in their tumor environment [25]. Moreover, metastatic cancer is a systemic disease that impacts multiple organs. It can alter metabolism through altered secretomes or directly colonize organs, compromising their function. Ultimately, it can lead to death, unlike primary tumors, which are typically curable with local therapies like radiation and surgery [23, 26]. A patient's response to systemic treatment for primary vs. metastatic illness can differ significantly. Due to acquired resistance of metastatic cancers to present therapy, most cases of clinically apparent metastasis cannot be cured. Figure 5.1 shows the metastasis cascade.

The three stages of metastasis, which can coexist, are dissemination, dormancy, and colonization. Throughout the metastatic cascade, cancer cells follow a series of actions to penetrate tissues, survive transit, and colonize organs [23, 27]. Tumor cells with oncogenic driver mutations spread across the body when they penetrate deeper layers of tissue via the basement membrane and learn to live without niche-specific growth hormones. After that, it moves into nearby blood arteries or lymphatics, followed by intravasation, and finally, extravasation into faraway organs by transendothelial migration, capillary disruption, migration via neurons, or direct local distribution into nearby regions like the pleural or peritoneal cavities [23, 27, 28]. As shown in mice models and deduced from the low quantity of CTCs in the

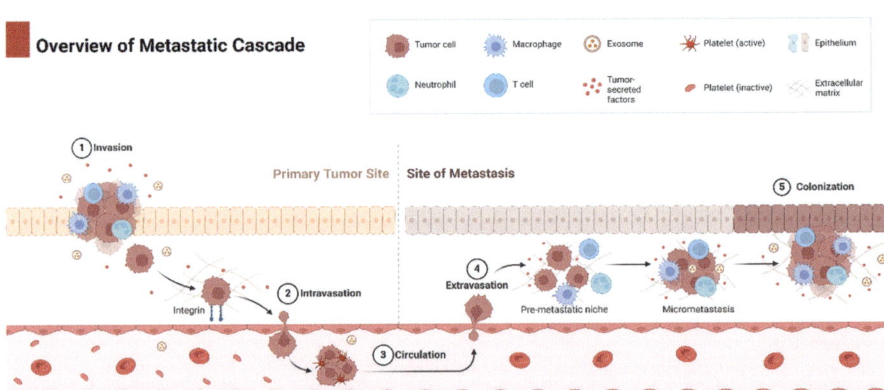

Fig. 5.1 The metastatic cascade (Biorender.com)

blood hours after the original tumor is removed, CTCs in circulation undergo significant attrition as a result of physical, redox, and immunological stress positions [29, 30]. Cancer cells circulate either singly or in microclusters that are rich in stem-like cancer cells and encased in platelets, neutrophils, or stromal cells generated from tumors. This coating enables CTC clusters to evade immune surveillance and gives them a higher metastatic potential than individual cells [29]. Disseminated tumor cells (DTCs) are further destroyed when they reach faraway organs due to factors like high oxidative stress, inadequate growth factors and nutrients, and aggressive immune defenses like infiltrating T cells, natural killer (NK) cells, tissue-specific macrophages, and others [25, 28]. Depending on their circumstances, DTCs that make it through the cell cycle can enter a dormant phase where they either stop replicating altogether or find a balance where immune system clearance or other stromal containment of proliferative clones by the tumor microenvironment (TME) keeps them from spreading too far [23, 31]. Due to the fact that DTCs cannot be detected through clinical imaging and patients are often unaware of subclinical disease, micrometastatic disease encompasses both dissemination and dormancy. After successfully adapting and co-opting their tumor microenvironment (TME), metastasis-initiating cells (MICs) might eventually permit outgrowth and organ colonization through the regenerative, angiogenic, and immune-suppressive programs. This is how clinically evident macrometastases are formed. Metastatic cascades are evolutionary processes that include clonal selection of cancer cell subpopulations that can endure selective microenvironmental stresses and continuous cellular and microenvironmental reprogramming [23]. This causes tumors to grow unchecked, which in turn causes organ failure, a breakdown in the organism's overall function, and eventually death. The concepts of metastasis are encompassed by this transformation continuum, which spans various areas.

In order for cells to complete each stage of the metastatic cascade, they need a wide variety of characteristics. Some of these characteristics start in the main tumor and are caused by mutations in genes that activate oncogenes and disrupt tumor suppressor genes. This allows the tumor to grow and spread uncontrollably, migrate, invade, and self-renew [32]. The great majority of cancer cells that exit the main tumor do not survive to create distant metastasis, even when these oncogenic features are present [23, 27, 33]. This means that metastasis is a huge evolutionary stumbling block. (1) Clones with metastasis-specific characteristics are selected from the genetically heterogeneous population of cancer cells in the main tumor, or (2) cells that exit the tumor undergo non-genetic dynamic adaptation to meet the demands of each stage of metastasis.

On a spectrum of phenotypic states, cancer cells go from residing in the initial lesion to invading the surrounding area, entering the bloodstream, and finally spreading to distant secondary locations [34]. Metastatic lesions form when a cell or cells have the ability to overcome a number of biophysical and molecular impediments that would be insurmountable for their original, non-metastasized selves [26, 35, 36]. Importantly, the fundamental tumor-establishing capacities may depend on cellular actions that are incompatible or inconsistent with several of these capabilities. For instance, whereas cells within the primary tumor mass can be dividing rapidly, numerous studies show that cells that have spread or are experiencing an epithelial-to-mesenchymal transition (EMT) essentially pause cell division [37–39]. Although there is a lack of link between the "grow" and "go" phenotypic states in metastatic cancer cells, these cells have the ability to resume proliferation after being quiescent for extended periods of time after they are halted at a secondary site [40, 41]. A metastatic patient cohort research found that tumors with a proliferative phenotype were more inflammatory, and those with a more EMT-like phenotype had elevated metabolism and stress responses [42]. Experimental and computational models of metastasis, both current and prospective, will need to incorporate the various steps of the process while accounting for this plasticity. Beginning with local invasion and metastasis, the next phases are to move to distant metastatic sites and colonize them, and finally, to evade the immune system, which is frequently shown as a state of dormancy. Figures 5.2 and 5.3 demonstrate EMT mechanism.

When cancer cells were found in the bone marrow of patients with early-stage disease, the idea that these cells had spread from advanced primary tumors to generate metastatic lesions was significantly rethought [43, 44]. Autochthonous animal models of breast cancer that metastasized spontaneously also showed these phenomena, with cells shed from premalignant lesions surviving in distal organs and eventually giving birth to micro-metastases [34]. Likewise, pancreatic cancer models have shown early spread beyond the preneoplastic lesion [45, 46]. It becomes

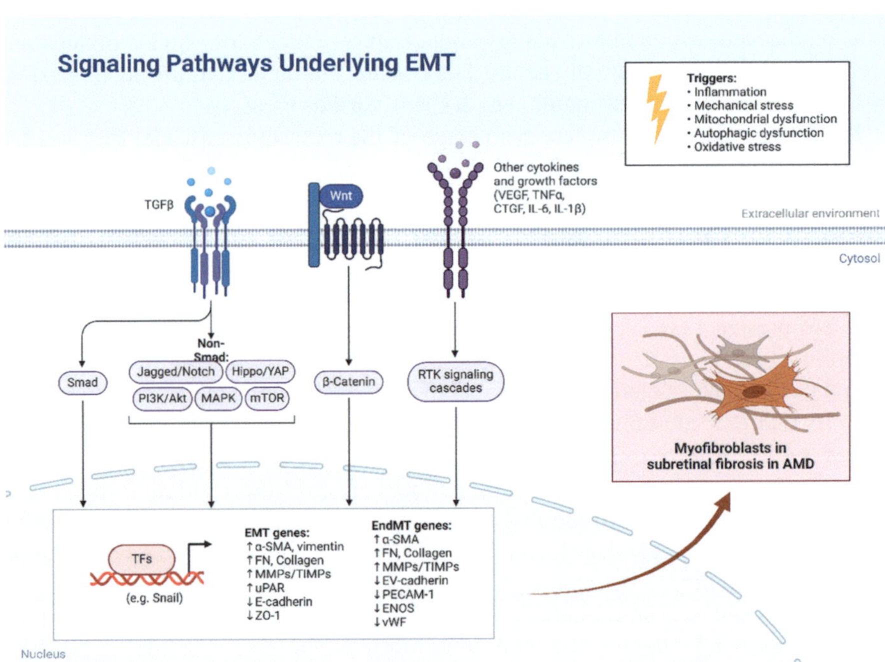

Fig. 5.2 EMT-related pathways (Biorender.com)

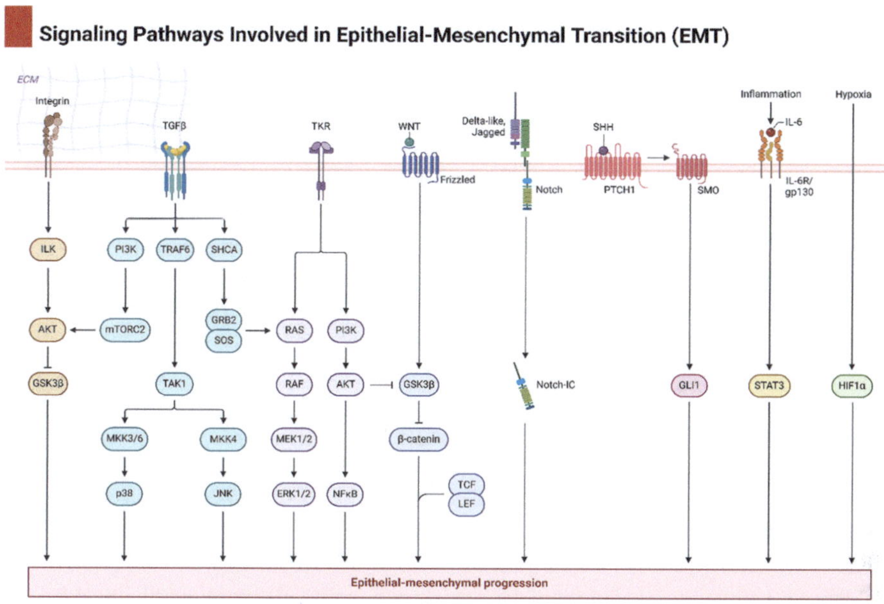

Fig. 5.3 EMT-related pathways (Biorender.com)

more difficult to diagnose, detect, and treat patients when micro-metastases appear in the early stages of disease.

Furthermore, new imaging techniques and meticulously designed in vitro systems have shown that cancer cells can use two or more pathways simultaneously to get away from a main lesion. It has been discovered that there are more types of invasive programs than was previously thought. For instance, there is evidence that either single cells or clusters of cells can spread from the main tumor mass. These programs can be either cell-intrinsic [47] or triggered by the extracellular microenvironment [48, 49]. The morphological adaptation of cancer cells to their microenvironmental physical restrictions includes the deformation of the hard nucleus. This process can result in chromosomal instability, altered gene expression, and metastasis [50]. A possible explanation for the observed increase in genomic heterogeneity at metastatic sites could be invasion-induced chromosomal instability. There has been some recent debate on whether or not epithelial cells can induce metastasis by first adopting an entirely mesenchymal phenotype. Researchers have demonstrated, using organoid cultures of primary breast cancer epithelial cells, that the leading cell maintains a positive stain for the basal epithelial marker cytokeratin 14 (K14) throughout the collective migration of epithelial cells [51]. Similarly, clusters of cancer cells exiting the tumor have been seen to preserve E-cadherin, as caught by intravital imaging [52]. Genetic reduction of transcription factors involved in EMT does not affect the rate of disease metastasis, according to studies in animal models of breast and pancreatic cancer [39]. On the other hand, new research suggests that pancreatic tumor metastasis requires the EMT transcription factor Zeb1 [53], and that epithelial cells and post-EMT mesenchymal-like cells work together to become metastatic through paracrine signaling [54].

Tissue microenvironments are more than just a cell-autonomous event; they play a significant role in metastasis initiation as well. It has long been known that tumor progression is significantly influenced by changes in tissue oxygen tension, the architecture of the surrounding extracellular matrix, immune cells, stromal fibroblasts, endothelial cells, and cancer cells interacting with one another. As the tumor's oxygen tension changes, stabilizing the transcription factor hypoxia-inducible factor (HIF) can cause a shift from collective to amoeboid migration, which in turn promotes the metastatic phenotype by stimulating reciprocal signaling between cancer cells and mesenchymal stem cells [55, 56]. Recent research suggests that tumor-associated macrophages (TAMs) trigger the early dispersion of Her2+ breast cancer cells [57] and that cancer cell-secreted lactate might activate TAMs to increase angiogenesis [58], a prerequisite for distant metastasis. Adding even more intricacy to the process, the microenvironment's effects on cancer cell invasion and migration are typically cell-autonomous as well as tissue context-dependent [59]. Integrating massive amounts of molecular characterization data obtained from in vitro and in vivo experimental models is necessary to understand the intricate interactions that cause metastasis, which involve cancer cells and the tumor microenvironment. For instance, in pancreatic cancer, data-driven modeling of protein phosphorylation helped shed light on the symbiotic molecular interactions between tumor cells and the surrounding stroma, which in turn allowed for a comprehensive elucidation of the function of heterotypic cell-cell interactions in tumor progression [60, 61].

Furthermore, it is a very inefficient method for dispersed tumor cells to colonize faraway tissues. There are surprisingly few clinically identifiable metastases, despite the high number of circulating tumor cells (CTCs) seen in cancer patients' blood (>1000 CTCs/mL of blood plasma) [62]. Once a metastasized cell has been effectively arrested in the vascular bed, it must extravasate and adapt to a new tissue milieu, which might or might not be favorable to its survival. Although kidney, heart, and stomach lesions are uncommon, those in the liver, lungs, bones, and brain are the most common locations for overt metastatic lesions [63]. Metastatic colonization, then, is not just the result of cancer cells growing outside of their original organ; it's the product of a complicated interaction between cancer cells that have spread and the microenvironments of many tissues throughout the body.

Despite the fact that there is a lack of data about the tissue tropism that different cancer subtypes exhibit, researchers are actively working to fill this knowledge gap. Researchers using a parabiosis mouse model found that the omentum is the preferred site of hematogenous metastasis for ovarian cancer, with this preference being controlled by a unique interaction between ligands and receptors in the two compartments [64]. On the other hand, breast cancer cells are able to more easily adhere to the lung parenchyma when the metastasis suppressor RARRES3 is downregulated [65]. One possible element in pre-metastatic niche conditioning is the presence of circulating cytokines and growth factors, along with microRNA-loaded exosomes. Research on animals has shown that exosomes can promote metastasis by increasing blood vessel permeability and preparing the cells already present at the metastatic site to form an environment that is both inflammatory and metabolically active [66–68]. More recent research has also pointed to a possible function for exosomes in tissue tropism through the use of exosome-specific integrin receptors [69]. While we have some idea of how exosomes work in the body, researchers do not yet know how they interact with recipient cells, how long their effects last, or if they target specific cells or organs. Incorporating intercellular communication explicitly into future computational and experimental systems biology models of metastasis will help incorporate dynamic multi-scale features of the metastatic cascade. Metastatic niche creation and the function of the initial tumor in deciding tumor tropism may be better understood with the use of this method.

5.2.1 Two Main Models of Metastasis

The first theory, sometimes known as the "phenotypic plasticity model," postulates that cells that start metastasis must go through extensive molecular changes in order to complete each step of the metastatic cascade [70]. Cancer cells must undergo EMT in order to exit the main tumor location. As a result, they can invade more deeply and move more quickly, taking advantage of oxygen and nutritional gradients supplied by the tumor's vasculature, which is frequently leaky, disorganized, and half-formed. While EMT may not be essential for metastasis to occur, it is crucial for chemoresistance acquisition, according to recent research [39].

To limit "epithelial plasticity" to cancer cells alone involving somatic mutations and (epi)genetic alterations is an oversimplification. The stroma, which consists of many cell types and extracellular matrix (ECM) components, plays a crucial role in the primary tumor's maintenance and progression from a restricted to an invasive condition [71]. A variety of stromal cell types, including fibroblasts, inflammatory cells, endothelial cells, and mesenchymal cells, can be "activated" by cancer cells. As a result, these biological components can facilitate the invasion and multiplication of cancer cells [72, 73]. Cancer cells are able to enter the bloodstream as CTCs due to a mix of environmental variables and molecular features on both the tumor and stromal sides [74]. This may be controversial because of the idea that EMT is irreversible [75] and because cancer cells need to undergo MET once they reach a metastatic site in order to resume their proliferative and metastatic activity. This would indicate alterations in the proteome and transcriptome that are not present in the DTCs of other malignancies that tend to originate from the epithelial cells [43, 76, 77]. A high level of epithelial-mesenchymal plasticity would be necessary for cancer cells with the potential to metastasize to move through the various stages of metastasis. It is yet unclear whether EMT-associated transcription factors have positive or negative metastatic effects, as some studies have found this to be the case [78–80].

The second approach, sometimes titled the "genetic" or "clonal" model, postulates that certain subsets of malignant cancer cells have a genetic predisposition to metastasize [81, 82]. Some metastases do not have a distinct phenotype, which was a clinical fact that our model attempted to address. In this paradigm, tumor-initiating cell clones or subpopulations are genetically modified to permanently activate EMT characteristics, making them metastatically suitable. Inherent (or "driver") mutations in these cancer subpopulations may have originated during tumorigenesis (when tumorigenic alterations reach a cell early in its differentiation process, like a tissue stem cell), or acquired (or "passenger") mutations may have resulted from exposure to environmental factors, such as the selective pressure exerted by chemotherapeutic agents. The fact that the CTCs also tend to cluster lends credence to an additional intriguing theory. Similar to how lung cancer cells may transport their own "cancer soil" as passenger soil, cancer cells, in this case, may enhance their capacity to dock and multiply [83].

In addition, initial seeding relies heavily on cell-cell interactions and cell adherence to the extracellular matrix (ECM). The extracellular matrix (ECM) of a developing tumor changes dramatically in terms of its biochemical composition and its physical characteristics, including its elasticity, tension, and stiffness [84]. Integrins bridge the gap between extracellular matrix (ECM) mechanical signals and intracellular signaling pathways, making them essential players in tumor growth [85].

Moreover, metastatic PCas exhibit elevated levels of active β1 integrin, which grants them two advantages: first, the ability to adhere to extracellular matrix molecules such as fibronectin and collagen type I, which improves their capacity to colonize distant organs. Second, they are more resistant to anoikis, a form of programmed cell death caused by inadequate adhesion to the growth substrate, which increases their chances of survival [86, 87].

The idea of "osteomimicry" by prostate cancer cells was proposed by Koeneman and colleagues [88] since cancer cells also express other integrins such as αv and β3, which enhance their adhesion to a wider range of extracellular matrix (ECM) proteins found in other organs. These proteins include osteopontin, thrombospondin, vitronectin, fibronectin, intracellular adhesion molecule (ICAM-1), and vascular adhesion molecule (VCAM-1) [89–91]. With the help of the chemokine- (C-X-C-motif) axis CXCL12/CXCR4, prostate cancer cells are able to homing to the bone and establish long-term dormancy by contacting the bone marrow niche. One of the many substances released by prostate cancer cells is the chemokine CXCL16, which enhances the recruitment of MSCs from the bone marrow. After MSCs undergo differentiation into CAFs, they release copious amounts of CXCL12, which enhance cancer cells' ability to undergo EMT and upregulate their expression of the corresponding receptor CXCR4 [92]. In order to aid in their extravasation and migration, cancer cells also increase the production of matrix metalloproteases [93]. Since this mechanism has been described for various cancers, it has gained interest as a potential therapeutic target for solid tumors [91].

5.3 Metastasis in Prostate Cancer

The presence of metastases has a direct impact on the prognosis and clinical outcome of prostate cancer [70]. Bone metastases are most commonly found in the spine, pelvis, and ribs [94]. A propensity toward the hematopoietic active red bone marrow is suggested by the increased involvement of the axial skeleton and the multifocal nature of this distribution. Clinical evidence supports this idea, showing that secondary (embryological) sources of hematopoiesis can become active and metastasize when axial skeleton metastases are substantial. This mechanism was believed to be supported by anatomical elements in the past, such as the venous Batson's plexus down the spine [95]. About 2.5 L of blood every minute flows through an adult human's bone marrow. Bone marrow is unique among organs in that its arterial supply terminates immediately in big arteries (sinusoids). A unique feature of sinusoids is the endothelium, which enables the endothelial cells to dynamically open their pores. The sinusoids have a sluggish and, in some spots, almost nonexistent blood flow. Not only do these characteristics make it easy for hematopoietic stem cells (HSCs) to enter the bloodstream, but they also make it easier for cancer cells to extravasate and lodge in the bone marrow. It is worth noting that the sinusoids, which are also located in the spleen, do not often serve as sites of metastasis. This raises doubts about the idea that the design of the sinusoids in the bone marrow has a solely orthostatic role in prostate cancer [96].

Up to 10% of patients already have bone metastases diagnosed at initial prostate cancer diagnosis, even though the main tumor is detected early. Further, between 20% and 30% of individuals who have radical prostatectomy (RP) for organ-confined prostate cancer (stage T1–T3) may experience a recurrence and ultimately die from advanced illness; within this group, 70–80% will have bone metastases. Almost certainly, most recurrences are brought on by hidden "micrometastases" or disseminated tumor cells (DTCs) that have previously invaded the target tissue prior to the first tumor's identification and treatment. This provides compelling evidence that a large percentage of PCa cases detected at an early stage have cancer cells within the main tumor that possess stem-like characteristics and can metastasize to other organs (MICs) [97]. Metastatic sites require microenvironments that are conducive to colonization and may include biological and molecular characteristics that aid in the homeostasis and proliferation of cancer cells.

Only a small fraction of DTCs, between 0.001% and 0.02%, are able to metastasize, meaning that tumors do not grow efficiently [20, 98]. A multi-stage process, the metastatic process begins with the initial tumor and culminates in the formation of tumors at distant sites. As an initial step toward dissemination, cells undergo epithelial-to-mesenchymal transition (EMT), a change from a sessile/epithelial to a mesenchymal/invasive phenotype. The development of invasive traits and the spread of cancer cells from the main tumor to nearby and faraway tissues depend on this "dedifferentiation" stage. The DTCs must exit the initial site, remain in circulation, adhere to the vasculature, migrate and colonize, enter dormancy, and then revive at the distant location in order to develop distant metastasis. The receptive microenvironment makes all this possible. Lots of research has gone into trying to figure out how these processes work so that we can pinpoint the optimal time to treat the cancer cells, the microenvironment, or both [99, 100].

In addition, the bone marrow is the primary location for metastases in prostate cancer [101]. In adults, hematopoiesis mostly occurs in bone marrow, where the high proliferative rates needed to maintain hematological homeostasis are temporally linked to the long-term, lifelong persistence of HSCs [102, 103]. Therefore, the bone marrow must have systems to sustain both activities. The bone marrow's unique vascular architecture has the properties that enable this function [104], and it is also a location of strong cellular trafficking [105–107].

There are multiple functional processes involved in prostate cancer metastasis [28, 108, 109]. Metastatic cancer begins at the tumor edge, where cells undergo an epithelial-mesenchymal transition (EMT) that gives them invasive characteristics. From there, the cells enter the bloodstream as either single cells or aggregates of many, activate survival programs, defend themselves from immune cell attacks, and eventually spread to other organs, most often bone, through extravasation and colonization [28]. Bone marrow metastatic niche access and stromal-derived factor 1/C-X-C receptor 4 (SDF1/CXCR4) interactions are prerequisites for prostate cancer cell bone tropism [110]. Bidirectional interactions occur between the disseminated tumor cells and cells in the tumor microenvironment that either build bone (osteoblasts) or break it down (osteoclasts). Mesenchymal cells promote the formation and survival of androgen-independent and chemotherapy-resistant cancer stem cells (CSCs), which populate the metastatic niche. CSCs also help recruit fibroblasts associated with cancer [92]. On top of that the expansion of bone metastases requires angiogenesis. The imbalance between osteoblast-mediated bone production and osteoclast-mediated bone resorption can lead to osteoblastic, osteoclastic, and mixed lesions, which are all considered PC-related metastases [111, 112]. Osteoblastic and osteolytic components coexist in many bone metastases.

The axis formed by members of the tumor necrosis factor (TNF)/tumor necrosis factor receptor (TNFR) superfamily and the receptor activator of nuclear factor-ĘB (RANK)/RANK ligand (RANKL)/osteoprotegerin OPG is an essential part of bone destruction and osteolytic metastasis. There are a number of factors that contribute to the breakdown of bone, including parathyroid hormone, RANKL, interleukin-1 (IL-1), IL-6, and tumor cell-secreted parathyroid hormone [111, 113]. The last effectors of osteolysis, including carboanhydrase II, H^+ ATPase, and cathepsin K, are stimulated by RANK/RANKL interactions, which activate NFğB signaling. The release of osteolysis factors like transforming growth factor β (TGFβ), insulin-like growth factor 1 (IGF1), and Ca^{2+} initiates a vicious cycle that promotes the proliferation of tumor cells and the creation of parathyroid hormone-related protein. Metastases that form as a result of osteoblastic activity can be accelerated by substances including endothelin 1, fibroblast growth factor (FGF), platelet-derived growth factor (PDGF), RANKL, and IGF1 [111, 113]. Latent TGFβ can be activated, inhibitory IGF binding proteins can release IGF1, and proteases such as urokinase can inactivate the osteolytic factor parathyroid hormone-related protein [111]. Paralysis, neurological impairments, chronic pain, spinal cord suppression, bone fractionation, and other skeletal-related events are linked to bone metastases [114].

In one investigation Yuan and colleagues demonstrated that SETD2 Integrates the EZH2 and AMPK Signaling Pathways to Limit Prostate Cancer Metastasis [115]. A negative correlation exists between the levels of H3K36me3 mediated by SETD2 and H3K27me3 catalyzed by EZH2. However, the exact molecular relationship between these two enzymatic processes is still unknown. According to this study, SETD2 inhibits the spread of prostate cancer (PCa) by acting on its substrate, EZH2. Scientific evidence suggests that SETD2 facilitates EZH2 breakdown via methylation. Metastatic characteristics can be acquired by cells when a Polycomb-repressive chromatin state is induced by SETD2 deficiency. On the other hand, mice with mutant EZH2 or SETD2 proteins that are unable to bind to EZH2 are more likely to develop metastatic PCa. In addition, we find that SETD2 expression is boosted by metformin-induced AMPK signaling, which converges at FOXO3.

In another research, Cheng and colleagues illustrated that SGK2 upregulates GPX4, which inhibits ferroptosis and increases the spread of prostate cancer [116]. The results of this study show that SGK2 prevents ferroptosis, a process that aids in the metastasis of prostate cancer. Patients with metastatic prostate cancer who had higher SGK2 expression had poorer clinical outcomes, as reported by the study's authors. In vivo and in vitro studies showed that SGK2 overexpression sped up prostate cancer metastasis by phosphorylating the Thr-24 and Ser-319 sites of fork-head box O1 (FOXO1), whereas SGK2 knockdown decreased this ability. By following this pathway, FOXO1 was able to displace GPX4 from its nuclear location to the cytoplasm, where it lost its ability to inhibit the enzyme.

Moreover, Guccini and collaborators exhibited that impaired TIMP1 function enhances prostate cancer metastasis via reprogramming aging cells [117]. The function of senescence in prostate cancer is controlled by a molecular switch that is identified in this study as the metalloproteinase inhibitor TIMP1. In mice, the growth of prostate cancer is limited by senescence induced by either chemotherapy or a PTEN deficit. Eliminating senescent cells using a senolytic BCL-2 inhibitor hinders metastasis, and TIMP1 deletion enables senescence to enhance metastasis. Senescent tumor cells undergo a mechanistic transformation when TIMP1 depletion activates matrix metalloproteinases (MMPs), reprogramming them to exhibit the senescence-associated secretory phenotype (SASP). Patients treated in an adjuvant setting for prostate cancer are more likely to experience the poorest clinical outcomes and docetaxel resistance when PTEN and TIMP1 are lost.

Furthermore, Luo and co-workers revealed that interactions between exosomal PGAM1 and ACTG1 enhance angiogenesis and metastasis in prostate cancer [118]. Researchers in this work used in vitro and in vivo methods to learn how exosomal PGAM1 contributes to angiogenesis in metastatic prostate cancer patients. To identify the mechanism by which exosomal PGAM1 affects prostate cancer, we administered Glutathione-*S*-transferase pulldown, co-immunoprecipitation, western blotting, and gelatin degradation experiments. Metastatic prostate cancer patients' plasma levels of exosomal PGAM1 were significantly higher than non-metastatic prostate cancer patients' levels, according to their findings. Exosomes transported by prostate cancer cells to HUVECs further demonstrated that PGAM1 was an important initiator of prostate cancer cell metastasis by boosting invadopodia formation. Furthermore, podosome production and neovascular sprouting in HUVECs can be enhanced when exosomal PGAM1 binds to γ-actin (ACTG1). Injection of prostate cancer cells into naked mice through the tail vein resulted in an increase in lung metastasis mediated by exosomal PGAM1.

5.4 Epithelial-Mesenchymal Transition (EMT) in Prostate Cancer

To commence, EMT has been found to play a role in a variety of physiological and pathological processes. Transdifferentiation (EMT) is originally a physiological process wherein epithelial cells transform into mesenchymal cells by means of a certain signaling pathway. Through epithelial-mesenchymal transition (EMT), epithelial cells acquire mesenchymal traits like anti-apoptosis, strong motility and invasion capabilities, and extracellular matrix disarray, while losing epithelial phenotypes like cell polarity and cell-cell adhesion. The adenocarcinoma-forming glandular epithelium of the prostate gland and its ductules is the original site of origin for prostate cancers. Recent investigations have shown that malignant tumor cells originating from the epithelium can leave the epithelium, invade the stroma region, and disseminate to distal organs by EMT [119], which castration can provoke.

The processes of EMT and MET (Mesenchymal-epithelial transition), which are reversible, involve several proteins. For EMT research, several biomarkers have been identified, such as E-cadherin, N-cadherin, Vimentin, Snail, Zeb1, Twist, and others [120]. One of these, E-cadherin, is found on the surface of epithelial cells and helps bind normal epithelial cells together through cell-cell adhesion. The presence of EMT and tumor invasion is inversely related to its expression level. In contrast, cytoskeletal markers Vimentin and cell surface markers N-cadherin are linked to EMT beginning and invasive carcinoma progression from well-differentiated adenomas. Furthermore, Twist, Snail, Slug, Zeb1, and Zeb2 can all down-regulate E-cadherin levels, which in turn triggers EMT [121].

Androgen deprivation causes EMT in prostate cancer [119]. Castration reduces levels of epithelial markers (such as E-cadherin) and increases expression of mesenchymal markers (such as N-cadherin, Zeb1, Twist1, and Slug) in normal mouse prostate tissue. Human LuCaP35 xenograft tumors that have been castrated show similar alterations. Furthermore, they demonstrate that EMT happens in ADT-treated human samples. Zeb1, a transcription factor and mesenchymal marker, promotes the progression of the EMT transition through a Zeb1–AR feedback loop [119]. Another group has also provided evidence that Zeb1 is involved in CRPC. Given to Graham and colleagues, insulin-like growth factor-I (IGF-I) is responsible for the overexpression of Zeb1, which is significantly increased in prostate cancer cells [122]. Alternately, Gleason score is significantly correlated with twist expression, and twist is an overexpressed transcription factor in prostate cancer. Twist inhibition raises E-cadherin levels and lowers androgen-independent prostate cancer cells' invasion and migratory capabilities [123, 124]. Another EMT transcription factor, Slug, is androgen-regulated, AR-cooperative, and promotes CRPC formation [125].

The N-cadherin expression in CRPC xenografts and primary and metastatic tumors of CRPC patients is significantly upregulated, according to Reiter and colleagues [126]. Exogenous N-cadherin has the potential to stimulate EMT, invasion, and migration in many prostate cancer cell lines both in laboratory settings and in living organisms. Blocking the path to castration-resistance by reducing the activity of AKT and IL-8 production, specific N-cadherin antibodies could limit EMT, tumor development, invasion, and migration. So, N-cadherin is a major contributor to prostate cancer metastasis and CRPC, according to this group's findings. Additional preclinical and clinical validation of therapeutics targeting this EMT component using monoclonal antibodies is being considered as a potentially fruitful strategy.

Additionally, in the past 10 years, numerous EMT biomarkers have been linked to the progression of prostate cancer. The progression of adenoma to carcinoma is accelerated when cell-cell adhesion is disrupted, as occurs when E-cadherin is lost or converted to N-cadherin [127]. Cadherin-11, an osteoblast cadherin, may improve the invasion and migratory capabilities of prostate cancer cells by associating them with osteoblasts [128]. Factor for zinc-finger transcription Snail has the potential to initiate EMT in prostate cancer and suppress E-cadherin transcription and expression [129]. These chemicals may be EMT markers for CRPC, even though they have only been studied for prostate cancer in general and not for CRPC specifically.

Together, these investigations provide strong evidence that EMT and its biomarkers have a role in prostate cancer treatment resistance [130]. The invasive and metastatic capacity of prostate cancer cells is regulated by E-cadherin, N-cadherin, Zeb1, Twist, Slug, Snail, and other EMT markers. Thus, potential future cancer treatments may include therapeutic approaches that aim to intervene in the EMT process or perhaps reverse EMT phenotypes.

A mesenchymal phenotype can be achieved through the induction of mesenchymal markers, as demonstrated in numerous in vitro and mouse investigations employing experimental EMT treatments of cancer cells [131–133]. The interactions between tumor cells, tumor-associated stromal components, and the tumor microenvironment (TME) can be better understood with the use of in vivo metastasis models [134]. In addition to shedding light on in vitro differentiation induction, organoid culturing techniques have offered great model systems for demonstrating how signals triggering EMT may impact immunological anti-tumor responses and treatment resistance [135].

By studying the effects of mesenchymal plasticity on prostate cancer metastatic potential, Ruscetti and colleagues [136] were able to better understand the in vivo function of EMT. The scientists created a sophisticated in vivo tracking system that they used to study the ability of mesenchymal-like EMT intermediate tumor cells to initiate tumors in comparison to mesenchymal cells that had finished EMT. They demonstrated that primary tumors could be initiated by both intermediate mesenchymal and tumor cells fully expressing EMT mesenchymal. Intravenous injection killed all save the mesenchymal-like intermediate tumor cells that made it into the bloodstream and lung tissue. While the fully expressed EMT tumor cells look like growing progenitor cells without stemness traits, the mesenchymal-like intermediate tumor cells seem like dormant stem cells. The authors note that mesenchymal-like intermediate tumors likely receive growth factors from the surrounding microenvironment at metastatic sites to keep them in their dormant quiescent state since these tumors typically cluster in the proximal region of the prostate gland, where stem cells are located [137].

In another research, Zhao and colleagues demonstrated that Ephrin-A2 enhances angiogenesis and induces EMT, which in turn promotes prostate cancer spread [138]. The study's authors found that prostate cancer cells' ectopic expression of ephrin-A2 enhanced cell motility and invasion in laboratory tests, tumor metastasis, and angiogenesis in living organisms, and that ephrin-A2 silencing entirely counteracted these effects. In contrast to its ineffectiveness in inhibiting tumor cell proliferation in vitro, ephrin-A2 markedly enhanced primary tumor growth in vivo. Additionally, in order to ascertain ephrin-A2's biological role, we evaluated the expression of EMT-related markers in well-established cell lines. Ephrin-A2 overexpression in prostate cancer cells was found to decrease epithelial marker expression (ZO-1, E-cadherin, and claudin-1) and increase mesenchymal marker expression (N-cadherin, β-catenin, vimentin, Slug, and Snail). Conversely, ephrin-A2 knockout had no effect on EMT marker expression.

Research with the PC3 prostate cancer cell line xenograft demonstrated that IL6 expression in prostate cancer stimulates a subset of cancer-associated fibroblasts, leading to EMT, invasiveness, and stemness [139]. Since FNPCs and other advanced prostate cancers tend to have overexpressed levels of this growth factor, FGF signals likely play a significant role in prostate cancer progression [12]. In addition to promoting prostate cancer progression via Sox9 and Wnt signaling, EMT appears to have a role in growth factor receptor (Fgfr1) expression [140]. This provides more evidence that IL6 and FGF may serve as indicators for prognosis.

An immunosuppressive tumor microenvironment (TME) is formed when prostate cancers interact intimately with tumor cells and stromal components around them [141, 142]. Regarding prostate cancer's tumor microenvironment (TME), early research on this subject emphasizes the function of cancer-associated fibroblasts (CAFs). The stemness features and EMT phenotype were enhanced, prostate cancer tumor cell motility and metastatic spread were accelerated, and CAFs were stimulated toward cooperative cellular activities by these TME cells interacting with polarized M2 macrophages [143].

Moreover, a key driver of lineage plasticity, which is characterized by heightened EMT and stemness potentials, was found to be Rb1 loss in research employing a PBCre4:Ptenf/f mouse model of prostate adenocarcinoma caused by Pten deletion. Based on transcriptomic profiling, the epigenetic reprogramming factors Sox2 and Ezh2 are the ones responsible for causing this phenotype in both mice and humans

[144]. Rb1 and Tp53 are tumor suppressor genes that approximately half of NEPCs deactivate. More research has revealed that androgen deprivation therapy resistance is caused by epigenetic modifications and the acquisition of lineage plasticity, which are both accompanied by the loss of Tp53 and Rb1 [144, 145]. Reduction of luminal epithelial cell markers and increase of basal and neuroendocrine markers, as demonstrated by Mu and collaborators demonstrates that a Sox2-mediated cellular plasticity is induced by loss of both Rb1 and Tp53 [145].

In a study, Hu and co-workers established that In prostate cancer, MIIP blocks EMT and cell invasion via the miR-181a/b-5p-KLF17 axis [146]. By preventing cell invasion and the epithelial-mesenchymal transition (EMT), the researchers in this work proved that MIIP suppresses prostate cancer. A decrease in EMT-inducing factors and an increase in E-cadherin and KLF17 were seen in vitro in response to overexpressing MIIP, which also inhibited cellular invasion of PC3 and DU145. When xenografted subcutaneously or injected into the tibia, a persistent MIIP knockdown in prostate cancer cells enhanced tumor development or bone osteolytic lesions. In terms of the molecular mechanism, MIIP inhibits the expression of two onco-miRNAs, miR-181a-5p, and miR-181b-5p, which eliminates the inhibitory effect of these miRNAs on their target, KLF17. KLF17 is a negative regulator of EMT because it directly suppresses the transcription of SNAIL1/2 and TWIST. Lastly, researchers showed that downregulation of MIIP was associated with downregulation of KLF17 and E-cadherin, but upregulation of miR-181a/b-5p, by comparing the expression of these genes in paired cancer samples vs. adjacent normal tissues from a cohort of human prostate cancer patients. Microarray immunohistochemistry analysis of prostate cancer tissues further validated the favorable association between MIIP and KLF17.

On top of that drug resistance in cancers, including CRPC, is mostly caused by EMT and CSCs, according to many research. Certain recent research has linked EMT features to CSC markers, which may explain why certain tumors recur and others develop therapeutic resistance.

Experimental evidence linking EMT to CSC development in breast cancer was recently found by Mani and co-workers [147]. Similar to how the expression of well-known E-cadherin transcription repressors, like Twist and Snail, induces EMT, they have shown that differentiated mammary epithelial cells undergo EMT after being treated with TGF-β, which is a possible inducer of EMT. These cells then develop into CD44high CD24low stem-like cells. Zeb1, a critical regulator of epigenetic modifications (EMT), is necessary for the upkeep of breast cancer stem cell properties and, critically, a new refined work by the Weinberg group shows that it is enough to transform cells from non-cancer stem cell to cancer stem cell status [148]. The case of pancreatic cancer is not dissimilar. The EMT signature ZEB1 inhibits the pluripotency genes (Bmi-1, Sox2, and Klf4) by repressing miR-200c, miR-203, and miR-128 [149]. Research has shown that EMT and CSCs are stem cells in breast and pancreatic cancers, and it is now being considered that these two processes may have a role in the development of prostate cancer and other malignancies. As anticipated, Kong and collaborators [150] also found that PC3 prostate cancer cells that are made to express PDGF-D exhibit EMT traits and cancer stem-like cell features following the activation of the polycomb repressor complex and over-expression of pluripotency genes like Nanog, Oct4, Sox2, Lin28, and others. This is linked to an increase in the cells' ability to form clones and prostaspheres in vitro and tumorigenicity in vivo. Importantly, miR-200b and miR-200c connect EMT phenotypes to CSCs markers throughout the process. Reversed EMT and decreased self-renewal ability are caused by over-expression of miR-200 family, which regulates the expression of Notch1 and/or Lin28B [150]. The link between EMT induction and the development of a prostate CSC-like phenotype after androgen deprivation has also been demonstrated by Sun and colleagues [119]. After castration, the gene expression profiles of the prostate tissues in normal and castrated mice show a reversal of E-cadherin expression and an upregulation of mesenchymal markers such N-cadherin, Zeb1, Twist, and slug. Several mesenchymal markers, such as Vimentin, Zeb1, Zeb2, Twist1, Snail1, and Slug, are shown to be greatly elevated in the Lin−CD44+CD133+Sca-1+CD117+ cells, according to microarray gene analysis. Mouse prostate non-stem cells, as contrasted with those Lin−CD44−CD133−Sca-1−CD117 [119].

In another investigation, Fang and colleagues illustrated that the Wnt/β-Catenin pathway is negatively regulated by β-ionone, which in turn inhibits the Epithelial-Mesenchymal Transition (EMT) in prostate cancer cells [151]. Human PC-3 prostate cancer cells (PC3) and Human 22RV1 prostate adenocarcinoma cells (22RV1) showed considerable inhibition of migration, invasion, and EMT after being treated with β-ionone. Also, naked mice that were given xenografts to grow under the skin showed no signs of tumor growth or EMT when given β-ionone. After being treated with β-ionone, the study also discovered that the EMT-promoting protein β-catenin was downregulated. Upstream migration, invasion, and EMT processes were impeded by β-ionone because it sped up the ubiquitination and degradation of β-catenin in PCa, according to additional mechanistic investigations.

A member of the immunoglobulin superfamily, Contactin1 (Cntn-1) is a glycoprotein found on neuronal membranes that aids in cell attachment. Several different forms of carcinoma have demonstrated that the protein uses EMT-dependent promotion to increase cell invasion, migration, and metastasis [152]. In prostate cancer cell lines and xenografts, downregulation of Cntn-1 led to reduced PI3K/Akt signaling activity and docetaxel resistance [153]. Given the substantial correlation between Pten loss and PI3K/AKT dysregulation with advanced prostate cancer and CRPC, our preclinical study highlights the possibility of a joint function between EMT and common driver mutations for prostate cancer.

Recent research reveals that restoring Pten in breast cancer models suppresses EMT and stemness CSCs activity via Abi1 (Abelson interactor 1) downregulation [154]. Previous studies have also demonstrated that Pten depletion promotes EMT. Actin cytoskeletal reorganization and intercellular adhesion have both been linked to the adaptor protein Abi1. Through its regulation of the EMT-WNT pathway, Abi1 recently regulated prostate cancer development and epithelial plasticity [154]. Activation of the FYN-STAT3 axis and the non-canonical WNT receptor Fzd2 were both identified as pathways by which Abi1 regulates EMT [154]. Another recognized EMT driver, TGF-β1, was found to increase progression through migration, invasion, and tumor initiation by means of an isoform that is produced through alternative splicing of CD44 [155]. Furthermore, NOTCH signaling activates the estrogen receptor, which makes it a key role in stem-like basal cells, and this pathway is involved in EMT and metastasis [156].

Moreover, Zhang and co-workers indicated that the NF-κB pathway is used by prostate cancer cells to halt EMT and proliferation when Notch-4 is silenced [157]. Notch-4 expression was shown to be significantly higher in the prostate cancer cell lines DU145, PC3, and LnCAP as compared to the non-malignant prostate epithelial cell line RWPE1, according to the current study. Reducing Notch-4 expression in DU145 and PC3 prostate cancer cell lines reduced their vitality and proliferation. A decrease in Notch-4 considerably enhanced apoptosis in PC3 cells, according to another research. Reductions in cell motility and invasion as well as changes to EMT marker expression were seen with Notch-4 silencing. Researchers tested the hypothesis that Notch-4 ablation reduces NF-κB activity by activating NF-κB p50 and p65 in PC3 cells with PMA. The findings show that PMA administration hindered the effects of Notch-4 ablation on PC3 cell biology, such as cell proliferation, cell death, migration, invasion, and EMT. The current study's findings demonstrate that prostate cancer progression can be inhibited by RNAi targeting Notch-4 expression.

When describing the tumor microenvironment (TME) and immune landscape, the genetic background plays a significant role. The immunological makeup of the tumor microenvironment (TME) in generated tumors varied significantly between genetically engineered mice models (GEMMs) bearing homozygous Pten deletion, according to research by Bezzi and co-workers. Correlating to the attraction of myeloid cells through distinct pathways, loss of the Zbtb7a gene in conjunction with Pten loss increased Cxcl5 expression, while loss of Tp53 in conjunction with Pten loss increased Clcl17 expression [158]. In addition, basal cells, secretory luminal cells, and uncommon neuroendocrine cells are encased in the gland by stroma and vasculature, according to classical investigations of the normal prostatic epithelium in mice [159]. Evidence of stem/progenitor cells in basal and luminal prostate epithelial lineages has been provided by a number of in vitro organoid-forming experiments [160] and stem cell enrichment tests [161–164].

5.5 Conclusion and Perspectives

Recent research on EMT has shown how crucial it is to decipher the relationships between stemness, cell plasticity, and therapeutic efficacy. Moreover, interactions with the tumor microenvironment (TME), migration, metastasis, and tumor invasiveness are all intricately tied to these processes. Several potential drivers and effectors of EMT have the potential to serve as biomarkers for prognosis in cases of metastatic illness. Much research into EMT's function in cancer development and treatment resistance has taken place within the previous decade. Additional research is required to determine the best targets for improving the therapy of CRPC in prostate cancer. Although Notch and Wnt signaling have a more significant role in cancer stemness phenotypes and EMT in prostate cancer, SNAIL appears to be an important driver of EMT in prostate cancer. For certain cancers, blocking both of these mechanisms might work. At the same time, it may be possible to anticipate EMT progression and treatment response by developing transcriptional markers of the disease in humans. Additionally, epigenetic modifications show potential; nonetheless, there is a risk that worldwide changes in methylation and histone modification can cause unanticipated changes in gene expression, which could result in undesirable side effects. Previous research on other malignancies has shown that targeting particular epigenetic effectors, including LSD1, that are known to be involved in EMT, may also have significant benefits for prostate cancer. Additionally, fresh perspectives for innovative treatment methods may emerge from a deeper comprehension of how EMT and stemness influence the immunological tumor microenvironment of prostate cancer.

Conflict of Interest The authors declare no conflict of interest.

References

1. Adekoya TO, Richardson RM. Cytokines and chemokines as mediators of prostate cancer metastasis. Int J Mol Sci. 2020;21(12):4449.
2. Shen MM, Abate-Shen C. Molecular genetics of prostate cancer: new prospects for old challenges. Genes Dev. 2010;24(18):1967–2000.
3. Feldman BJ, Feldman D. The development of androgen-independent prostate cancer. Nat Rev Cancer. 2001;1(1):34–45.
4. Litwin MS, Tan HJ. The diagnosis and treatment of prostate cancer: a review. JAMA. 2017;317(24):2532–42.
5. Karantanos T, Corn PG, Thompson TC. Prostate cancer progression after androgen deprivation therapy: mechanisms of castrate resistance and novel therapeutic approaches. Oncogene. 2013;32(49):5501–11.
6. Wang Q, et al. Androgen receptor regulates a distinct transcription program in androgen-independent prostate cancer. Cell. 2009;138(2):245–56.
7. Wang G, et al. Genetics and biology of prostate cancer. Genes Dev. 2018;32(17–18):1105–40.
8. Sartor O, de Bono JS. Metastatic prostate cancer. N Engl J Med. 2018;378(7):645–57.
9. Teo MY, Rathkopf DE, Kantoff P. Treatment of advanced prostate cancer. Annu Rev Med. 2019;70:479–99.
10. Adekoya TO, et al. Activator of G protein signaling 3 modulates prostate tumor development and progression. Carcinogenesis. 2019;40(12):1504–13.
11. Ghosh PM, et al. Signal transduction pathways in androgen-dependent and -independent prostate cancer cell proliferation. Endocr Relat Cancer. 2005;12(1):119–34.
12. Bluemn EG, et al. Androgen receptor pathway-independent prostate cancer is sustained through FGF signaling. Cancer Cell. 2017;32(4):474–489.e6.
13. Tangen CM, et al. Ten-year survival in patients with metastatic prostate cancer. Clin Prostate Cancer. 2003;2(1):41–5.
14. Logothetis CJ, Lin SH. Osteoblasts in prostate cancer metastasis to bone. Nat Rev Cancer. 2005;5(1):21–8.

15. Jin JK, Dayyani F, Gallick GE. Steps in prostate cancer progression that lead to bone metastasis. Int J Cancer. 2011;128(11):2545–61.
16. Datta K, et al. Mechanism of lymph node metastasis in prostate cancer. Future Oncol. 2010;6(5):823–36.
17. Vinjamoori AH, et al. Atypical metastases from prostate cancer: 10-year experience at a single institution. AJR Am J Roentgenol. 2012;199(2):367–72.
18. Testa U, Castelli G, Pelosi E. Cellular and molecular mechanisms underlying prostate cancer development: therapeutic implications. Medicines (Basel). 2019;6(3):82.
19. Taichman RS, et al. The evolving biology and treatment of prostate cancer. J Clin Invest. 2007;117(9):2351–61.
20. Berish RB, et al. Translational models of prostate cancer bone metastasis. Nat Rev Urol. 2018;15(7):403–21.
21. Luzzi KJ, et al. Multistep nature of metastatic inefficiency: dormancy of solitary cells after successful extravasation and limited survival of early micrometastases. Am J Pathol. 1998;153(3):865–73.
22. Li P, Yang R, Gao W-Q. Contributions of epithelial-mesenchymal transition and cancer stem cells to the development of castration resistance of prostate cancer. Mol Cancer. 2014;13(1):55.
23. Gerstberger S, Jiang Q, Ganesh K. Metastasis. Cell. 2023;186(8):1564–79.
24. Massagué J, Ganesh K. Metastasis-initiating cells and ecosystems. Cancer Discov. 2021;11(4):971–94.
25. Talmadge JE, Fidler IJ. AACR centennial series: the biology of cancer metastasis: historical perspective. Cancer Res. 2010;70(14):5649–69.
26. Quail DF, Joyce JA. Microenvironmental regulation of tumor progression and metastasis. Nat Med. 2013;19(11):1423–37.
27. Alečković M, McAllister SS, Polyak K. Metastasis as a systemic disease: molecular insights and clinical implications. Biochim Biophys Acta Rev Cancer. 2019;1872(1):89–102.
28. Lambert AW, Pattabiraman DR, Weinberg RA. Emerging biological principles of metastasis. Cell. 2017;168(4):670–91.
29. Obenauf AC, Massagué J. Surviving at a distance: organ-specific metastasis. Trends Cancer. 2015;1(1):76–91.
30. Ring A, et al. Biology, vulnerabilities and clinical applications of circulating tumour cells. Nat Rev Cancer. 2023;23(2):95–111.
31. Ganesh K, Massagué J. Targeting metastatic cancer. Nat Med. 2021;27(1):34–44.
32. Risson E, et al. The current paradigm and challenges ahead for the dormancy of disseminated tumor cells. Nat Cancer. 2020;1(7):672–80.
33. Hanahan D, Weinberg RA. Hallmarks of cancer: the next generation. Cell. 2011;144(5):646–74.
34. Fidler IJ. Metastasis: quantitative analysis of distribution and fate of tumor emboli labeled with 125 I-5-iodo-2′-deoxyuridine. J Natl Cancer Inst. 1970;45(4):773–82.
35. Suhail Y, et al. Systems biology of cancer metastasis. Cell Syst. 2019;9(2):109–27.
36. Wang C, et al. Longitudinally collected CTCs and CTC-clusters and clinical outcomes of metastatic breast cancer. Breast Cancer Res Treat. 2017;161(1):83–94.
37. Aceto N, et al. Circulating tumor cell clusters are oligoclonal precursors of breast cancer metastasis. Cell. 2014;158(5):1110–22.
38. Rojas-Puentes L, et al. Epithelial-mesenchymal transition, proliferation, and angiogenesis in locally advanced cervical cancer treated with chemoradiotherapy. Cancer Med. 2016;5(8):1989–99.
39. Vega S, et al. Snail blocks the cell cycle and confers resistance to cell death. Genes Dev. 2004;18(10):1131–43.
40. Zheng X, et al. Epithelial-to-mesenchymal transition is dispensable for metastasis but induces chemoresistance in pancreatic cancer. Nature. 2015;527(7579):525–30.
41. Giese A, et al. Dichotomy of astrocytoma migration and proliferation. Int J Cancer. 1996;67(2):275–82.

42. Hatzikirou H, et al. 'Go or grow': the key to the emergence of invasion in tumour progression? Math Med Biol. 2012;29(1):49–65.
43. Robinson DR, et al. Integrative clinical genomics of metastatic cancer. Nature. 2017;548(7667):297–303.
44. Schardt JA, et al. Genomic analysis of single cytokeratin-positive cells from bone marrow reveals early mutational events in breast cancer. Cancer Cell. 2005;8(3):227–39.
45. Klein CA, et al. Comparative genomic hybridization, loss of heterozygosity, and DNA sequence analysis of single cells. Proc Natl Acad Sci U S A. 1999;96(8):4494–9.
46. Muzumdar MD, et al. Clonal dynamics following p53 loss of heterozygosity in Kras-driven cancers. Nat Commun. 2016;7:12685.
47. Rhim AD, et al. EMT and dissemination precede pancreatic tumor formation. Cell. 2012;148(1–2):349–61.
48. Alexander S, et al. Dynamic imaging of cancer growth and invasion: a modified skin-fold chamber model. Histochem Cell Biol. 2008;130(6):1147–54.
49. Hofschröer V, et al. Extracellular protonation modulates cell-cell interaction mechanics and tissue invasion in human melanoma cells. Sci Rep. 2017;7:42369.
50. Wolf K, et al. Multi-step pericellular proteolysis controls the transition from individual to collective cancer cell invasion. Nat Cell Biol. 2007;9(8):893–904.
51. Bakhoum SF, et al. Chromosomal instability drives metastasis through a cytosolic DNA response. Nature. 2018;553(7689):467–72.
52. Cheung KJ, et al. Collective invasion in breast cancer requires a conserved basal epithelial program. Cell. 2013;155(7):1639–51.
53. Friedl P, Gilmour D. Collective cell migration in morphogenesis, regeneration and cancer. Nat Rev Mol Cell Biol. 2009;10(7):445–57.
54. Krebs AM, et al. The EMT-activator Zeb1 is a key factor for cell plasticity and promotes metastasis in pancreatic cancer. Nat Cell Biol. 2017;19(5):518–29.
55. Neelakantan D, et al. EMT cells increase breast cancer metastasis via paracrine GLI activation in neighbouring tumour cells. Nat Commun. 2017;8:15773.
56. Lehmann S, et al. Hypoxia induces a HIF-1-dependent transition from collective-to-amoeboid dissemination in epithelial cancer cells. Curr Biol. 2017;27(3):392–400.
57. Chaturvedi P, et al. Hypoxia-inducible factor-dependent breast cancer-mesenchymal stem cell bidirectional signaling promotes metastasis. J Clin Invest. 2013;123(1):189–205.
58. Linde N, et al. Macrophages orchestrate breast cancer early dissemination and metastasis. Nat Commun. 2018;9(1):21.
59. Colegio OR, et al. Functional polarization of tumour-associated macrophages by tumour-derived lactic acid. Nature. 2014;513(7519):559–63.
60. Spill F, et al. Impact of the physical microenvironment on tumor progression and metastasis. Curr Opin Biotechnol. 2016;40:41–8.
61. Tape CJ. Systems biology analysis of heterocellular signaling. Trends Biotechnol. 2016;34(8):627–37.
62. Tape CJ, et al. Oncogenic KRAS regulates tumor cell signaling via stromal reciprocation. Cell. 2016;165(4):910–20.
63. Nagrath S, et al. Isolation of rare circulating tumour cells in cancer patients by microchip technology. Nature. 2007;450(7173):1235–9.
64. Fidler IJ. The pathogenesis of cancer metastasis: the 'seed and soil' hypothesis revisited. Nat Rev Cancer. 2003;3(6):453–8.
65. Pradeep S, et al. Hematogenous metastasis of ovarian cancer: rethinking mode of spread. Cancer Cell. 2014;26(1):77–91.
66. Morales M, et al. RARRES3 suppresses breast cancer lung metastasis by regulating adhesion and differentiation. EMBO Mol Med. 2014;6(7):865–81.
67. Becker A, et al. Extracellular vesicles in cancer: cell-to-cell mediators of metastasis. Cancer Cell. 2016;30(6):836–48.

68. Costa-Silva B, et al. Pancreatic cancer exosomes initiate pre-metastatic niche formation in the liver. Nat Cell Biol. 2015;17(6):816–26.
69. Schillaci O, et al. Exosomes from metastatic cancer cells transfer amoeboid phenotype to non-metastatic cells and increase endothelial permeability: their emerging role in tumor heterogeneity. Sci Rep. 2017;7(1):4711.
70. Hoshino A, et al. Tumour exosome integrins determine organotropic metastasis. Nature. 2015;527(7578):329–35.
71. Manna F, et al. Metastases in prostate cancer. Cold Spring Harb Perspect Med. 2019;9(3):a033688.
72. van der Pluijm G. Epithelial plasticity, cancer stem cells and bone metastasis formation. Bone. 2011;48(1):37–43.
73. Mueller MM, Fusenig NE. Friends or foes—bipolar effects of the tumour stroma in cancer. Nat Rev Cancer. 2004;4(11):839–49.
74. Bhowmick NA, Moses HL. Tumor-stroma interactions. Curr Opin Genet Dev. 2005;15(1):97–101.
75. Carmeliet P, Jain RK. Principles and mechanisms of vessel normalization for cancer and other angiogenic diseases. Nat Rev Drug Discov. 2011;10(6):417–27.
76. Thiery JP. Epithelial-mesenchymal transitions in tumour progression. Nat Rev Cancer. 2002;2(6):442–54.
77. Braun S, et al. Cytokeratin-positive cells in the bone marrow and survival of patients with stage I, II, or III breast cancer. N Engl J Med. 2000;342(8):525–33.
78. Dasgupta A, Lim AR, Ghajar CM. Circulating and disseminated tumor cells: harbingers or initiators of metastasis? Mol Oncol. 2017;11(1):40–61.
79. Yang J, Weinberg RA. Epithelial-mesenchymal transition: at the crossroads of development and tumor metastasis. Dev Cell. 2008;14(6):818–29.
80. Ocaña OH, et al. Metastatic colonization requires the repression of the epithelial-mesenchymal transition inducer Prrx1. Cancer Cell. 2012;22(6):709–24.
81. Vanharanta S, Massagué J. Origins of metastatic traits. Cancer Cell. 2013;24(4):410–21.
82. Nowell PC. The clonal evolution of tumor cell populations. Science. 1976;194(4260):23–8.
83. Ruiz C, et al. Advancing a clinically relevant perspective of the clonal nature of cancer. Proc Natl Acad Sci U S A. 2011;108(29):12054–9.
84. Duda DG, et al. Malignant cells facilitate lung metastasis by bringing their own soil. Proc Natl Acad Sci U S A. 2010;107(50):21677–82.
85. Miles FL, Sikes RA. Insidious changes in stromal matrix fuel cancer progression. Mol Cancer Res. 2014;12(3):297–312.
86. Friedland JC, Lee MH, Boettiger D. Mechanically activated integrin switch controls alpha5beta1 function. Science. 2009;323(5914):642–4.
87. Lee YC, et al. Targeting constitutively activated β1 integrins inhibits prostate cancer metastasis. Mol Cancer Res. 2013;11(4):405–17.
88. Jin JK, et al. Talin1 phosphorylation activates β1 integrins: a novel mechanism to promote prostate cancer bone metastasis. Oncogene. 2015;34(14):1811–21.
89. Koeneman KS, Yeung F, Chung LW. Osteomimetic properties of prostate cancer cells: a hypothesis supporting the predilection of prostate cancer metastasis and growth in the bone environment. Prostate. 1999;39(4):246–61.
90. Thalmann GN, et al. Osteopontin: possible role in prostate cancer progression. Clin Cancer Res. 1999;5(8):2271–7.
91. Zhao Y, et al. Tumor alphavbeta3 integrin is a therapeutic target for breast cancer bone metastases. Cancer Res. 2007;67(12):5821–30.
92. Schneider JG, Amend SR, Weilbaecher KN. Integrins and bone metastasis: integrating tumor cell and stromal cell interactions. Bone. 2011;48(1):54–65.
93. Jung Y, et al. Recruitment of mesenchymal stem cells into prostate tumours promotes metastasis. Nat Commun. 2013;4:1795.

94. Sun YX, et al. Skeletal localization and neutralization of the SDF-1(CXCL12)/CXCR4 axis blocks prostate cancer metastasis and growth in osseous sites in vivo. J Bone Miner Res. 2005;20(2):318–29.
95. Kakhki VR, et al. Pattern and distribution of bone metastases in common malignant tumors. Nucl Med Rev Cent East Eur. 2013;16(2):66–9.
96. Batson OV. The function of the vertebral veins and their role in the spread of metastases. Ann Surg. 1940;112(1):138–49.
97. Hensel J, Thalmann GN. Biology of bone metastases in prostate cancer. Urology. 2016;92:6–13.
98. Valastyan S, Weinberg RA. Tumor metastasis: molecular insights and evolving paradigms. Cell. 2011;147(2):275–92.
99. Schneider A, et al. Bone turnover mediates preferential localization of prostate cancer in the skeleton. Endocrinology. 2005;146(4):1727–36.
100. Sterling JA, et al. Advances in the biology of bone metastasis: how the skeleton affects tumor behavior. Bone. 2011;48(1):6–15.
101. Weilbaecher KN, Guise TA, McCauley LK. Cancer to bone: a fatal attraction. Nat Rev Cancer. 2011;11(6):411–25.
102. Bubendorf L, et al. Metastatic patterns of prostate cancer: an autopsy study of 1,589 patients. Hum Pathol. 2000;31(5):578–83.
103. Mendelson A, Frenette PS. Hematopoietic stem cell niche maintenance during homeostasis and regeneration. Nat Med. 2014;20(8):833–46.
104. Calvi LM, Link DC. The hematopoietic stem cell niche in homeostasis and disease. Blood. 2015;126(22):2443–51.
105. Nombela-Arrieta C, et al. Quantitative imaging of haematopoietic stem and progenitor cell localization and hypoxic status in the bone marrow microenvironment. Nat Cell Biol. 2013;15(5):533–43.
106. Méndez-Ferrer S, et al. Haematopoietic stem cell release is regulated by circadian oscillations. Nature. 2008;452(7186):442–7.
107. Mazo IB, Massberg S, von Andrian UH. Hematopoietic stem and progenitor cell trafficking. Trends Immunol. 2011;32(10):493–503.
108. Casanova-Acebes M, et al. Rhythmic modulation of the hematopoietic niche through neutrophil clearance. Cell. 2013;153(5):1025–35.
109. Weidle UH, et al. The functional role of prostate cancer metastasis-related micro-RNAs. Cancer Genomics Proteomics. 2019;16(1):1–19.
110. Manca P, et al. Determinants of bone specific metastasis in prostate cancer. Crit Rev Oncol Hematol. 2017;112:59–66.
111. Conley-LaComb MK, et al. Pharmacological targeting of CXCL12/CXCR4 signaling in prostate cancer bone metastasis. Mol Cancer. 2016;15(1):68.
112. Mundy GR. Metastasis to bone: causes, consequences and therapeutic opportunities. Nat Rev Cancer. 2002;2(8):584–93.
113. Loberg RD, et al. Pathogenesis and treatment of prostate cancer bone metastases: targeting the lethal phenotype. J Clin Oncol. 2005;23(32):8232–41.
114. Dushyanthen S, Cossigny DA, Quan GM. The osteoblastic and osteoclastic interactions in spinal metastases secondary to prostate cancer. Cancer Growth Metastasis. 2013;6:61–80.
115. Luo J, Beer TM, Graff JN. Treatment of nonmetastatic castration-resistant prostate cancer. Oncology (Williston Park). 2016;30(4):336–44.
116. Yuan H, et al. SETD2 restricts prostate cancer metastasis by integrating EZH2 and AMPK signaling pathways. Cancer Cell. 2020;38(3):350–365.e7.
117. Cheng L, et al. SGK2 promotes prostate cancer metastasis by inhibiting ferroptosis via upregulating GPX4. Cell Death Dis. 2023;14(1):74.
118. Guccini I, et al. Senescence reprogramming by TIMP1 deficiency promotes prostate cancer metastasis. Cancer Cell. 2021;39(1):68–82.e9.

119. Luo JQ, et al. Exosomal PGAM1 promotes prostate cancer angiogenesis and metastasis by interacting with ACTG1. Cell Death Dis. 2023;14(8):502.
120. Sun Y, et al. Androgen deprivation causes epithelial-mesenchymal transition in the prostate: implications for androgen-deprivation therapy. Cancer Res. 2012;72(2):527–36.
121. Zeisberg M, Neilson EG. Biomarkers for epithelial-mesenchymal transitions. J Clin Invest. 2009;119(6):1429–37.
122. Singh A, Settleman J. EMT, cancer stem cells and drug resistance: an emerging axis of evil in the war on cancer. Oncogene. 2010;29(34):4741–51.
123. Graham TR, et al. Insulin-like growth factor-I-dependent up-regulation of ZEB1 drives epithelial-to-mesenchymal transition in human prostate cancer cells. Cancer Res. 2008;68(7):2479–88.
124. Qin Q, et al. Normal and disease-related biological functions of Twist1 and underlying molecular mechanisms. Cell Res. 2012;22(1):90–106.
125. Kwok WK, et al. Up-regulation of TWIST in prostate cancer and its implication as a therapeutic target. Cancer Res. 2005;65(12):5153–62.
126. Wu K, et al. Slug, a unique androgen-regulated transcription factor, coordinates androgen receptor to facilitate castration resistance in prostate cancer. Mol Endocrinol. 2012;26(9):1496–507.
127. Tanaka H, et al. Monoclonal antibody targeting of N-cadherin inhibits prostate cancer growth, metastasis and castration resistance. Nat Med. 2010;16(12):1414–20.
128. Gravdal K, et al. A switch from E-cadherin to N-cadherin expression indicates epithelial to mesenchymal transition and is of strong and independent importance for the progress of prostate cancer. Clin Cancer Res. 2007;13(23):7003–11.
129. Huang CF, et al. Cadherin-11 increases migration and invasion of prostate cancer cells and enhances their interaction with osteoblasts. Cancer Res. 2010;70(11):4580–9.
130. Baritaki S, et al. Pivotal roles of snail inhibition and RKIP induction by the proteasome inhibitor NPI-0052 in tumor cell chemoimmunosensitization. Cancer Res. 2009;69(21):8376–85.
131. Nauseef JT, Henry MD. Epithelial-to-mesenchymal transition in prostate cancer: paradigm or puzzle? Nat Rev Urol. 2011;8(8):428–39.
132. Robinton DA, Daley GQ. The promise of induced pluripotent stem cells in research and therapy. Nature. 2012;481(7381):295–305.
133. Kleiman RJ, Engle SJ. Human inducible pluripotent stem cells: realization of initial promise in drug discovery. Cell Stem Cell. 2021;28(9):1507–15.
134. Chaves LP, et al. Epithelial-mesenchymal transition signaling and prostate cancer stem cells: emerging biomarkers and opportunities for precision therapeutics. Genes (Basel). 2021;12(12):1900.
135. Gómez-Cuadrado L, et al. Mouse models of metastasis: progress and prospects. Dis Model Mech. 2017;10(9):1061–74.
136. Lambert AW, Weinberg RA. Linking EMT programmes to normal and neoplastic epithelial stem cells. Nat Rev Cancer. 2021;21(5):325–38.
137. Ruscetti M, et al. Tracking and functional characterization of epithelial-mesenchymal transition and mesenchymal tumor cells during prostate cancer metastasis. Cancer Res. 2015;75(13):2749–59.
138. Salm SN, et al. TGF-{beta} maintains dormancy of prostatic stem cells in the proximal region of ducts. J Cell Biol. 2005;170(1):81–90.
139. Zhao Y, et al. Ephrin-A2 promotes prostate cancer metastasis by enhancing angiogenesis and promoting EMT. J Cancer Res Clin Oncol. 2021;147(7):2013–23.
140. Giannoni E, et al. Reciprocal activation of prostate cancer cells and cancer-associated fibroblasts stimulates epithelial-mesenchymal transition and cancer stemness. Cancer Res. 2010;70(17):6945–56.
141. Acevedo VD, et al. Inducible FGFR-1 activation leads to irreversible prostate adenocarcinoma and an epithelial-to-mesenchymal transition. Cancer Cell. 2007;12(6):559–71.

142. Melo CM, et al. The role of somatic mutations on the immune response of the tumor microenvironment in prostate cancer. Int J Mol Sci. 2021;22(17):9550.
143. Kwon JTW, Bryant RJ, Parkes EE. The tumor microenvironment and immune responses in prostate cancer patients. Endocr Relat Cancer. 2021;28(8):T95–107.
144. Comito G, et al. Cancer-associated fibroblasts and M2-polarized macrophages synergize during prostate carcinoma progression. Oncogene. 2014;33(19):2423–31.
145. Ku SY, et al. Rb1 and Trp53 cooperate to suppress prostate cancer lineage plasticity, metastasis, and antiandrogen resistance. Science. 2017;355(6320):78–83.
146. Mu P, et al. SOX2 promotes lineage plasticity and antiandrogen resistance in TP53- and RB1-deficient prostate cancer. Science. 2017;355(6320):84–8.
147. Hu W, et al. MIIP inhibits EMT and cell invasion in prostate cancer through miR-181a/b-5p-KLF17 axis. Am J Cancer Res. 2020;10(2):630–47.
148. Mani SA, et al. The epithelial-mesenchymal transition generates cells with properties of stem cells. Cell. 2008;133(4):704–15.
149. Chaffer CL, et al. Poised chromatin at the ZEB1 promoter enables breast cancer cell plasticity and enhances tumorigenicity. Cell. 2013;154(1):61–74.
150. Wellner U, et al. The EMT-activator ZEB1 promotes tumorigenicity by repressing stemness-inhibiting microRNAs. Nat Cell Biol. 2009;11(12):1487–95.
151. Kong D, et al. Epithelial to mesenchymal transition is mechanistically linked with stem cell signatures in prostate cancer cells. PLoS One. 2010;5(8):e12445.
152. Fang Q, et al. β-ionone inhibits epithelial-mesenchymal transition (EMT) in prostate cancer cells by negatively regulating the Wnt/β-catenin pathway. Front Biosci (Landmark Ed). 2022;27(12):335.
153. Liang Y, et al. The role of contactin 1 in cancers: what we know so far. Front Oncol. 2020;10:574208.
154. Chen B, et al. CNTN-1 promotes docetaxel resistance and epithelial-to-mesenchymal transition via the PI3K/Akt signaling pathway in prostate cancer. Arch Med Sci. 2021;17(1):152–65.
155. Nath D, et al. Abi1 loss drives prostate tumorigenesis through activation of EMT and non-canonical WNT signaling. Cell Commun Signal. 2019;17(1):120.
156. Chen Q, et al. TGF-β1 promotes epithelial-to-mesenchymal transition and stemness of prostate cancer cells by inducing PCBP1 degradation and alternative splicing of CD44. Cell Mol Life Sci. 2021;78(3):949–62.
157. Shen Y, et al. Estrogen receptor α-NOTCH1 axis enhances basal stem-like cells and epithelial-mesenchymal transition phenotypes in prostate cancer. Cell Commun Signal. 2019;17(1):50.
158. Zhang J, et al. Notch-4 silencing inhibits prostate cancer growth and EMT via the NF-κB pathway. Apoptosis. 2017;22(6):877–84.
159. Bezzi M, et al. Diverse genetic-driven immune landscapes dictate tumor progression through distinct mechanisms. Nat Med. 2018;24(2):165–75.
160. Isaacs JT, Coffey DS. Etiology and disease process of benign prostatic hyperplasia. Prostate. 1989;15(S2):33–50.
161. Drost J, et al. Organoid culture systems for prostate epithelial and cancer tissue. Nat Protoc. 2016;11(2):347–58.
162. Kahounová Z, et al. Slug-expressing mouse prostate epithelial cells have increased stem cell potential. Stem Cell Res. 2020;46:101844.
163. Karthaus WR, et al. Regenerative potential of prostate luminal cells revealed by single-cell analysis. Science. 2020;368(6490):497–505.
164. Stoyanova T, et al. Prostate cancer originating in basal cells progresses to adenocarcinoma propagated by luminal-like cells. Proc Natl Acad Sci U S A. 2013;110(50):20111–6.

Part III
Molecular Events

Chapter 6
Prostate Cancer and WNT/STAT3 Signaling

Sareh Etemad, Mahdokht Sadat Manavi, Mahsa Haji Heidari Varnousafaderani, Ferdos Faghihkhorasani, Hajarossadat Ghaderi, Seddigheh Eslamparast Kordmahalleh, Nasim Ebrahimi, Mostafa Haji-Fatahaliha, and Amir Reza Aref

Abstract Globally, prostate cancer remains a major health problem, needing a thorough knowledge of the underlying molecular processes that govern its development. In this chapter, we dig into the complex functions of the Wnt and STAT3 signaling pathways in prostate cancer, illuminating their involvement in the progression and metastasis of the illness. The WNT and STAT3 signaling pathways are

S. Etemad
Department of Pathology, Faculty of Anatomical Pathology, Ghaem Hospital, University of Medicine, Mashhad, Iran

M. S. Manavi
Otolaryngology Department, Tehran University of Medical Science, Tehran, Iran

M. H. H. Varnousafaderani
Faculty of Medicine, University of Debrecen, Debrecen, Hungary

F. Faghihkhorasani
Medical Campus, Xi'an Jiaotong University, Xi'an, Shaanxi Province, China

H. Ghaderi
Laboratory of Regenerative and Medical Innovation, Pasteur Institute of Iran, Tehran, Iran

S. E. Kordmahalleh
School of Medicine, Guilan University of Medical Science, Rasht, Iran

N. Ebrahimi (✉)
Genetics Division, Department of Cell and Molecular Biology and Microbiology, Faculty of Science and Technology, University of Isfahan, Isfahan, Iran

M. Haji-Fatahaliha
Department of Immunology, Faculty of Medicine, Tabriz University of Medical Sciences, Tabriz, Iran

A. R. Aref (✉)
Mass General Cancer Center, Department of Surgery, Massachusetts General Hospital, Harvard Medical School, Boston, MA, USA

Broad Institute of MIT and Harvard, Harvard Medical School, Cambridge, MA, USA
e-mail: aaref@mgh.harvard.edu

G. Sethi et al. (eds.), *Prostate Cancer: Molecular Events and Therapeutic Modalities*, https://doi.org/10.1007/978-981-97-4612-5_6

thoroughly discussed at the beginning of the chapter, emphasizing both their critical roles in healthy cellular activities and the dysregulation of these pathways in prostate cancer. Both routes are known to exert substantial influence on cellular growth, survival, migration, and differentiation during carcinogenesis. In addition, we investigate the crucial yet unresolved interaction among the WNT and STAT3 pathways in prostate cancer. Understanding the complex regulatory mechanisms driving prostate cancer growth may be revealed by examining the molecular and cellular interactions between different pathways. The potential of WNT and STAT3 as therapeutic targets in the treatment of prostate cancer is covered in great detail in this chapter. Targeting these pathways presents interesting opportunities for creating tailored therapeutics intended to slow disease progression and enhance patient outcomes due to their significant roles in tumor formation and metastasis. The importance of the WNT and STAT3 signaling pathways in prostate cancer and their value as possible therapeutic targets are highlighted in Chap. 6's conclusion. It may be possible to develop efficient precision medicines for patients with prostate cancer by better understanding their interactions and focusing on these pathways, thereby advancing oncology and enhancing clinical outcomes.

Keywords Tumorigenesis · Epithelial-mesenchymal transition (EMT) · Therapeutic targets · NF-κB signaling pathway · Tumor microenvironment (TME)

6.1 Introduction

Prostate cancer is a prevalent malignancy, which influences the male population worldwide. Despite advancements in screening techniques and therapeutic options, prostate cancer remains a significant cause of morbidity and mortality [1]. Understanding the molecular mechanisms underlying its progression is crucial for the development of more efficient therapeutic strategies. Among the intricate network of signaling pathways involved in cancer progression, the Wnt and STAT3 pathways have emerged as key players in various malignancies, including prostate cancer. The Wnt signaling pathway has a substantial role in development of embryos, tissue homeostasis, and cell fate determination [2]. Irregular triggering of the Wnt pathway has been reported in different kinds of malignancies, such as prostate cancer. Wnt pathway in its canonical route, mediated by β-catenin, controls the gene transcription of target molecules associated with cellular growth, cell survival, and cell differentiation. Aberrant activity of Wnt signaling can lead to uncontrolled cellular growth, evasion of apoptosis, and increased metastatic potential, all of which are hallmarks of cancer [3]. Similarly, the STAT3 (signal transducer and activator of transcription 3) pathway has been implicated in prostate cancer progression. STAT3 is a transcription factor that is activated by various cytokines, growth factors, and oncogenic kinases [4]. Upon activation, STAT3 translocates to the nucleus and regulates the expression of genes involved in cell survival, proliferation, angiogenesis, and immune evasion. Persistent activation of STAT3 has been reported in various cancer types, including prostate cancer, associated with tumor invasion, progression, and therapy resistance [5].

The interplay between the Wnt and STAT3 pathways in prostate cancer has been investigated. However, studies have indicated that Wnt signaling could induce STAT3 activity, resulting in an increased rate of tumor cell survival and proliferation. Conversely, STAT3 activation can modulate Wnt signaling by regulating the transcription of staple elements of the pathway. These reciprocal interactions between Wnt and STAT3 signaling pathways create a positive feedback loop, amplifying the oncogenic signals and promoting cancer progression [6].

The potential of targeting the Wnt/STAT3 signaling pathway for cancer treatment has sparked considerable interest in the scientific community. Inhibition of Wnt signaling components or downstream effectors has shown promising anticancer effects in preclinical models of prostate cancer [7]. Similarly, targeted inhibition of STAT3 has demonstrated efficacy in suppressing tumor proliferation and enhancing the sensitivity of cancerous cells to conventional treatments [8].

In this chapter, we delved into the intricate relationship between the Wnt and STAT3 pathways and prostate cancer progression. We discussed the mechanisms through which these pathways influence each other and contribute to the development and maintenance of the malignant phenotype. Furthermore, we explored the therapeutic potential of targeting the Wnt/STAT3 pathway for prostate cancer treatment. By gaining a comprehensive understanding of the Wnt/STAT3 signaling roles in prostate cancer, this chapter aimed to provide insights that may lead to the development of novel therapeutic approaches and improve patient outcomes.

6.2 An Overview of Wnt Signaling Pathway

The Wnt family consists of 19 secreted lipoglycoproteins rich in cysteine, which play a significant role in regulating cell proliferation, self-renewal of stem cells, cell differentiation, and cell migration during the development of embryos and organ formation [9]. Wnts bind to frizzled receptors (FZDs) and various co-receptors, including low-density lipoprotein receptor-related proteins (LRP-4, -5, and -6), the inactive tyrosine-protein kinase membrane receptors (ROR-1 and -2), and the tyrosine-protein kinase RYK38, to trigger canonical (β-catenin-dependent) and non-canonical (β-catenin-independent) signaling pathways [10, 11]. The canonical route of Wnt signaling is characterized by the nuclear stabilization and translocation of β-catenin protein. When WNT ligands are not present, β-catenin is captured and degraded by a destruction complex consisting of adenomatous polyposis coli (APC), axin, glycogen synthase kinase-3 (GSK3), and casein kinase 1 (CK1) [2]. Binding of Wnt to frizzled receptors and LRP5/6 co-receptors leads to secondary phosphorylation by CK1 and GSK3, as well as recruitment of axin and Disheveled to the plasma membrane, thus, causing a disruption in the assembly of the destruction complex [12]. This interruption causes the stabilization of β-catenin, leading to its accumulation within the cytoplasm and its translocation into the nucleus. β-catenin interacts with transcription factor family members, such as histone acetyltransferase p300 (p300 HAT), CREB-binding protein (CBP), B-cell lymphoma 9 protein (BCL9), BCL9-like protein (BCL9L), and lymphoid enhancer-binding factor 1 (LEF-1), in the nucleus to regulate the transcription of Wnt target genes [13] (Fig. 6.1).

A novel branch of Wnt signaling, known as Wnt-STOP, was identified about 10 years ago. During this pathway, the signaling process is initiated when Wnt binds to LRP6. However, its impacts are independent of transcription and involve the inclusion of cyclin-Y instead of β-catenin. Wnt-STOP signals lead to protein stabilization during the mitotic phase. These signals play a role in endolysosomal biogenesis, cell cycle progression, DNA repair, and cellular architecture, thus potentially playing a noteworthy function in the initiation and progression of cancer [14].

6.3 Role of Wnt in Prostate Cancer Progression

The Wnt/β-catenin pathway contribution to tumorigenesis and cancer growth has been extensively studied across various cancer types [15–18]. Different levels of regulation, including extracellular inhibitors, genetic mutations, and nuclear transcriptional factors, can modulate the Wnt/β-catenin pathway. Any disruption in

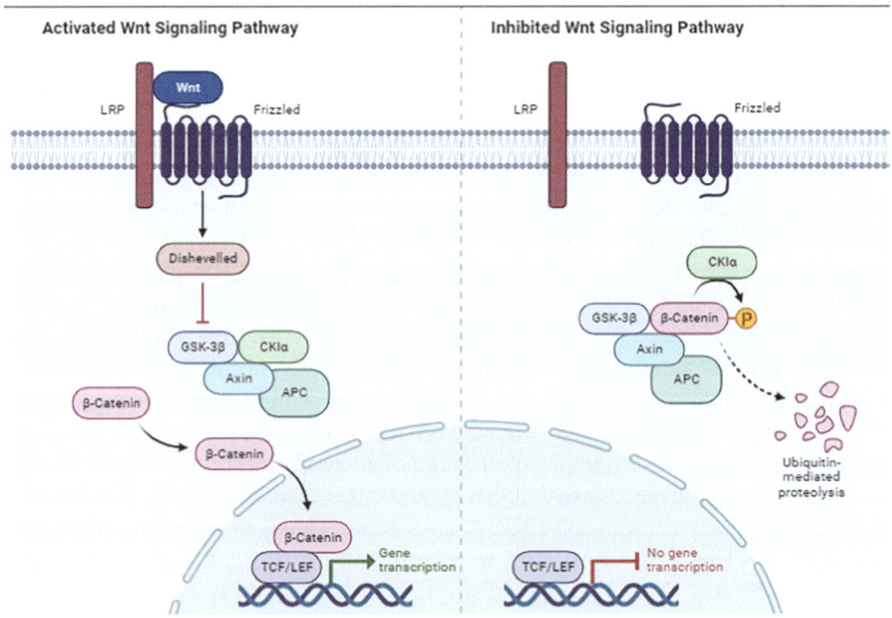

Fig. 6.1 Activation and inactivation of Wnt signaling pathway

these regulatory levels can lead to cancer initiation and progression. Additionally, dysregulation of downstream genes of the Wnt/β-catenin pathway in the cytoplasm or nucleus, such as Cyclin D1 and C-myc, may also contribute to cancer development. Numerous pieces of evidence have studied the role of the Wnt/β-catenin signaling in prostate cancer. Although this signaling pathway is predominantly known as an oncogenic pathway, not all of its downstream genes are capable of promoting cancer. However, Foxa2, a gene in the downstream of Wnt/β-catenin signaling cascade, is induced by its activity and could have an important involvement in the occurrence of bone metastasis during prostate cancer [19]. Similarly, Foxb2, another tissue-specific activator of the Wnt/β-catenin pathway, has been implicated in the progression of prostate cancer, according to the study by Mupparapu et al. [20].

One aspect that links the Wnt/β-catenin pathway to prostate cancer is the interaction of β-catenin with the androgen receptor pathway. Thus, mutations in the β-catenin gene can play a role in the advancement and growth of prostate cancer [21]. Recent studies have focused on identifying cancer-associated mutations related to the Wnt/β-catenin pathway using single-strand conformational polymorphism (SSCP) analysis. Voller et al. reported five mutations in the regulatory regions of these genes in prostate cancer. The results of this study revealed that the majority of these mutations (4 out of 5 reported mutations) were associated with phosphorylation sites [21].

In conclusion, the Wnt/β-catenin pathway has been extensively studied for its involvement in cancer development, particularly in prostate cancer. Dysregulation of various factors within this pathway can contribute to tumorigenesis, and understanding these molecular events may offer possible candidates for therapeutic strategies in the treatment of prostate cancer. Mutation at the integration site of Mouse Mammary Tumor Virus (MMTV) or Wnt-1 has been rarely reported in primary prostate epithelial cells. However, further studies have shown a significantly elevated expression of Wnt-1 in cellular and tissue levels of prostate cancer. Particularly, this mutation has been more frequently observed in bone the spread of prostate cancer to lymph nodes [22]. Moreover, in hormone-resistant and metastatic prostate cancer, an upregulation of Wnt-1 has been indicated by Taille and colleagues' study [23]. Similarly, Thiel and coworkers demonstrated high levels of Wnt-1 in human prostate cancer cell line (DU145) [24]. Additionally, increased expression of Wnt-2 has been reported in primary prostate cancer tumors and prostate cancer metastases in studies by Katoh and Hall et al. [25, 26], respectively. Furthermore, research has indicated that Wnt3a results in increased expression of β-catenin in both the nucleus and cytoplasm, consequently enhancing activity of androgen receptor and ultimately promoting prostate cancer progression [27].

Unlike most genes associated with the Wnt/β-catenin pathway, which plays an oncogenic role, Wnt5a is predominantly known as a tumor suppressor gene in certain cancers. However, in prostate cancer, it acts as a proto-oncogene according to studies conducted [28]. Zhao and colleagues in their study indicated that miR-26a can prevent prostate cancer progression by suppressing the expression of Wnt-5a, highlighting its role in prostate cancer advancement [29]. On the other hand, some studies have shown that increased activity of matrix metalloproteinase-1 (MMP-1) and activation of JNK leads to elevated Wnt-5 expression, enhancing the invasive potential of prostate cancer cells [28]. Additionally, Wnt-6 expression has been remarkably upregulated in occult breast cancer tissues in comparison to normal tissues [30]. Moreover, higher-grade prostate tumors have reported an increase in Wnt-11 expression. Furthermore, this Wnt protein is also upregulated in hormone-independent prostate cancers [31]. Conversely, Wnt-10b expression decreases in localized prostate cancer tissues compared to benign tissues [32]. In any case, genomic alterations and mutations related to the Wnt/β-catenin pathway, which leads to the occurrence of prostate cancer, have been extensively described in reference [33].

6.4 An Overview of STAT3 Signaling Pathway

Over the course of the last 20 years, it has become clear that Interleukin-6 (IL-6) activates a molecular pathway involved in immune modulation within the liver. Because of the resemblances of IL-6 in both structure and function with the STAT family, this pathway was designated as STAT3. In addition to IL-6, several cytokines and growth factors, including Epidermal Growth Factor (EGF), IL-11, G-CSF, and Oncostatin M have been identified to trigger STAT3 signaling [34, 35]. STAT3 consists of six key domains, with the most significant ones being: (1) The N-terminal domain responsible for binding to DNA and modulation of proteins nuclear translocation. (2) The central domain, DNA-binding domain, is essential for the transcription factor's binding to DNA. (3) The linker domain, which is responsible for the stability and strength of STAT3's binding to DNA. (4) The alpha-helical coiled-coil domain, which manages STAT3's interaction with other proteins. (5) The C-terminal domain, which facilitates the STAT3 activation through phosphorylation at tyrosine 705 and serine 727 sites [36, 37]. Multiple pieces of evidence indicate that STAT3 exhibits pleiotropic activities and multiple functions through its various isoforms, including STAT3α, STAT3β, STAT3γ, and STAT3δ. The STAT3α isoform is essential for pro-inflammatory actions mediated by IL-6 [37, 38]. Conversely, STAT3β acts as an inhibitor of pro-inflammatory factor production. Similar to the Wnt pathway, the STAT3 signaling pathway also comprises canonical and non-canonical signaling routes. IL-6 is the most well-known STAT3 signaling inducer. The following stages for triggering STAT3 are carried out through its phosphorylation on tyrosine 705 and serine 727 after JAKs have been stimulated and phosphorylated as a result of interactions between cytokines and growth factors and receptors on the surface of cell membranes [39]. Following the phosphorylation of the mentioned residues, the SH2 domains interact, leading to the dimerization of STAT3. In this dimerized state, STAT3 translocates into the nucleus, where it modulates the expression of target genes and affects various transcription factors [40]. Given that a wide spectrum of genes can be influenced by STAT3 activity, diverse cellular mechanisms, including cell death, autophagy, apoptosis, cell migration, and cell differentiation, can be regulated by this pathway. Consequently, aberrant STAT3 expression can be associated with the development of different malignancies, promoting growth and metastasis. Moreover, uncontrolled activation of the STAT3 signaling pathway has been linked to drug resistance and radioresistance in cancers. Therefore, the inhibition and targeting of this pathway in cancer treatment could hold significant importance in preventing cancer progression and enhancing therapeutic outcomes [41, 42].

One crucial aspect of studying the STAT3 pathway is its interaction with other cellular signaling pathways and its mode of action, especially in different types of cancers [43]. For instance, under hypoxic conditions, elevated levels of MAFF induced by excessive IL-11 expression via HIF-1α function can trigger STAT3 signaling, fostering the progression and metastasis of cancer cells [44]. Additionally, SLCO1B3 activation can lead to cancer initiation and enhanced migratory capacity of colorectal tumor cells through the activation of the STAT3 pathway [45]. The findings from these studies collectively suggest that STAT3 pathway activation is correlated with prostate cancer progression and tumor growth.

6.5 The STAT3 Involvement in the Prostate Cancer Advancement

Based on the studies conducted so far, multiple roles of STAT3 in the progression of prostate cancer have been identified. Prostate cancer cells, similar to other types of cancer cells, require a rich energy source to accelerate their proliferation rate, achieved through alterations in cellular metabolism. During this metabolic shift, cancer cells opt for glycolysis as their preferred method for energy supply [46]. Notably, fructose serves as a fuel in glycolysis, making increased fructose uptake by cancer cells crucial. This uptake is facilitated by the glucose transporter 5 (GLUT5). In prostate cancer, IL-6 acts as an upstream mediator and causes the STAT3 activation, which, in turn, enhances the expression of GLUT5. Consequently, fructose uptake increases, fostering the growth of prostate tumors [47].

According to the findings, there is a positive correlation between elevated serum cholesterol levels and the high possibility of prostate cancer, as cholesterol serves as a precursor for androgens leading to prostate cancer progression [48]. Low-density lipoprotein cholesterol (LDL) can activate the STAT3 signaling pathway, leading to increased growth of prostate tumor cells. Inhibition of the LDL/STAT3 axis has been indicated to reduce the survival time of prostate tumor cells [49–52]. Leptin, as an adipokine associated with obesity, can also induce STAT3 signaling, thereby enhancing the rate of prostate cancer proliferation. Additionally, a high percentage of leptin has been found to be correlated with poor prognosis in prostate cancer patients [52].

STAT3 also plays a role in the progression of prostate cancer through its effects on the tumor microenvironment (TME). Within the TME, various cancer cells, immune cells, macrophages, normal cells, and fibroblasts interact in complex ways. Particularly, tumor-associated macrophages (TAMs) have a significant impact on cancer progression, drug resistance, and disease prognosis during their interaction with tumor cells [53]. TAMs are classified as M2 polarized macrophages, one of two types of macrophages with distinct biological characteristics that play a critical role in controlling the course of cancer [54–57]. Prostate cancer cells that are treated with LINC00467 proliferate and proceed through the cell cycle. LINC00467 scavenges miR-494-3p to activate STAT3 signaling, causing macrophages to become polarized M2, which promotes the progression of prostate cancer [58]. HepaCAM has the ability to block STAT3 phosphorylation, preventing prostate tumor cells from spreading [59]. Preventing and escaping apoptosis are other strategies employed by prostate cancer cells to increase their proliferation and expansion. Overexpression of IL-8 causes the induction of the STAT3/Akt signaling pathway and ultimately results in increased expression of NF-κB, leading to the inhibition of apoptosis and enhanced proliferation of prostate cancer cells [60].

In addition to what has been mentioned so far, the role of long non-coding RNAs (lncRNAs) is also significant in the progression of prostate cancer, particularly through communications with signaling pathways including Wnt and STAT3 pathways [61]. For instance, it has been shown that LINC00473 acts as a sponge, inhibiting the expression of miR-195-5p, thereby activating the JAK/STAT3/SEPT2 axis and promoting increased proliferation of prostate cancer cells [62]. Furthermore, LncRNA AC245100.4 triggers the oncogenic STAT3/NR4A3 axis, leading to the stimulation of prostate cancer growth [63]. Conversely, LncRNA MAGI2-AS3 acts as a sponge for miR-424-5p, suppressing the STAT3 signaling pathway, and thus functioning as a tumor suppressor [64].

In addition to cell growth and proliferation, the STAT3 pathway also has an involvement in enhancing the invasiveness of prostate tumor cells and their metastasis. Numerous investigations have indicated a reduction in KLF5 expression during prostate cancer, which is correlated with an enhanced risk of metastasis. The downregulation of KLF5 leads to elevated levels of STAT3 and IGF1 expression, which are commonly observed in aggressive prostate tumors [65]. Consequently, the suppression of STAT3 has been shown to inhibit the progression and metastasis of prostate tumor cells. Moreover, STAT3 interacts with the NF-κB pathway, where the activation of this pathway induces STAT3 activity and promotes prostate metastasis. Some investigations have shown that the disruption of the NF-κB/STAT3 pathway through inhibition and suppression effectively halts the progression and metastasis of prostate tumors in experimental and animal model studies [66]. Furthermore, conditions of oxidative stress and high levels of reactive oxygen species (ROS) enhance STAT3 signaling activity. In this context, STAT3 induces overexpression of TWIST1 triggered by EGF, leading to EMT in prostate tumor cells and consequently enhancing their invasive potential and metastasis [67]. On the other hand, research has shown that vitamin D can suppress STAT3 signaling, thus inhibiting prostate tumor cell metastasis [68]. Castration has been seen as a viable treatment because of the function that androgens play in the development of prostate cancer. However, castration may accelerate prostate cancer metastasis via an EMT mechanism. Prostate cancer treated with metformin had less castration-mediated EMT. Metformin inhibits STAT3 signaling to block EMT and reduce metastasis of prostate tumor cells by down-regulating COX2/PGE2 [69]. In summary, understanding the intricate involvement of the STAT3 pathway in prostate cancer metastasis opens up new avenues for targeted therapies aimed at controlling tumor progression and metastatic spread [70].

6.6 Crosstalk Between the Wnt and STAT3 Signaling Pathways

As previously mentioned, both the STAT3 and the Wnt signaling pathways have a fundamental role in various types of tumors. Moreover, both pathways are involved in proliferation of normal and cancer stem cells, particularly in the establishment of stemness properties in cancer-initiating cells, leading to tumor proliferation and metastasis [71–73]. Despite the involvement of both the Wnt and STAT3 pathways in cancer metastasis, the molecular and cellular crosstalk, and coordination between these pathways during cancer progression remain unclear. Although the Wnt and STAT3 pathways individually involved in tumor progression and metastasis in various kinds of cancers, the precise molecular and cellular interplay between these two pathways during cancer advancement is not well understood. Further investigation is required to elucidate the intricate relationship and communication between these pathways, which could potentially offer valuable insights for targeted therapeutic approaches in cancer treatment. In this regard, Kim et al. used basal-like p53-null syngeneic mice models of three negative breast cancer together with a lentiviral-based signaling reporter system to explore the demographic changes generated from both STAT3 and Wnt pathways in primary tumors and metastases [74]. In this study, they describe different subpopulations in basal-like p53-null mammary cancers and changes in distribution of cells among primary tumors and their corresponding metastases. These subpopulations are generated from the activation of STAT3 and/or Wnt signaling pathways. Significantly, the variation among clones obtained from these pathways varies as metastatic lesions advance in comparison to matched initial tumors, with a growing overlap in populations driven by both STAT3 and Wnt pathways [74].

Prostate cancer usually involves activation of the Wnt signaling system, which promotes tumor development, growth, and resistance to treatment [75]. Recent research suggests that treating prostate cancer by focusing on the Wnt pathway may be successful. The functional effects of activating the Wnt pathway at various phases of prostate cancer growth are yet unknown, though [75]. On the other hand, prostate cancer triggers STAT3 signaling activity, which encourages the malignant nature of cancerous cells. The STAT3 signaling stimulation boosts glycolysis, promotes cell growth, and inhibits apoptosis in prostate cancer cells. Additionally, STAT3 signaling activates the EMT pathway, leading to promotion of cancer metastasis [6]. Other cancer forms, such as gastric cancer, have shown interactions between the STAT3 and Wnt signaling pathways, where Wnt overexpression results in STAT3 activation in a galectin-3-dependent route [76]. Although there is no direct evidence of interactions between Wnt and STAT3 signaling in prostate cancer, the importance of both pathways in the development of the disease raises the possibility that they do interact. Prostate cancer cell populations that initiate tumors as well as differentiated cell populations may both be affected by STAT3 signaling inhibition [77]. The capacity of prostate cancer cells to start developing prostatic adenocarcinoma was severely hampered by STAT3 knockdown [78]. Additionally, inhibiting STAT3 in conjunction with several therapies has shown potential to halt tumor growth and metastasis [79]. In summary, interaction between the Wnt and STAT3 signaling pathways is essential for prostate cancer progression. Potential treatment approaches for treating prostate cancer may include targeting these mechanisms, either alone or together. In order to create efficient targeted medicines, further study is required to clarify the specific processes of interaction between these pathways.

6.7 Potential of Targeting Wnt and STAT3 Pathways in Prostate Cancer Therapy

There is hope for prostate cancer treatment by focusing on the Wnt and STAT3 signaling pathways. The prostate cancer etiology, cancer progression, and treatment resistance are all significantly influenced by the Wnt/β-catenin signaling pathway [7]. Abnormal Wnt pathway activation may promote tumor development, growth, and treatment resistance in prostate tumors [75]. On the other hand, prostate cancer also activates the STAT3 signaling pathway, which encourages tumor cells to behave malignantly [48]. Recent research suggests that prostate cancer treatment that targets the Wnt pathway may be effective [75]. To find efficient treatment options and biomarkers that may assist inform treatment choices and enhance patient care, preclinical research into the regarding the potential of addressing Wnt signaling as a therapeutic approach for managing prostate cancer, encompassing both primary tumors and metastatic sites, is essential [75]. In non-cancerous cells, there is evidence pointing to a connection between STAT3 and Wnt signaling [6]. However, little research has been done on the interplay between the Wnt and STAT3 pathways in response to cellular damage and safeguarding mechanisms. Understanding the interactions between these pathways might provide important insights for creating emerging treatment approaches.

Prostate cancer development may be stopped by suppressors that target complexes of Wnt receptors at the cell surface or obstruct the β-catenin interaction with androgen receptor and the LEF-1 [79]. Phase I studies for certain Wnt signaling inhibitors are ongoing, however, patients with prostate cancer have not yet been included [6]. Additionally, focusing on the STAT3 signaling pathway has shown promise as a treatment for a variety of cancers [80]. Within the tumor environment, STAT3 is widely hyperactivated in both malignant and non-cancerous cells. It is essential for the synthesis of immunosuppressive factors and for suppressing the expression of critical immune activation regulators.

6.8 Conclusion

In conclusion, prostate cancer treatment may benefit from focusing on the STAT3 and Wnt signaling pathways. In order to create efficient treatment plans and biomarkers to inform therapy choices and enhance patient care, further study is required to understand how these pathways interact.

References

1. Rawla P. Epidemiology of prostate cancer. World J Oncol. 2019;10(2):63–89.
2. Liu J, Xiao Q, Xiao J, Niu C, Li Y, Zhang X, et al. Wnt/β-catenin signalling: function, biological mechanisms, and therapeutic opportunities. Signal Transduct Target Ther. 2022;7(1):3.
3. Zhang Y, Wang X. Targeting the Wnt/β-catenin signaling pathway in cancer. J Hematol Oncol. 2020;13(1):165.
4. Aggarwal BB, Kunnumakkara AB, Harikumar KB, Gupta SR, Tharakan ST, Koca C, et al. Signal transducer and activator of transcription-3, inflammation, and cancer: how intimate is the relationship? Ann N Y Acad Sci. 2009;1171:59–76.
5. Yu H, Pardoll D, Jove R. STATs in cancer inflammation and immunity: a leading role for STAT3. Nat Rev Cancer. 2009;9(11):798–809.
6. Fragoso MA, Patel AK, Nakamura RE, Yi H, Surapaneni K, Hackam AS. The Wnt/β-catenin pathway cross-talks with STAT3 signaling to regulate survival of retinal pigment epithelium cells. PLoS One. 2012;7(10):e46892.
7. Wang C, Chen Q, Xu H. Wnt/β-catenin signal transduction pathway in prostate cancer and associated drug resistance. Discov Oncol. 2021;12(1):40.
8. Yang PL, Liu LX, Li EM, Xu LY. STAT3, the challenge for chemotherapeutic and radiotherapeutic efficacy. Cancers (Basel). 2020;12(9):2459.
9. Cadigan KM, Nusse R. Wnt signaling: a common theme in animal development. Genes Dev. 1997;11(24):3286–305.
10. Pfister AS, Kühl M. Of Wnts and ribosomes. Prog Mol Biol Transl Sci. 2018;153:131–55.
11. MacDonald BT, He X. Frizzled and LRP5/6 receptors for Wnt/β-catenin signaling. Cold Spring Harb Perspect Biol. 2012;4(12):a007880.
12. Nusse R, Clevers H. Wnt/β-catenin signaling, disease, and emerging therapeutic modalities. Cell. 2017;169(6):985–99.
13. Shang S, Hua F, Hu ZW. The regulation of β-catenin activity and function in cancer: therapeutic opportunities. Oncotarget. 2017;8(20):33972–89.
14. García de Herreros A, Duñach M. Intracellular signals activated by canonical Wnt ligands independent of GSK3 inhibition and β-catenin stabilization. Cells. 2019;8(10):1148.
15. Arend RC, Londoño-Joshi AI, Straughn JM Jr, Buchsbaum DJ. The Wnt/β-catenin pathway in ovarian cancer: a review. Gynecol Oncol. 2013;131(3):772–9.
16. Tian J, He H, Lei G. Wnt/β-catenin pathway in bone cancers. Tumour Biol. 2014;35(10):9439–45.
17. Chiurillo MA. Role of the Wnt/β-catenin pathway in gastric cancer: an in-depth literature review. World J Exp Med. 2015;5(2):84–102.

18. Liu C, Takada K, Zhu D. Targeting Wnt/β-catenin pathway for drug therapy. Med Drug Discov. 2020;8:100066.
19. Yu X, Wang Y, DeGraff DJ, Wills ML, Matusik RJ. Wnt/β-catenin activation promotes prostate tumor progression in a mouse model. Oncogene. 2011;30(16):1868–79.
20. Moparthi L, Pizzolato G, Koch S. Wnt activator FOXB2 drives the neuroendocrine differentiation of prostate cancer. Proc Natl Acad Sci USA. 2019;116(44):22189–95.
21. Voeller HJ, Truica CI, Gelmann EP. Beta-catenin mutations in human prostate cancer. Cancer Res. 1998;58(12):2520–3.
22. Chen G, Shukeir N, Potti A, Sircar K, Aprikian A, Goltzman D, et al. Up-regulation of Wnt-1 and beta-catenin production in patients with advanced metastatic prostate carcinoma: potential pathogenetic and prognostic implications. Cancer. 2004;101(6):1345–56.
23. de la Taille A, Rubin MA, Chen MW, Vacherot F, de Medina SG, Burchardt M, et al. Beta-catenin-related anomalies in apoptosis-resistant and hormone-refractory prostate cancer cells. Clin Cancer Res. 2003;9(5):1801–7.
24. Thiele S, Rauner M, Goettsch C, Rachner TD, Benad P, Fuessel S, et al. Expression profile of WNT molecules in prostate cancer and its regulation by aminobisphosphonates. J Cell Biochem. 2011;112(6):1593–600.
25. Katoh M. Frequent up-regulation of WNT2 in primary gastric cancer and colorectal cancer. Int J Oncol. 2001;19(5):1003–7.
26. Hall CL, Bafico A, Dai J, Aaronson SA, Keller ET. Prostate cancer cells promote osteoblastic bone metastases through Wnts. Cancer Res. 2005;65(17):7554–60.
27. Verras M, Brown J, Li X, Nusse R, Sun Z. Wnt3a growth factor induces androgen receptor-mediated transcription and enhances cell growth in human prostate cancer cells. Cancer Res. 2004;64(24):8860–6.
28. Yokoyama NN, Shao S, Hoang BH, Mercola D, Zi X. Wnt signaling in castration-resistant prostate cancer: implications for therapy. Am J Clin Exp Urol. 2014;2(1):27–44.
29. Zhao S, Ye X, Xiao L, Lian X, Feng Y, Li F, et al. MiR-26a inhibits prostate cancer progression by repression of Wnt5a. Tumour Biol. 2014;35(10):9725–33.
30. Sandsmark E, Hansen AF, Selnæs KM, Bertilsson H, Bofin AM, Wright AJ, et al. A novel non-canonical Wnt signature for prostate cancer aggressiveness. Oncotarget. 2017;8(6):9572–86.
31. Zhu H, Mazor M, Kawano Y, Walker MM, Leung HY, Armstrong K, et al. Analysis of Wnt gene expression in prostate cancer: mutual inhibition by WNT11 and the androgen receptor. Cancer Res. 2004;64(21):7918–26.
32. Madueke I, Hu WY, Hu D, Swanson SM, Vander Griend D, Abern M, et al. The role of WNT10B in normal prostate gland development and prostate cancer. Prostate. 2019;79(14):1692–704.
33. Schneider JA, Logan SK. Revisiting the role of Wnt/β-catenin signaling in prostate cancer. Mol Cell Endocrinol. 2018;462(Pt A):3–8.
34. Nikolskii AA, Shilovskiy IP, Barvinskaia ED, Korneev AV, Sundukova MS, Khaitov MR. Role of STAT3 transcription factor in pathogenesis of bronchial asthma. Biochemistry (Mosc). 2021;86(11):1489–501.
35. Hillmer EJ, Zhang H, Li HS, Watowich SS. STAT3 signaling in immunity. Cytokine Growth Factor Rev. 2016;31:1–15.
36. Chen Q, Lv J, Yang W, Xu B, Wang Z, Yu Z, et al. Targeted inhibition of STAT3 as a potential treatment strategy for atherosclerosis. Theranostics. 2019;9(22):6424–42.
37. Garg M, Shanmugam MK, Bhardwaj V, Goel A, Gupta R, Sharma A, et al. The pleiotropic role of transcription factor STAT3 in oncogenesis and its targeting through natural products for cancer prevention and therapy. Med Res Rev. 2020;
38. Szelag M, Piaszyk-Borychowska A, Plens-Galaska M, Wesoly J, Bluyssen HA. Targeted inhibition of STATs and IRFs as a potential treatment strategy in cardiovascular disease. Oncotarget. 2016;7(30):48788–812.
39. Yang R, Song Y, Shakoor K, Yi W, Peng C, Liu S. Insights into the role of STAT3 in intrahepatic cholangiocarcinoma (Review). Mol Med Rep. 2022;25(5):171.

40. Chalikonda G, Lee H, Sheik A, Huh YS. Targeting key transcriptional factor STAT3 in colorectal cancer. Mol Cell Biochem. 2021;476(9):3219–28.
41. Ashrafizadeh M, Gholami MH, Mirzaei S, Zabolian A, Haddadi A, Farahani MV, et al. Dual relationship between long non-coding RNAs and STAT3 signaling in different cancers: new insight to proliferation and metastasis. Life Sci. 2021;270:119006.
42. Hussain Y, Mirzaei S, Ashrafizadeh M, Zarrabi A, Hushmandi K, Khan H, et al. Quercetin and its nano-scale delivery systems in prostate cancer therapy: paving the way for cancer elimination and reversing chemoresistance. Cancers (Basel). 2021;13(7):1602.
43. Geethadevi A, Nair A, Parashar D, Ku Z, Xiong W, Deng H, et al. Oncostatin M receptor-targeted antibodies suppress STAT3 signaling and inhibit ovarian cancer growth. Cancer Res. 2021;81(20):5336–52.
44. Xiong W, Chen Y, Zhang C, Li J, Huang H, Zhu Y, et al. Pharmacologic inhibition of IL11/STAT3 signaling increases MHC-I expression and T cell infiltration. J Transl Med. 2023;21(1):416.
45. Zhi L, Zhao L, Zhang X, Liu W, Gao B, Wang F, et al. SLCO1B3 promotes colorectal cancer tumorigenesis and metastasis through STAT3. Aging (Albany NY). 2021;13(18):22164–75.
46. Li M, Chen X, Wang X, Wei X, Wang D, Liu X, et al. RSL3 enhances the antitumor effect of cisplatin on prostate cancer cells via causing glycolysis dysfunction. Biochem Pharmacol. 2021;192:114741.
47. Huang X, Fang J, Lai W, Hu Y, Li L, Zhong Y, et al. IL-6/STAT3 axis activates Glut5 to regulate fructose metabolism and tumorigenesis. Int J Biol Sci. 2022;18(9):3668–75.
48. Sadrkhanloo M, Paskeh MDA, Hashemi M, Raesi R, Motahhary M, Saghari S, et al. STAT3 signaling in prostate cancer progression and therapy resistance: an oncogenic pathway with diverse functions. Biomed Pharmacother. 2023;158:114168.
49. Jung YY, Ko JH, Um JY, Chinnathambi A, Alharbi SA, Sethi G, et al. LDL cholesterol promotes the proliferation of prostate and pancreatic cancer cells by activating the STAT3 pathway. J Cell Physiol. 2021;236(7):5253–64.
50. Philp LK, Rockstroh A, Sadowski MC, Taherian Fard A, Lehman M, Tevz G, et al. Leptin antagonism inhibits prostate cancer xenograft growth and progression. Endocr Relat Cancer. 2021;28(5):353–75.
51. Burton AJ, Gilbert R, Tilling K, Langdon R, Donovan JL, Holly JMP, et al. Circulating adiponectin and leptin and risk of overall and aggressive prostate cancer: a systematic review and meta-analysis. Sci Rep. 2021;11(1):320.
52. Gorrab A, Pagano A, Ayed K, Chebil M, Derouiche A, Kovacic H, et al. Leptin promotes prostate cancer proliferation and migration by stimulating STAT3 pathway. Nutr Cancer. 2021;73(7):1217–27.
53. Chen X, Zhou J, Li X, Wang X, Lin Y, Wang X. Exosomes derived from hypoxic epithelial ovarian cancer cells deliver microRNAs to macrophages and elicit a tumor-promoted phenotype. Cancer Lett. 2018;435:80–91.
54. Tang X, Mo C, Wang Y, Wei D, Xiao H. Anti-tumour strategies aiming to target tumour-associated macrophages. Immunology. 2013;138(2):93–104.
55. Binnemars-Postma K, Storm G, Prakash J. Nanomedicine strategies to target tumor-associated macrophages. Int J Mol Sci. 2017;18(5):979.
56. Anfray C, Ummarino A, Andón FT, Allavena P. Current strategies to target tumor-associated-macrophages to improve anti-tumor immune responses. Cells. 2019;9(1):46.
57. Tian X, Wu Y, Yang Y, Wang J, Niu M, Gao S, et al. Long noncoding RNA LINC00662 promotes M2 macrophage polarization and hepatocellular carcinoma progression via activating Wnt/β-catenin signaling. Mol Oncol. 2020;14(2):462–83.
58. Jiang H, Deng W, Zhu K, Zeng Z, Hu B, Zhou Z, et al. LINC00467 promotes prostate cancer progression via M2 macrophage polarization and the miR-494-3p/STAT3 Axis. Front Oncol. 2021;11:661431.

59. Tan B, Chen X, Fan Y, Yang Y, Yang J, Tan L. STAT3 phosphorylation is required for the HepaCAM-mediated inhibition of castration-resistant prostate cancer cell viability and metastasis. Prostate. 2021;81(9):603–11.
60. Guo Y, Zang Y, Lv L, Cai F, Qian T, Zhang G, et al. IL-8 promotes proliferation and inhibition of apoptosis via STAT3/AKT/NF-κB pathway in prostate cancer. Mol Med Rep. 2017;16(6):9035–42.
61. Mirzaei S, Paskeh MDA, Okina E, Gholami MH, Hushmandi K, Hashemi M, et al. Molecular landscape of LncRNAs in prostate cancer: a focus on pathways and therapeutic targets for intervention. J Exp Clin Cancer Res. 2022;41(1):214.
62. Xing Z, Li S, Liu Z, Zhang C, Meng M, Bai Z. The long non-coding RNA LINC00473 contributes to cell proliferation via JAK-STAT3 signaling pathway by regulating miR-195-5p/SEPT2 axis in prostate cancer. Biosci Rep. 2020;40(9):BSR20191850.
63. Liu C, Lin P, Zhao J, Xie H, Li R, Yang X, et al. Knockdown of long noncoding RNA AC245100.4 inhibits the tumorigenesis of prostate cancer cells via the STAT3/NR4A3 axis. Epigenomics. 2021;13(20):1591–605.
64. Wei X, Hou Y, Zhang Y, Zhang H, Sun Z, Meng X, et al. Long non-coding RNA MAGI2-AS3 inactivates STAT3 pathway to inhibit prostate cancer cell proliferation via acting as a microRNA-424-5p sponge. J Cancer. 2022;13(1):343–53.
65. Ma J-B, Bai J-Y, Zhang H-B, Jia J, Shi Q, Yang C, et al. KLF5 inhibits STAT3 activity and tumor metastasis in prostate cancer by suppressing IGF1 transcription cooperatively with HDAC1. Cell Death Dis. 2020;11(6):466.
66. Sikka S, Shanmugam MK, Siveen KS, Ong TH, Yang MH, Lee JH, et al. Diosgenin attenuates tumor growth and metastasis in transgenic prostate cancer mouse model by negatively regulating both NF-κB/STAT3 signaling cascades. Eur J Pharmacol. 2021;906:174274.
67. Cho KH, Choi MJ, Jeong KJ, Kim JJ, Hwang MH, Shin SC, et al. A ROS/STAT3/HIF-1α signaling cascade mediates EGF-induced TWIST1 expression and prostate cancer cell invasion. Prostate. 2014;74(5):528–36.
68. Grant WB. Vitamin D may reduce prostate cancer metastasis by several mechanisms including blocking Stat3. Am J Pathol. 2008;173(5):1589–90.
69. Tong D, Liu Q, Liu G, Xu J, Lan W, Jiang Y, et al. Metformin inhibits castration-induced EMT in prostate cancer by repressing COX2/PGE2/STAT3 axis. Cancer Lett. 2017;389:23–32.
70. Babaei G, Khadem Ansari MH, Aziz SG, Bazl MR. Alantolactone inhibits stem-like cell phenotype, chemoresistance and metastasis in PC3 cells through STAT3 signaling pathway. Res Pharm Sci. 2020;15(6):551–62.
71. Vanharanta S, Massagué J. Origins of metastatic traits. Cancer Cell. 2013;24(4):410–21.
72. Jacob LS, Vanharanta S, Obenauf AC, Pirun M, Viale A, Socci ND, et al. Metastatic competence can emerge with selection of preexisting oncogenic alleles without a need of new mutations. Cancer Res. 2015;75(18):3713–9.
73. Malanchi I, Santamaria-Martínez A, Susanto E, Peng H, Lehr HA, Delaloye JF, et al. Interactions between cancer stem cells and their niche govern metastatic colonization. Nature. 2011;481(7379):85–9.
74. Kim SJ, Garcia-Recio S, Creighton CJ, Perou CM, Rosen JM. Alterations in Wnt- and/or STAT3 signaling pathways and the immune microenvironment during metastatic progression. Oncogene. 2019;38(31):5942–58.
75. Koushyar S, Meniel VS, Phesse TJ, Pearson HB. Exploring the Wnt pathway as a therapeutic target for prostate cancer. Biomol Ther. 2022;12(2):309.
76. Kim SJ, Kang HG, Kim K, Kim H, Zetterberg F, Park YS, et al. Crosstalk between WNT and STAT3 is mediated by galectin-3 in tumor progression. Gastric Cancer. 2021;24(5):1050–62.
77. Han Z, Wang X, Ma L, Chen L, Xiao M, Huang L, et al. Inhibition of STAT3 signaling targets both tumor-initiating and differentiated cell populations in prostate cancer. Oncotarget. 2014;5(18):8416–28.
78. Bishop JL, Thaper D, Zoubeidi A. The multifaceted roles of STAT3 signaling in the progression of prostate cancer. Cancers (Basel). 2014;6(2):829–59.

79. Murillo-Garzón V, Kypta R. WNT signalling in prostate cancer. Nat Rev Urol. 2017;14(11):683–96.
80. Zou S, Tong Q, Liu B, Huang W, Tian Y, Fu X. Targeting STAT3 in cancer immunotherapy. Mol Cancer. 2020;19(1):145.

Chapter 7
Prostate Cancer and EZH2 Signaling

Mohammed Kavei, Siavash Seifollahy Fakhr, Afsaneh Mousaei, Bita Ghaffari, Nazanin Fatemeh Fadavinia, Tara Noroozi Yeganeh, Nasim Ebrahimi, Mostafa Haji-Fatahaliha, and Amir Reza Aref

Abstract Enhancer of zeste homolog 2 (EZH2), a member of the Polycomb group (PcG) proteins, functions as a fundamental component of the polycomb repressive complex 2 (PRC2), with two other core subunits. The enzyme has histone methyl-

---

M. Kavei
Department of Biology, Faculty of Science, Arak University, Arak, Iran

S. S. Fakhr
Department of Biotechnology, Faculty of Applied Ecology, Agricultural Science and Biotechnology, Campus Hamar, Inland Norway University of Applied Sciences, Hamar, Norway

A. Mousaei
Department of Biology, College of Science, Qaemshahr Branch, Islamic Azad University, Qaem Shahr, Mazandaran, Iran

B. Ghaffari
Department of Cell and Molecular Biology, Faculty of Science, Kharazmi University, Karaj, Iran

N. F. Fadavinia
Department of Basic Sciences, Garmsar Branch, Islamic Azad University, Garmsar, Iran

T. N. Yeganeh
Medical Genomics Research Center, Tehran Medical Sciences Islamic Azad University, Tehran, Iran

N. Ebrahimi (✉)
Genetics Division, Department of Cell and Molecular Biology and Microbiology, Faculty of Science and Technology, University of Isfahan, Isfahan, Iran

M. Haji-Fatahaliha
Department of Immunology, Faculty of Medicine, Tabriz University of Medical Sciences, Tabriz, Iran

A. R. Aref (✉)
Mass General Cancer Center, Department of Surgery, Massachusetts General Hospital, Harvard Medical School, Boston, MA, USA

Broad Institute of MIT and Harvard, Harvard Medical School, Cambridge, MA, USA
e-mail: aaref@mgh.harvard.edu

G. Sethi et al. (eds.), *Prostate Cancer: Molecular Events and Therapeutic Modalities*, https://doi.org/10.1007/978-981-97-4612-5_7

transferase (MTase) activity, which selectively facilitates the methylation of histone 3 lysine 27 (H3K27) on promoters of target genes. PRC2 functions as epigenetic silencers that have considerable importance in maintaining cellular identity and preserving the pluripotency of embryonic stem cells. Over the course of the last 20 years, a growing body of data has provided support for the presence of mutations in the EZH2 gene and/or its upregulation in several hematological malignancies and solid tumors, particularly prostate cancer. Moreover, EZH2 is known as one of the most increased genes in neuroendocrine prostate tumors, which exhibit increased abundance as a result of the therapeutic administration of high-affinity inhibitors targeting the androgen receptor system. Numerous studies have shown the epigenetic roles of EZH2 in the silencing of tumor suppressor factors and the facilitation of carcinogenesis. However, there have been reports of inconsistencies between EZH2 and H3K27 methylation. Moreover, the effectiveness of enzyme inhibitors targeting EZH2 in prostate cancer has been demonstrated to have constraints, highlighting the need for a more thorough understanding of the many activities of EZH2. In this chapter, we will begin by examining the regulatory mechanisms that govern the classical activities of EZH2 as a histone methyltransferase (MTase). Additionally, we will provide an overview of the multiple mechanisms engaged in bringing the PRC2 to the chromatin. Furthermore, in this chapter, we provide a comprehensive overview of other substrates of EZH2 that are not histones. Additionally, we examine the impact of post-translational changes on EZH2, which may influence its substrate selectivity. In conclusion, we provide a summary of the additional roles of EZH2 that go beyond its role as an MTase and/or a component of the PRC2. Specifically, we highlight its involvement as a transcriptional cofactor and explore the potential for therapeutic targeting of EZH2 in the context of prostate cancer.

Keywords Androgen receptor · Neuroendocrine prostate cancer · Post-translational modifications · Polycomb repressive complex · Epigenetic regulation

7.1 Introduction

Transcription and its regulation represent pivotal processes determining cellular fate, and it is evident that disruptions in the factors involved in transcription participate in the progression of cancer. Genetic or epigenetic alterations in transcription result in the onset and advancement of cancer. Enhancer of zeste homolog 2 (EZH2), a crucial member of the Polycomb group (PcG) gene family due to its determinative role in transcriptional repression, holds particular significance in cancer-related studies. The polycomb repressive complex 2 (PRC2) is a nuclear protein complex of PcG that silences transcription and gene expression through chromatin structure modulation [1]. Within this complex, EZH2 acts as the catalytic subunit, resulting in trimethylation of Lys-27 on histone 3 (H3K27me3) [1, 2]. This epigenetic alteration modifies chromatin structure, leading to suppression of gene transcription. In general, the process of H3K27me3 represents a highly critical and determinant epigenetic event in the fate of stem cells and tissue development [3].

One of the additional roles of PRC2 includes the methylation of non-histone proteins such as the transcription factor GATA binding protein 4 (GATA4) [4]. It is noteworthy that EZH2 can also independently interact with other proteins and participate in the activation of downstream genes or methylation of non-histone targets apart from PRC2 [5–7]. As mentioned earlier, EZH2 orchestrates the regulation of autophagy, apoptosis [8], and cell cycle progression [9]. Additionally, it is involved in DNA repair, cell senescence inhibition [10], cellular lineage determination, and signaling pathway modulation [11]. Thus, the diverse roles of EZH2 in various cellular processes are associated with many cancers, including prostate cancer [12].

Given the significant role of EZH2 in cancer, it has garnered attention as a target for targeted therapies and novel treatment strategies. This chapter delves into the role of EZH2 in the initiation and progression of prostate cancer, metastasis, drug resistance, and immune regulation, in addition to its potential as a therapeutic target in emerging approaches, such as EZH2 methyltransferase (MTase) activity inhibitors, EZH2 degradation inducers, and combination therapies with other treatment modalities.

7.2 An Overview of EZH2

7.2.1 The Structure of EZH2

The EZH2 gene consists of 20 exons, ultimately encoding a 746 amino acid protein, located at position 7q35 [13]. The EZH2 protein is composed of five domains, namely Domain I, II, EED-interaction domain (EID), C-terminal suppressor of variegation 39, enhancer of zeste and trithorax domain ([su(var)3-9, enhancer-of-zeste and trithorax] SET domain), and cysteine-rich domain (CXC domain) [2, 14]. The SET domain is predominantly essential for the histone methyltransferase activity of EZH2. The N-terminal domains serve as the primary sites for protein-protein interactions, contributing to the assembly of partner subunits and the proper function of PRC2 [2].

7.2.2 EZH2 Action Modes

With the help of its SET domain, EZH2 primarily functions as a histone methyltransferase, and in either a PRC2-dependent or independent manner, it may co-activate or inhibit transcription.

Contrary to the previous notion of histones solely acting as packaging proteins in the nucleosome core, histones establish dynamic interactions between DNA and other cellular components. Histone modifications and alterations lead to changes in chromosome structure and the positioning or exposure of target sequences to transcription factors, ultimately resulting in the activation or repression of target genes. The cellular enzyme, which catalyzes histone modification, may transmit the data it contains to the chromosomal regulator, which ultimately results in a change in the expression of genes [15].

As previously mentioned, PRC2, through its EZH2 subunit, leads to the trimethylation of H3K27, resulting in the formation of H3K27me3 within the nucleus. At this stage, PRC1 interacts with H3K27me3 and monoubiquitinates histone H2A at lysine 119. In this state, chromatin compaction increases, and the transcription of downstream genes is repressed [16]. One of the important downstream genes in this pathway is p21, known as a key tumor suppressor gene. This gene inhibits the function of cell cycle CDKs (cyclin-dependent kinases). During its activity, EZH2 binds to the p21 promoter and, through the modulation of H3K27me3, suppresses the transcription of the p21 gene, thereby enhancing the cell cycle and cell proliferation [17]. In some cases, EZH2, in association with PRC2, can methylate non-histone proteins. The cardiac transcription factor GATA4 is usually methylated at lysine 299 by the telomerase activity of EZH2. As a result, the acetylation of GATA4 through p300 is reduced, leading to the repression of GATA4 expression [4].

EZH2 can also independently activate downstream genes through direct methylation of non-histone proteins, even in the absence of PRC2. For instance, EZH2 can activate STAT3 by methylating its sequence. However, for this process to occur, EZH2 needs to be phosphorylated, which is carried out by AKT (or protein kinase B (PKB)) at serine 21 [5]. The role of EZH2 in gene activation, independent of PRC2, was first reported in castration-resistant prostate cancer. It was revealed that phosphorylated EZH2 leads to increased expression of the androgen receptor (AR) transcription factor through a methylation-dependent mechanism. Ultimately, AR activation results in the upregulation of downstream genes and promotes the proliferation of cancer cells [6]. The most recent research, however, showed that EZH2 might function non-catalytically in castration-resistant prostate cancer cells in a manner that was independent of PRC2 and methylation. By occupying the AR gene's promoter, EZH2 could directly trigger transcription of the gene, which was unaffected by a compound that inhibits the enzyme EZH2 [7].

7.3 EZH2 Involvement in Cancer Progression

Various members of the PcG family, such as EZH2, have significant influences on cancer progression [18]. As previously mentioned, EZH2 regulates the expression of downstream genes and proteins through both PRC2-dependent and PRC2-independent mechanisms involving methylation. These are the fundamental ways by which it operates and exhibits the numerous roles previously indicated. However, aberrant expression, such as overexpression, downregulation, and expression loss, as well as mutations, are linked to the onset, spread, and metastasis of cancer. Numerous pieces of evidence have demonstrated a significant role for EZH2 in various cancer processes [19]. Interestingly, while many studies have shown its oncogenic role in different cancers, such as breast cancer, gastric cancer, thyroid carcinoma, and endometrial carcinoma, some research has reported a tumor suppressor role for EZH2.

Additionally, an in vivo investigation supports the significance of EZH2 in the spread of cancer cells [20]. While melanoma-positive lymph nodes and distant lung metastases often arise in control melanoma model mice, these conditions are significantly reduced and almost absent in EZH2 conditional knockout mice [21]. The earliest and crucial step in cell invasion and metastasis is the epithelial-mesenchymal transition (EMT). Exogenous EZH2 overexpression increased mesenchymal marker Vimentin expression while decreasing epithelial marker E-cadherin level in an experiment with pancreatic cancer cells, whereas EZH2 knockdown decreased Vimentin expression while increasing E-cadherin expression [22]. These findings demonstrated EZH2's potential to induce EMT in pancreatic cancer cells. A significant factor in tumor metastasis is tumor angiogenesis, and EZH2 is a crucial factor for this process regulation. The activation of vascular endothelial growth factor (VEGF) via a paracrine circuit which stimulates angiogenesis by methylating and silencing vasohibin1 is directly responsible for the rise in endothelial EZH2 [23].

7.4 EZH2 and Prostate Cancer Progression

Recent investigations have demonstrated that the expression of EZH2 significantly increases in aggressive prostate cancer, thus playing a crucial role in the progression of prostate cancer. Inhibition or reduction of EZH2 expression leads to cell cycle arrest. Furthermore, it induces reduced invasiveness and cellular proliferation under laboratory conditions. Additionally, its downregulation can halt tumor growth within the body [24–28]. Based on the aforementioned, the oncogenic behaviors of EZH2 are due to its epigenetic silencing of tumor suppressor genes [29]. Moreover, studies have indicated that EZH2 has non-histone substrates, including forkhead box A1 (FOXA1) [30]. EZH2 leads to the methylation of FOXA1, resulting in the recruitment of deubiquitinase and prevention of FOXA1 degradation, thereby increasing the protein level of FOXA1 in the cell. Elevated expression of both FOXA1 and EZH2 is correlated to poor prognosis in patients with prostate cancer. Furthermore, FOXA1 overexpression makes PCa cells more vulnerable to EZH2 MTase inhibitors that prevent FOXA1 protein degradation. These enzymatic EZH2 inhibitors' growth-inhibitory effects may be reversed by re-expressing FOXA1. However, the effectiveness of these enzymatic EZH2 inhibitors in prostate cancer is often considerably less than what is observed in hematologic malignancies, pointing to the presence of essential EZH2 target genes that are resistant to PRC2 MTase activity [31]. EZH2 demonstrates an oncogenic activity in polycomb-independent and androgen-refractory prostate cancer cell lines, involving EZH2's capacity to operate as an androgen receptor activator [6].

The operational role of the androgen receptor's activation depends on the phosphorylation of EZH2. Additionally, the presence of the intact methyltransferase domain is essential for this functionality [7]. It has recently been revealed that EZH2 directly associates with the androgen receptor promoter, enhancing its expression through increased and strengthened transcriptional induction. Therefore, it can be stated that EZH2 leads to heightened androgen receptor transcription in prostate cancer cell lines, amplifying its signaling and conferring resistance of cancer cells to enzymatic EZH2 inhibitors. Structural analysis of EZH2 has uncovered a disordered domain bearing significant resemblance to the transcriptional activator domain of the p53 protein, suggesting a potentially pivotal role in the inducible gene expression of EZH2 [32]. While the aforementioned function of EZH2 operates independently of PRC2, in some instances, a small fraction of PRC2 also contributes to gene silencing by EZH2. This alignment is congruent with the established role of EZH2 in the repression of growth regulators and enhancement of stemness attributes [29]. Therefore, it has been established that the androgen receptor level in prostate cancer cells marginally increases as a consequence of enzymatic EZH2 inhibition [7]. However, following EZH2 knockdown, the total androgen receptor protein level decreases, indicating the predominant role of EZH2 in androgen receptor transcriptional activation is epigenetic in nature at the androgen receptor promoter. These findings call for the creation of EZH2-degrading substances that will not only eliminate EZH2's epigenetic activity but also its PRC2-independent function in activating androgen receptor [33]. Although the utilization of androgen receptor pathway inhibitors (ARPIs), including enzalutamide, has witnessed an increased inclination toward combinatorial approaches, approximately one-fifth of prostate cancer patients encounter treatment-induced neuroendocrine prostate cancer (NEPC). In these patients, androgen receptor expression is suppressed, rendering NEPC essentially refractory to intervention. Resistance to all forms of hormonal therapies and the loss of neuroendocrine differentiating features within NEPC tumors are prevalent. Neuroendocrine markers such as chromogranin A, neuron-specific enolase (NSE), CD56, and synaptophysin are employed for characterizing these tumors [34, 35].

In general, the overall median survival of patients diagnosed with NEPC is estimated to be less than 1 year [36–38]. The compromised clinical outcomes of NEPC patients have been attributed to the upregulation of genes involved in cell cycle dysregulation and uncontrolled cellular proliferation [39]. Data analysis from RNA-seq has revealed a significantly higher expression of EZH2 in NEPC tumors compared to castration-resistant prostate cancer (CRPC) tumors [40, 41]. Comparative genotyping of patient-derived xenografts with prostate tumors and NEPC models demonstrated substantial genetic distinctions. For instance, the tumor suppressor gene Retinoblastoma (Rb) was found to be absent in NEPC patients [42]. Additionally, mutations leading to the functional loss of p53 and Rb1 contribute to the development of NEPC in genetically engineered mice [43, 44]. Forty percent of NEPC tumors have increased N-Myc proto-oncogene (MYCN) gene, which produces the N-Myc protein, in contrast to 5% of prostate adenocarcinoma tumors [40]. Therefore, it has become evident that the elevated expression level of MYCN is significantly associated with the occurrence of NEPC tumors compared to CRPC. EZH2, serving as a chromatin regulator, exhibits a distinct expression pattern in NEPC in contrast to CRPC, indicating the epigenetic nature of neuroendocrine differentiation (NED). Furthermore, it was shown that the suppressed genes in NEPC mouse models had a higher concentration of PRC2 target genes and were linked to unfavorable outcomes [41]. This implies that the overexpression of EZH2 has a functional importance in this context. The N-Myc-downregulated genes in the MYCN-driven NEPC models have a notable enrichment of epigenetic targets associated with EZH2/PRC2 [45, 46]. Based on the acquired evidence, N-Myc interacts with SUZ12 polycomb repressive complex 2 subunit (SUZ12) and EZH2, altering the activity pathway of PRC2 to suppress androgen receptor signaling and thereby contributing to the emergence of NED. It is worth noting that an increase in the expression of EZH2 has been found in tumors that originate from prostate basal cells with overexpression of N-Myc and myrAKT1 [6, 47]. Moreover, the upregulation of EZH2 in NEPC tumors was confirmed in a more extensive collection of patient tumors and in organoids obtained from needle biopsies of metastatic lesions originating from end-stage prostate cancer patients [48, 49]. The endeavor to comprehend the molecular functioning of EZH2 in NEPC tumors has been pursued through various studies. An intriguing observation lies in the concurrent elevation of H3K27me3 alongside overexpression of EZH2 in NEPC tumors, indicating the epigenetic regulatory role of EZH2 in these tumors. One direct objective of EZH2 in NEPC tumors, subject to epigenetic silencing, is the inhibition of a pro-angiogenic inhibitor known as thrombospondin 1 (TSP1), as the reduction in TSP1 expression correlates with heightened EZH2 markers and NED [50, 51]. Given the more pronounced role of EZH2 in NEPC models compared to CRPC tumors, enzymatic EZH2 inhibitors exhibit improved efficacy in NEPC tumors [48]. Nevertheless, in order to achieve a 50% growth inhibition, the therapy still requires the administration of large dosages of the inhibitors, roughly 5 μM. This observation implies that methylation-independent PRC2 activities may play a significant part in the process. Notably, several studies have shown a clear association between the androgen receptor and EZH2-mediated epigenetic suppression in NEPC cells lacking the androgen receptor. Furthermore, it has been indicated that utilizing EZH2 inhibitors reinstates the transcription of the androgen receptor [52, 53]. While the reduction of EZH2 and its enzymatic inhibitors elicit contrasting effects in androgen receptor-positive cells, both of these alterations lead to an increase in androgen receptor levels within NEPC cells. It appears that as prostate cancer progresses to NEPC, the role of androgen receptor activation mediated by EZH2 diminishes, which could contribute to the emergence of the AR-negative nature of NEPC cells. However, recent findings indicate that EZH2 inhibitors have the potential to restore the sensitivity of NEPC cells to ARPI, hence confirming the rationale for their combined administration. The concurrent administration of GSK503 and enzalutamide had a synergistic impact on the inhibition of tumor development in post-castration double knockout (DKO) models with Pten and Rb1 deletion [7].

Given the rising prevalence of NEPC tumors in the field, there is a pressing need for enhanced treatment approaches. Notably, the overexpression of EZH2 in NEPC tumors presents an opportunity to promptly integrate these improved therapies into clinical practice. While the majority of research has shown that the main function of

EZH2 in NEPC is epigenetic, there is at least one study that has shown a different role [7]. This work has proven that the function of EZH2 may be shifted from modifying H3K27 to modifying a non-histone substrate called STAT3. In this case, the methylation of STAT3 by EZH2 enhances neuroendocrine differentiation in NEPC induced by enzalutamide [54, 55]. The divergent mechanistic findings described in this study highlight the need for additional investigation into the functions of EZH2. Specifically, it is important to define the non-histone substrates and interacting partners of EZH2 in NEPC. This knowledge will provide valuable guidance for the utilization of existing EZH2 inhibitors in combination treatments and will also contribute to the development of novel PRC2 inhibitors that can effectively block all functions of EZH2.

7.5 Therapeutic Effects of EZH2 in Cases of Prostate Cancer

Due to the high potential of small molecule inhibitors of EZH2, research and investigation into these matters, along with new therapeutic approaches including methods targeting EZH2 inhibition, have garnered significant attention in recent years [56]. Tazemetostat, also known by its trade name EPZ-6438, serves as an orally administered small molecule and represents the first inhibitor of EZH2 enzymatic activity to have obtained Food and Drug Administration (FDA) approval [57–59]. Given the prevalence of gain-of-function mutations in EZH2 in epithelioid sarcomas and follicular lymphomas, Tazemetostat received FDA approval for the treatment of these conditions in early 2020 [60]. Furthermore, this small molecule inhibitor is being utilized in laboratory studies for other solid tumors, including prostate tumors and various forms of lymphomas. DS-3201, also known as Valemetostat (commercial name), serves as a dual inhibitor of EZH1/2 and is utilized against both solid and hematologic tumors. This orally administered inhibitor exhibits a remarkably high level of specificity and is currently being employed in phase I/II clinical trials [61–63]. Other EZH2 inhibitor drugs that are applied for metastatic prostate cancer clinical trials are summarized in Table 7.1.

The exploration of protein breakdown has emerged as a potentially fruitful direction for the advancement of therapeutic interventions [64–66]. Currently, there are a minimum of two distinct proteolysis-targeting chimeras (PROTACs) in clinical development by Arvinas. These PROTACs are being investigated for their potential therapeutic efficacy in the management of prostate and breast cancer. As previously mentioned, EZH2 exhibits both histone and non-histone methylation activity, along with methylation-independent mechanisms that facilitate the development of cancer and cellular proliferation. While the inhibition of EZH2 would effectively suppress methylation activity, such as H3K27me3, the enzymatic inhibitors would have little impact on the non-canonical methylation-independent activities of EZH2. Therefore, the degradation of EZH2 may be a feasible strategy for addressing the non-canonical functions of EZH2 that are independent of methylation. In pursuit of this objective, a recent study documented the identification of the first specific inhibitor of EZH2

Table 7.1 Clinical studies of drugs targeting EZH2 in prostate cancer

Drug name	Status	Phase	Mechanism of action	NCT number
Tazemetostat/ Prednisone/ Abiraterone/ Enzalutamide	Recruiting	Phase I	EZH2 inhibitor in metastatic prostate cancer	NCT04179864
CPI-1205/Abiraterone/ Enzalutamide/ Prednisone	Recruiting	Phase I/II	EZH2 inhibitor in metastatic prostate cancer	NCT03480646
PF-06821497	Recruiting	Phase I	EZH2 inhibitor in metastatic prostate cancer and metastatic castration-resistant prostate cancer	NCT03460977
SHR3680/SHR2554	Recruiting	Phase I/II	EZH2 inhibitor in metastatic prostate cancer and metastatic castration-resistant prostate cancer	NCT03741712

[67]. The chemical MS1943, which was documented in 2020, has shown the ability to promote degradation of EZH2 in many cancer cell lines, including the PNT2 cell line, which is a non-malignant prostate cancer cell line [68]. The study revealed that the induction of apoptosis by MS1943 was attributed, in part, to the initiation of endoplasmic reticulum (ER) stress and the robust activation of the unfolded protein response (UPR) pathway. Given the current absence of enzymatic inhibitors targeting EZH2 in prostate cancer, drugs that degrade EZH2 have significant potential for future investigation [67].

In addition, Liap et al. explored the effects of inhibiting the activity of the methyltransferase EZH2 in prostate cancer treatment. EZH2 inhibitors are currently undergoing clinical trials for treating non-Hodgkin lymphomas characterized by EZH2 gain-of-function mutations [69, 70]. The study shows that these inhibitors block the EZH2 transactivation activity and inhibit the proliferation of CRPC cells. The research demonstrates that the expression of DNA damage response (DDR) genes in various kinds of solid tumors with normal types of EZH2 is remarkably associated with EZH2 reliance and higher sensitivity to EZH2 blockers. When CRPC cells are treated with EZH2 blockers, their sensitivity to genotoxic stress is dramatically enhanced. This reveals a previously unrecognized way in which EZH2 inhibitors function and provides a foundation for possible synergistic cancer treatment approaches [70].

Prostate cancers are categorized as immunologically "cold" tumors due to the limited number of patients exhibiting a positive reaction to checkpoint inhibitor (CPI) treatment. Recent findings have indicated that the presence of interferon-stimulated genes (ISGs) predicts a favorable response to checkpoint inhibitor treatment across various disease sites. The EZH2 is excessively expressed in prostate cancer and is known for its suppressive effect on interferon-stimulated genes [71]. In this current investigation, Morel et al. illustrated that inhibiting EZH2 in prostate cancer models triggers a stress response involving double-stranded

RNA–STING–ISG activation, leading to an increase in genes associated with antigen presentation, Th1 chemokine signaling, and interferon response [72, 73]. This includes the upregulation of programmed cell death protein 1 (PD-L1), which is reliant on stimulator of interferon genes (STING) activation. Consequently, EZH2 inhibition significantly enhances the migration of activated $CD8^+$ T cells within tumors and boosts the presence of M1 tumor-associated macrophages, effectively overturning resistance to PD-1 CPI treatment. Their research highlights EZH2's substantial role as a suppressor of anti-tumor immunity and its impact on the effectiveness of CPI treatment. These findings propose EZH2 inhibition as a viable therapeutic approach for augmenting the response of prostate cancer to PD-1 CPI treatment [74].

CRPC arises subsequent to androgen deprivation therapy and persists as an untreatable condition owing to the absence of efficacious treatment regimens [75]. The administration of enzalutamide, a second-generation antagonist of the androgen receptor, provides a primary therapeutic effect but is thereafter met with the development of drug resistance and the recurrence of tumors [76]. The enhancer of EZH2 plays a significant role as a coactivator in the inhibition of androgen receptor-mediated gene expression, and its carcinogenic activity is known to escalate under conditions of castration. There exists a hypothesis suggesting that the simultaneous targeting of EZH2 and androgen receptor may provide significant efficacy in the treatment of CRPC [77, 78]. The objective of Shankar et al.'s research was to evaluate the efficacy of a combination therapy using the EZH2 inhibitor GSK126 and the antiandrogen enzalutamide in the treatment of CRPC cells. The co-administration of GSK126 and enzalutamide showed a synergistic effect in suppressing cell proliferation, inducing cell cycle arrest, and significantly enhancing cell death in 22Rv1 and C4–2B CRPC cells. The combination treatment demonstrated a notable reduction in the expression of androgen receptor and androgen receptor-v7, a declination in prostate-specific antigen (PSA) and protein kinase B (AKT) activity, a decrease in EZH2 and other members of the PRC2 complex (SUZ12 and EED), along with a simultaneous loss of H3K27 trimethylation and dissociation between androgen receptor and PRC2 complex members, as compared to the individual treatment. This work offers preclinical evidence to support the notion that the combination administration of an EZH2 inhibitor and an androgen receptor antagonist yields synergistic anticancer effects, thereby presenting novel therapeutic prospects for the treatment of CRPC tumors [79].

7.6 Future Perspective and Conclusion

In this, we have examined the activities of EZH2, including its histone and non-histone substrates. Furthermore, it has been demonstrated that EZH2 can function independently of the PRC2 complex in certain non-catalytic activities. Additionally, we have investigated the role of EZH2 in the progression of prostate cancer. In brief, EZH2 serves as an epigenetic modulator that exhibits robust and enduring upregulation in both clinical specimens and murine models of aggressive prostate cancer, including CRPC and NEPC. EZH2 has been well recognized as a crucial factor in the process of epigenetic reprogramming and lineage plasticity of neuroendocrine prostate cancer cells. Furthermore, it has been shown that a significant number of PRC2-target genes experience dysregulation in neuroendocrine prostate cancer. Nevertheless, the current enzymatic inhibitors targeting EZH2 have shown little efficacy in treating NEPC, a subtype characterized by the absence of androgen receptor expression. This implies that there may be other non-epigenetic targets of EZH2 that play a significant role in neuroendocrine prostate cancer pathogenesis. The aforementioned discoveries serve as a catalyst for future research endeavors aimed at discovering non-histone substrates of EZH2 and elucidating the non-epigenetic functions of EZH2 in prostate cancer, particularly in the context of NEPC, where its expression is significantly elevated. A comprehensive comprehension of this knowledge will play a crucial role in providing guidance for the utilization of catalytic inhibitors of EZH2 in combination therapy regimens, as well as in the advancement of innovative strategies to efficiently target EZH2 in advanced stages of prostate cancer.

References

1. Pasini D, Di Croce L. Emerging roles for polycomb proteins in cancer. Curr Opin Genet Dev. 2016;36:50–8.
2. Simon JA, Lange CA. Roles of the EZH2 histone methyltransferase in cancer epigenetics. Mutat Res. 2008;647(1–2):21–9.
3. Yin X, Yang S, Zhang M, Yue Y. The role and prospect of JMJD3 in stem cells and cancer. Biomed Pharmacother. 2019;118:109384.
4. He A, Shen X, Ma Q, Cao J, von Gise A, Zhou P, et al. PRC2 directly methylates GATA4 and represses its transcriptional activity. Genes Dev. 2012;26(1):37–42.
5. Kim E, Kim M, Woo DH, Shin Y, Shin J, Chang N, et al. Phosphorylation of EZH2 activates STAT3 signaling via STAT3 methylation and promotes tumorigenicity of glioblastoma stem-like cells. Cancer Cell. 2013;23(6):839–52.
6. Xu K, Wu ZJ, Groner AC, He HH, Cai C, Lis RT, et al. EZH2 oncogenic activity in castration-resistant prostate cancer cells is polycomb-independent. Science. 2012;338(6113):1465–9.
7. Kim J, Lee Y, Lu X, Song B, Fong KW, Cao Q, et al. Polycomb- and methylation-independent roles of EZH2 as a transcription activator. Cell Rep. 2018;25(10):2808–20.e4.
8. Yao Y, Hu H, Yang Y, Zhou G, Shang Z, Yang X, et al. Downregulation of Enhancer of Zeste Homolog 2 (EZH2) is essential for the induction of autophagy and apoptosis in colorectal cancer cells. Genes (Basel). 2016;7(10):83.
9. Nutt SL, Keenan C, Chopin M, Allan RS. EZH2 function in immune cell development. Biol Chem. 2020;401(8):933–43.
10. Ito T, Teo YV, Evans SA, Neretti N, Sedivy JM. Regulation of cellular senescence by polycomb chromatin modifiers through distinct DNA damage- and histone methylation-dependent pathways. Cell Rep. 2018;22(13):3480–92.
11. Batool A, Jin C, Liu YX. Role of EZH2 in cell lineage determination and relative signaling pathways. Front Biosci (Landmark Ed). 2019;24(5):947–60.
12. Yuan H, Han Y, Wang X, Li N, Liu Q, Yin Y, et al. SETD2 restricts prostate cancer metastasis by integrating EZH2 and AMPK signaling pathways. Cancer Cell. 2020;38(3):350–65.e7.

13. Cardoso C, Mignon C, Hetet G, Grandchamps B, Fontes M, Colleaux L. The human EZH2 gene: genomic organisation and revised mapping in 7q35 within the critical region for malignant myeloid disorders. Eur J Hum Genet. 2000;8(3):174–80.
14. Laible G, Wolf A, Dorn R, Reuter G, Nislow C, Lebersorger A, et al. Mammalian homologues of the polycomb-group gene enhancer of zeste mediate gene silencing in Drosophila heterochromatin and at S. cerevisiae telomeres. EMBO J. 1997;16(11):3219–32.
15. Wang R, Xin M, Li Y, Zhang P, Zhang M. The functions of histone modification enzymes in cancer. Curr Protein Pept Sci. 2016;17(5):438–45.
16. Cao R, Zhang Y. The functions of E(Z)/EZH2-mediated methylation of lysine 27 in histone H3. Curr Opin Genet Dev. 2004;14(2):155–64.
17. Xu J, Wang Z, Lu W, Jiang H, Lu J, Qiu J, Ye G. EZH2 promotes gastric cancer cells proliferation by repressing p21 expression. Pathol Res Pract. 2019;215(6):152374.
18. Duan R, Du W, Guo W. EZH2: a novel target for cancer treatment. J Hematol Oncol. 2020;13(1):104.
19. Kleer CG, Cao Q, Varambally S, Shen R, Ota I, Tomlins SA, et al. EZH2 is a marker of aggressive breast cancer and promotes neoplastic transformation of breast epithelial cells. Proc Natl Acad Sci USA. 2003;100(20):11606–11.
20. Mallen-St Clair J, Soydaner-Azeloglu R, Lee KE, Taylor L, Livanos A, Pylayeva-Gupta Y, et al. EZH2 couples pancreatic regeneration to neoplastic progression. Genes Dev. 2012;26(5):439–44.
21. Zingg D, Debbache J, Schaefer SM, Tuncer E, Frommel SC, Cheng P, et al. The epigenetic modifier EZH2 controls melanoma growth and metastasis through silencing of distinct tumour suppressors. Nat Commun. 2015;6:6051.
22. Ma J, Zhang J, Weng YC, Wang JC. EZH2-mediated microRNA-139-5p regulates epithelial-mesenchymal transition and lymph node metastasis of pancreatic cancer. Mol Cells. 2018;41(9):868–80.
23. Lu C, Han HD, Mangala LS, Ali-Fehmi R, Newton CS, Ozbun L, et al. Regulation of tumor angiogenesis by EZH2. Cancer Cell. 2010;18(2):185–97.
24. Tang X, Milyavsky M, Shats I, Erez N, Goldfinger N, Rotter V. Activated p53 suppresses the histone methyltransferase EZH2 gene. Oncogene. 2004;23(34):5759–69.
25. Bracken AP, Kleine-Kohlbrecher D, Dietrich N, Pasini D, Gargiulo G, Beekman C, et al. The polycomb group proteins bind throughout the INK4A-ARF locus and are disassociated in senescent cells. Genes Dev. 2007;21(5):525–30.
26. Bryant RJ, Cross NA, Eaton CL, Hamdy FC, Cunliffe VT. EZH2 promotes proliferation and invasiveness of prostate cancer cells. Prostate. 2007;67(5):547–56.
27. Yu J, Cao Q, Mehra R, Laxman B, Yu J, Tomlins SA, et al. Integrative genomics analysis reveals silencing of beta-adrenergic signaling by polycomb in prostate cancer. Cancer Cell. 2007;12(5):419–31.
28. Min J, Zaslavsky A, Fedele G, McLaughlin SK, Reczek EE, De Raedt T, et al. An oncogene-tumor suppressor cascade drives metastatic prostate cancer by coordinately activating Ras and nuclear factor-kappaB. Nat Med. 2010;16(3):286–94.
29. Jain P, Di Croce L. Mutations and deletions of PRC2 in prostate cancer. BioEssays. 2016;38(5):446–54.
30. Park SH, Fong KW, Kim J, Wang F, Lu X, Lee Y, et al. Posttranslational regulation of FOXA1 by polycomb and BUB3/USP7 deubiquitin complex in prostate cancer. Sci Adv. 2021;7(15):eabe2261.
31. Chinaranagari S, Sharma P, Chaudhary J. EZH2 dependent H3K27me3 is involved in epigenetic silencing of ID4 in prostate cancer. Oncotarget. 2014;5(16):7172–82.
32. Jiao L, Shubbar M, Yang X, Zhang Q, Chen S, Wu Q, et al. A partially disordered region connects gene repression and activation functions of EZH2. Proc Natl Acad Sci USA. 2020;117(29):16992–7002.

33. Aggarwal R, Huang J, Alumkal JJ, Zhang L, Feng FY, Thomas GV, et al. Clinical and genomic characterization of treatment-emergent small-cell neuroendocrine prostate cancer: a multi-institutional prospective study. J Clin Oncol. 2018;36(24):2492–503.
34. Wang W, Epstein JI. Small cell carcinoma of the prostate. A morphologic and immunohistochemical study of 95 cases. Am J Surg Pathol. 2008;32(1):65–71.
35. Mjønes P, Sagatun L, Nordrum IS, Waldum HL. Neuron-specific enolase as an immunohistochemical marker is better than its reputation. J Histochem Cytochem. 2017;65(12):687–703.
36. Alanee S, Moore A, Nutt M, Holland B, Dynda D, El-Zawahry A, McVary KT. Contemporary incidence and mortality rates of neuroendocrine prostate cancer. Anticancer Res. 2015;35(7):4145–50.
37. Zaffuto E, Pompe R, Zanaty M, Bondarenko HD, Leyh-Bannurah SR, Moschini M, et al. Contemporary incidence and cancer control outcomes of primary neuroendocrine prostate cancer: a SEER database analysis. Clin Genitourin Cancer. 2017;15(5):e793–800.
38. Zhu J, Liang X, Wu D, Chen S, Yang B, Mao W, Shen D. Clinicopathological characteristics and survival outcomes in neuroendocrine prostate cancer: a population-based study. Medicine (Baltimore). 2021;100(15):e25237.
39. Parimi V, Goyal R, Poropatich K, Yang XJ. Neuroendocrine differentiation of prostate cancer: a review. Am J Clin Exp Urol. 2014;2(4):273–85.
40. Beltran H, Rickman DS, Park K, Chae SS, Sboner A, MacDonald TY, et al. Molecular characterization of neuroendocrine prostate cancer and identification of new drug targets. Cancer Discov. 2011;1(6):487–95.
41. Dardenne E, Beltran H, Benelli M, Gayvert K, Berger A, Puca L, et al. N-Myc induces an EZH2-mediated transcriptional program driving neuroendocrine prostate cancer. Cancer Cell. 2016;30(4):563–77.
42. Tan HL, Sood A, Rahimi HA, Wang W, Gupta N, Hicks J, et al. Rb loss is characteristic of prostatic small cell neuroendocrine carcinoma. Clin Cancer Res. 2014;20(4):890–903.
43. Ku SY, Rosario S, Wang Y, Mu P, Seshadri M, Goodrich ZW, et al. Rb1 and Trp53 cooperate to suppress prostate cancer lineage plasticity, metastasis, and antiandrogen resistance. Science. 2017;355(6320):78–83.
44. Chen J, Shi M, Chuen Choi SY, Wang Y, Lin D, Zeng H, Wang Y. Genomic alterations in neuroendocrine prostate cancer: a systematic review and meta-analysis. BJUI Compass. 2023;4(3):256–65.
45. Clermont P-L, Lin D, Crea F, Wu R, Xue H, Wang Y, et al. Polycomb-mediated silencing in neuroendocrine prostate cancer. Clin Epigenetics. 2015;7(1):40.
46. Park SH, Fong KW, Mong E, Martin MC, Schiltz GE, Yu J. Going beyond polycomb: EZH2 functions in prostate cancer. Oncogene. 2021;40(39):5788–98.
47. Lee JK, Phillips JW, Smith BA, Park JW, Stoyanova T, McCaffrey EF, et al. N-Myc drives neuroendocrine prostate cancer initiated from human prostate epithelial cells. Cancer Cell. 2016;29(4):536–47.
48. Puca L, Bareja R, Prandi D, Shaw R, Benelli M, Karthaus WR, et al. Patient derived organoids to model rare prostate cancer phenotypes. Nat Commun. 2018;9(1):2404.
49. Beshiri M, Agarwal S, Yin JJ, Kelly K. Prostate organoids: emerging experimental tools for translational research. J Clin Invest. 2023;133(10):e169616.
50. Zhang Y, Zheng D, Zhou T, Song H, Hulsurkar M, Su N, et al. Androgen deprivation promotes neuroendocrine differentiation and angiogenesis through CREB-EZH2-TSP1 pathway in prostate cancers. Nat Commun. 2018;9(1):4080.
51. Merkens L, Sailer V, Lessel D, Janzen E, Greimeier S, Kirfel J, et al. Aggressive variants of prostate cancer: underlying mechanisms of neuroendocrine transdifferentiation. J Exp Clin Cancer Res. 2022;41(1):46.
52. Kleb B, Estécio MR, Zhang J, Tzelepi V, Chung W, Jelinek J, et al. Differentially methylated genes and androgen receptor re-expression in small cell prostate carcinomas. Epigenetics. 2016;11(3):184–93.

53. Schade AE, Kuzmickas R, Rodriguez CL, Mattioli K, Enos M, Gardner A, Cichowski K. Combating castration-resistant prostate cancer by co-targeting the epigenetic regulators EZH2 and HDAC. PLoS Biol. 2023;21(4):e3002038.
54. Luo J, Wang K, Yeh S, Sun Y, Liang L, Xiao Y, et al. LncRNA-p21 alters the antiandrogen enzalutamide-induced prostate cancer neuroendocrine differentiation via modulating the EZH2/STAT3 signaling. Nat Commun. 2019;10(1):2571.
55. Slabáková E, Kahounová Z, Procházková J, Souček K. Regulation of neuroendocrine-like differentiation in prostate cancer by non-coding RNAs. Noncoding RNA. 2021;7(4):75.
56. Tomassi S, Romanelli A, Zwergel C, Valente S, Mai A. Polycomb repressive complex 2 modulation through the development of EZH2-EED interaction inhibitors and EED binders. J Med Chem. 2021;64(16):11774–97.
57. Knutson SK, Warholic NM, Wigle TJ, Klaus CR, Allain CJ, Raimondi A, et al. Durable tumor regression in genetically altered malignant rhabdoid tumors by inhibition of methyltransferase EZH2. Proc Natl Acad Sci USA. 2013;110(19):7922–7.
58. Kuntz KW, Campbell JE, Keilhack H, Pollock RM, Knutson SK, Porter-Scott M, et al. The importance of being me: magic Methyls, methyltransferase inhibitors, and the discovery of tazemetostat. J Med Chem. 2016;59(4):1556–64.
59. Kurmasheva RT, Sammons M, Favours E, Wu J, Kurmashev D, Cosmopoulos K, et al. Initial testing (stage 1) of tazemetostat (EPZ-6438), a novel EZH2 inhibitor, by the Pediatric Preclinical Testing Program. Pediatr Blood Cancer. 2017;64(3)
60. Fan W, Morinaga H, Kim JJ, Bae E, Spann NJ, Heinz S, et al. FoxO1 regulates Tlr4 inflammatory pathway signalling in macrophages. EMBO J. 2010;29(24):4223–36.
61. Dou F, Tian Z, Yang X, Li J, Wang R, Gao J. Valemetostat: first approval as a dual inhibitor of EZH1/2 to treat adult T-cell leukemia/lymphoma. Drug Discov Ther. 2022;16(6):297–9.
62. Morishima S, Ishitsuka K, Izutsu K, Kusumoto S, Makiyama J, Utsunomiya A, et al. First-in-human study of the EZH1/2 dual inhibitor valemetostat in relapsed or refractory Non-Hodgkin Lymphoma (NHL)—updated results focusing on Adult T-Cell Leukemia-Lymphoma (ATL). Blood. 2019;134(Supplement_1):4025.
63. Kung PP, Bingham P, Brooun A, Collins M, Deng YL, Dinh D, et al. Optimization of orally bioavailable Enhancer of Zeste Homolog 2 (EZH2) inhibitors using ligand and property-based design strategies: identification of development candidate (R)-5,8-dichloro-7-(methoxy(oxetan-3-yl)methyl)-2-((4-methoxy-6-methyl-2-oxo-1,2-dihydropyridin-3-yl) methyl)-3,4-dihydroisoquinolin-1(2H)-one (PF-06821497). J Med Chem. 2018;61(3):650–65.
64. Cromm PM, Crews CM. Targeted protein degradation: from chemical biology to drug discovery. Cell Chem Biol. 2017;24(9):1181–90.
65. Nalawansha DA, Crews CM. PROTACs: an emerging therapeutic modality in precision medicine. Cell Chem Biol. 2020;27(8):998–1014.
66. Pettersson M, Crews CM. PROteolysis TArgeting Chimeras (PROTACs)—past, present and future. Drug Discov Today Technol. 2019;31:15–27.
67. Ma A, Stratikopoulos E, Park KS, Wei J, Martin TC, Yang X, et al. Discovery of a first-in-class EZH2 selective degrader. Nat Chem Biol. 2020;16(2):214–22.
68. Eich ML, Athar M, Ferguson JE 3rd, Varambally S. EZH2-targeted therapies in cancer: hype or a reality. Cancer Res. 2020;80(24):5449–58.
69. Yang YA, Yu J. EZH2, an epigenetic driver of prostate cancer. Protein Cell. 2013;4(5):331–41.
70. Yiji L, Chen-Hao C, Neel S, Tengfei X, Avery F, Mei Y, et al. A non-canonical EZH2 function sensitizes solid tumors to genotoxic stress. bioRxiv. 2020:2020.09.11.291534.
71. Burr ML, Sparbier CE, Chan KL, Chan YC, Kersbergen A, Lam EYN, et al. An evolutionarily conserved function of polycomb silences the MHC class I antigen presentation pathway and enables immune evasion in cancer. Cancer Cell. 2019;36(4):385–401.e8.
72. Peng D, Kryczek I, Nagarsheth N, Zhao L, Wei S, Wang W, et al. Epigenetic silencing of TH1-type chemokines shapes tumour immunity and immunotherapy. Nature. 2015;527(7577):249–53.

73. Ennishi D, Takata K, Béguelin W, Duns G, Mottok A, Farinha P, et al. Molecular and genetic characterization of MHC deficiency identifies EZH2 as therapeutic target for enhancing immune recognition. Cancer Discov. 2019;9(4):546–63.
74. Morel KL, Sheahan AV, Burkhart DL, Baca SC, Boufaied N, Liu Y, et al. EZH2 inhibition activates a dsRNA-STING-interferon stress axis that potentiates response to PD-1 checkpoint blockade in prostate cancer. Nat Cancer. 2021;2(4):444–56.
75. Singer EA, Golijanin DJ, Messing EM. Androgen deprivation therapy for advanced prostate cancer: why does it fail and can its effects be prolonged? Can J Urol. 2008;15(6):4381–7.
76. Kolinsky MP, Rescigno P, Bianchini D, Zafeiriou Z, Mehra N, Mateo J, et al. A phase I dose-escalation study of enzalutamide in combination with the AKT inhibitor AZD5363 (capivasertib) in patients with metastatic castration-resistant prostate cancer. Ann Oncol. 2020;31(5):619–25.
77. Barnard M, Mostaghel EA, Auchus RJ, Storbeck KH. The role of adrenal derived androgens in castration resistant prostate cancer. J Steroid Biochem Mol Biol. 2020;197:105506.
78. Feng Q, He B. Androgen receptor signaling in the development of castration-resistant prostate cancer. Front Oncol. 2019;9:858.
79. Shankar E, Franco D, Iqbal O, Moreton S, Kanwal R, Gupta S. Dual targeting of EZH2 and androgen receptor as a novel therapy for castration-resistant prostate cancer. Toxicol Appl Pharmacol. 2020;404:115200.

Chapter 8
Prostate Cancer and PTEN/PI3K/AKT/mTOR Signaling

Mahshid Seyed Karimi, Ferdos Faghihkhorasani, Al-Hasnawi Rasool Riyadh Abdulwahid, Sahar Mohammadi, Atiyeh Tavakoli, Parisa Osati, Nasim Ebrahimi, Mostafa Haji-Fatahaliha, and Amir Reza Aref

Abstract Despite the generally positive prognosis seen in patients with localized prostate cancer after surgical intervention and their excellent response to androgen-deprivation treatment, it's crucial to emphasize that about one-third of these indi-

---

The original version of the chapter has been revised. A correction to this chapter can be found at https://doi.org/10.1007/978-981-97-4612-5_15

M. Seyed Karimi
Department of Surgery and Anesthesiology, Shariati Hospital, Tehran University of Medical Sciences, Tehran, Iran

F. Faghihkhorasani · A.-H. R. R. Abdulwahid
Medical Campus, Xi'an Jiaotong University, Xi'an, Shaanxi Province, China

S. Mohammadi
Department of Biology, Islamic Azad University, Parand Branch, Tehran, Iran

A. Tavakoli
Department of Biology, Faculty of Basic Sciences, Islamic Azad University, Damghan Branch, Damghan, Iran

P. Osati
Department of Chemical Engineering, Fouman Faculty of Engineering, College of Engineering, University of Tehran, Tehran, Iran

N. Ebrahimi (✉)
Division of Genetics, Department of Cell and Molecular Biology and Microbiology, Faculty of Biological Science and Technology, University of Isfahan, Isfahan, Iran

M. Haji-Fatahaliha
Department of Immunology, Faculty of Medicine, Tabriz University of Medical Sciences, Tabriz, Iran

A. R. Aref (✉)
Mass General Cancer Center, Department of Surgery, Massachusetts General Hospital, Harvard Medical School, Boston, MA, USA

Broad, Institute of MIT and Harvard, Cambridge, MA, USA
e-mail: aaref@mgh.harvard.edu

G. Sethi et al. (eds.), *Prostate Cancer: Molecular Events and Therapeutic Modalities*, https://doi.org/10.1007/978-981-97-4612-5_8

viduals inevitably experience recurrence and subsequently develop castration-resistant prostate cancer (CRPC). Generally, the effectiveness of prostate cancer treatment is limited, highlighting the need to develop alternative treatments that might improve the outcomes of hormone administration and/or surgical castration. The abnormal regulation of the phosphoinositide 3-kinase (PI3K) pathway has become a subject of increasing interest in the context of prostate cancer. This is primarily because of the regular occurrences of post-translational modifications, epigenetic alterations, and genetic mutations affecting both PI3K and phosphatase and tensin homolog (PTEN). These alterations have been entangled in the development and advancement of prostate cancer and in the resistance to conventional androgen-deprivation treatment. In this chapter, we provide a comprehensive overview of the cellular activities of the key components involved in this cascade, as well as their dysregulation in prostate cancer. We also summarize the findings from both preclinical and clinical investigations, including inhibitors of PI3K signaling, and examine the non-genomic factors contributing to the lack of success in these therapeutic interventions.

Keywords Targeted therapy · Castration-resistant prostate cancer · PTEN inhibitors · Protein kinase · PTEN deletion

8.1 Introduction

Phosphoinositide 3-kinase (PI3K) and associated factors in its downstream serve as a central molecular hub, activating a wide spectrum of growth factors, thereby regulating virtually all cellular functions including survival, angiogenesis, cellular metabolism, cell cycle progression, and proliferation [1]. Given the vital roles of PI3K in cellular physiology and its intricate cross-talk with other cellular signaling pathways, it is evident that disruptions in its expression, function, or even its regulatory factors can lead to various dysfunctions and diseases, including cancer [2, 3]. Notably, the PI3K pathway and its key components, recognized as pro-oncogenic factors in cells, exhibit high drugability, making them a prime focus of research since the 1990s for targeted therapies and the discovery of novel drugs in the battle against cancer [4]. Consequently, now a significant quantity of medications targeting the PI3K pathway are available for preclinical studies, reflecting the substantial effort invested in this area for potential clinical application [5].

Prostate cancer, recognized as a medically heterogeneous cancer, is the most prevalent malignancy identified in men and consequently stands being the primary reason for cancer-related deaths among males. A substantial percentage of prostate cancers are androgen-dependent, thus surgical or pharmacological castration is employed as a therapy approach, leading to androgen deprivation and subsequently enhancing patient survival and their overall quality of life. However, in many instances, mere tumor excision or complete removal is insufficient. In nearly all cases, following surgical castration in patients with localized prostate cancer and a favorable prognosis, cancer relapse occurs, transforming into metastatic castration-resistant prostate cancer (CRPC) [6–8]. The deregulation of the PI3K pathway in prostate tumors, caused by genetic mutations like deletions or activating mutations of phosphatase and tensin homolog (PTEN), serine/threonine kinase 1 (also known as protein kinase B) (AKT1), and phosphatidylinositol-4,5-bisphosphate 3-kinase catalytic subunit alpha (PIK3CA), along with post-translational and epigenetic modifications, are consistently linked to the progression of cancer. Consequently, the PI3K cascade has become an appealing target for therapeutic interventions in prostate cancer [9]. Unfortunately, the achievements of these endeavors have often encountered obstacles, mostly stemming from the formation of resistance caused by acute resurgence and/or interaction with the androgen receptor (AR) or alternate signaling pathways. This chapter provides a summary of the roles performed by the principal participants within the PI3K signaling cascade, as well as an examination of their dysregulation within the framework of prostate cancer. In addition, we analyze the findings of preclinical and clinical investigations using inhibitors of PI3K signaling. Our emphasis is on the specific medications and pharmacological targets that have been implicated in their potential influence on prostate cancer. We emphasize the significance of employing combination medications in the management and treatment of this cancer.

8.2 An Overview of PI3K/AKT/mTOR Pathway

The PI3K/AKT/mechanistic target of rapamycin kinase (mTOR) pathway is among the central signaling pathways within cells, and its heightened activity has been documented within a broad spectrum of tumors and malignant progressions, including gastric, colorectal, breast, endometrial, glioblastoma, ovarian, and prostate cancers [1]. The activation of PI3K kinase serves as a pivotal hub between upstream and downstream signals, governing oncogenic processes. Various cellular mechanisms, encompassing protein synthesis, metabolism, cell survival, inflammation, progression, and invasion, can be under the control of this pathway. Mechanistically, PI3K, as a significant member of the large lipid enzyme family, phosphorylates the 3′-OH of inositol phosphatidylinositols located in the plasma membrane. Almost three decades have passed since the discovery of PI3K, initially reported for its ability to transform viral oncoproteins. Currently, three classes of PI3Ks have been identified in mammals, including Class I, Class II, and Class III, each serving distinct roles. Kinases of Class IA comprise a regulatory subunit and a catalytic unit. The catalytic subunits, known as p110-alpha, p110-beta, and p110-gamma, are derived from the transcription of the genes PIK3C-A, PIK3C-B, and PIK3C-D, respectively [10]. On the other hand, the regulatory subunits encompass p85-alpha, p85-beta, and p55-gamma, encoded by the genes PIK3R1, PIK3R2, and PIK3R3. In contrast, Class IB exhibits less diversity and is composed of two regulatory subunits, namely p101 and p84, along with a catalytic subunit named P110-gamma [10]. Among Class II PI3K proteins, three isoforms exist as monomers [11]. Despite extensive studies on these proteins and the elucidation of insights into their roles in cellular signaling, their functions remain largely unknown [12]. Class III has a sole member known as vacuolar protein sorting 34 (Vps34), expressed in all eukaryotic organisms. This protein, first identified in yeast, is involved in nutritional status alterations and integration of cellular responses [11]. Various signals primarily trigger PI3K activity via receptor tyrosine kinases

(RTKs), oncogenes such as Ras (directly binding to p110), and G protein-coupled receptors (GPCRs). Once triggered, PI3K promptly converts phosphatidylinositol 4,5-bisphosphate (PIP2) to phosphatidylinositol 3,4,5-trisphosphate (PIP3) via its catalytic subunit. PIP3 functions as a secondary messenger in the cellular context by facilitating the recruitment of a cascade of proteins that possess a homology domain similar to the pleckstrin homology (PH) domain found in the cell membrane. The unregulated activation of PI3K signaling is a prevalent occurrence in cancer, mostly attributed to the distinct functions shown by p110α and p110β, which are its catalytic subunits. The presence of genetic alterations in the PI3KA sequence, which encodes p110α, has been seen in cancerous cells originating from several organs including the brain, colon, liver, prostate, and lung [11, 13]. PI3KA plays a crucial role in promoting angiogenesis in endothelial cells. Angiogenesis is essential in creating a network of blood vessels that enables the transportation of oxygen and nutrients. Additionally, this gene is involved in cell cycle regulation and growth. Its involvement in these processes is significant as it can potentially facilitate the metastasis of cancer cells from the primary lesion. During oncogenesis, particularly in tumors initiated by RTKs and oncogenes, the isoform p110α is essential. In addition to its involvement in downstream signaling of GPCR pathways, p110β also plays a crucial role in high-grade prostatic intraepithelial neoplasia (HG-PIN) development within the epithelial prostate [14]. In an animal model of prostate cancer resulting from PTEN deficiency, the reduction of p110β hindered tumor formation and inhibited AKT phosphorylation, whereas reducing p110α did not yield such effects [15]. The available data from recent investigations consistently indicate that the inhibition of p110α has no impact on the progression of PTEN-null CRPC. However, the genetic or pharmacological interference with p110β significantly impedes the onset and advancement of CRPC, as shown by many studies [15, 16].

One of the key regulators of the PI3K/AKT pathway is the PTEN molecule, which is known as a well-studied tumor suppressor, catalyzes the dephosphorylation of PIP3 to PIP2, resulting in a reduction of PI3K/AKT pathway activity. PTEN not only acts on proteins but also on lipids, preventing tumor growth by inducing apoptosis and inhibiting cellular proliferation. Thus, mutations in PTEN lead to its inactivity and consequently promote tumorigenesis. Two major genetic alterations have been detected in the phosphatase subunit of PTEN. The initial one disturbs phosphatase operations on lipids and proteins, whereas the second one hinders phosphatase activity on protein substrates. In addition to the aforementioned roles, PTEN dysfunction is associated with various tumor-related processes, including tumor cell neoplastic transformation, cellular migration, genomic instability, and metastasis. Furthermore, PTEN occupies a central position in governing the tumor microenvironment [17]. In various types of cancers, including ovarian, breast, endometrial, prostate, melanoma, lymphoma, colon, and glioblastoma, these mutations in the PTEN sequence have been reported [18]. Additionally, animal studies have revealed that just a deletion in one copy of the PTEN gene can suffice to disrupt cellular signaling and consequently lead to unrestrained cell proliferation [19].

The second key factor in the discussed pathway is AKT, also known as protein kinase B (PKB), which becomes active as a result of PI3K activation and subsequent phosphorylation. AKT, belonging to the AGC family of serine/threonine kinases, has the following three isoforms with similar structures described: AKT, AKT1, and AKT2. These isoforms all possess a pleckstrin homology (PH) domain, wherein despite differences in amino acid sequences, the tertiary structure is conserved and binds to PIP3. Another domain of these isoforms is the lineage genes (LIN) domain, consisting of 39 acid amine residues and exhibiting the lowest degree of conservation. Remarkably, in humans, no other protein shares significant homology with LIN (17–46% identical). This domain acts as a linker, thus bridging between the PH domain and the domain with catalytic activity. The kinase domain spans amino acids 148 to 411 and concludes with a hydrophobic regulatory motif known as the C-terminal domain (CTD), which is responsible for adenosine triphosphate (ATP) binding. The ATP-binding region, consisting of 25 acid amines, exhibits a high degree of similarity, ranging from 96% to 100%, throughout the three isoforms. The conservation of the C-terminal hydrophobic domain is seen in all AGC family members of kinases. The hydrophobic amino acids are of utmost importance in facilitating the full activation of AKT for the process of substrate phosphorylation. Embedded inside the structure is an additional crucial residue responsible for the activation of the enzyme, known as Ser473. Despite structural similarities among the AKT isoforms, they exhibit distinct expression patterns in different tissues. Specifically, AKT1 is highly expressed in almost all organs except for the kidney, spleen, and liver, whereas AKT2 is prominently expressed in insulin-sensitive tissues, including skeletal muscles, adipose tissue, and the liver. Conversely, AKT3 is present in all tissues but shows lower expression levels in skeletal muscles and the liver. Thus, different AKT isoforms demonstrate diverse roles. For instance, while excessive AKT2 expression leads to cell motility and invasion, upregulation of AKT3 is associated with invasion in hormone-sensitive tumors [20]. Upon phosphorylation and activation, AKT identifies and phosphorylates threonine and serine residues on various substrates. Some important substrates of AKT include forkhead box transcription factors (FOXO), p21-activated protein kinase (Pak1), inducible nitric oxide synthase (iNOS), caspase-9, cyclin-dependent kinase inhibitor 1 (also known as p21) (p21WAF1/CIPK1), tuberous sclerosis complex 2 (TSC2), BCL2 associated agonist of cell death (BAD), and glycogen synthase kinase 3 (GSK3). All of these are involved in crucial cellular processes, cell life and death, angiogenesis, and metabolism. The overactivation of AKT has been documented in several types of cancers, such as lung cancer, multiple myeloma, breast cancer, glioblastoma, and prostate cancer [21]. mTOR kinase is widely recognized as the most extensively investigated downstream substrate of AKT. The AKT protein has the ability to phosphorylate and thereby activate mTOR. Additionally, AKT may indirectly activate mTOR by phosphorylation and deactivating tuberin also known as tuberous sclerosis 2 (TSC2). Tuberin typically functions to inhibit mTOR. The stimulation of mTOR leads to an augmentation in protein translation [22]. Recent investigations have shown that the activity of AKT could be effectively suppressed by the PH domain of leucine repeat sequence-rich phosphatase (PHLPP). Precisely, PHLPP has the ability to dephosphorylate the AKT's hydrophobic motif, with Ser473 in AKT1 being the particular target [23].

On the other side, mTOR is a serine/threonine kinase that governs several cellular activities, encompassing the synthesis of proteins, proliferation, cell growth, cell motility, cell survival, and transcription. The mTOR pathway acts as a key regulator of energy homeostasis and body weight, being responsive to many metabolic signals like amino acids, insulin, glucose, and other metabolic hormones. An important point based on recent studies is that mTOR, in addition to acting as a critical substrate of AKT, also serves as a significant activator of it. Activated mTOR typically constructs a complex with the protein rapamycin-insensitive companion of mTOR (RICTOR) and, through phosphorylation at Ser473, activates the AKT protein [24]. The sequestration of recently generated mTOR proteins inside cells after long-term rapamycin therapies might potentially be elucidated by the activation of TORC2. This medication has high efficacy in causing cell death through the apoptosis pathway and inhibiting the proliferation of cells with upregulated AKT due to its ability to disrupt the reassembly of the complex by binding to it over a period of time [25].

8.3 Involvement of PI3K/AKT/mTOR-PTEN Signaling in Prostate Cancer

Anomalously heightened PI3K signaling has been shown in 40% of prostate cancer cases that are identified at an early stage and in over 70% of cases that have progressed to an advanced stage [26–29]. The loss of PTEN is seen in about 30% of primary prostate cancers and 60% of CRPCs. This genetic alteration is often found in tumors with a high Gleason score and is considered a significant characteristic in both hormone-naïve and CRPCs [28]. In accordance with previous research, the activation of signaling pathways downstream of PI3K is correlated with resistance to androgen ablation therapy, progression to hormone-resistant illness, and worse clinical outcomes [29].

In accordance with the significance of this pathway in oncology, a substantial quantity of small molecule suppressors targeting PI3K, AKT, and/or mTOR have been under development since the 1990s. These inhibitors are designed to selectively target either singular or multiple kinases. The pioneering chemicals wortmannin and LY294002, which were the first inhibitors of PI3K, have had a profound impact in unraveling the intricacies of the PI3K pathway ever since their identification in the 1990s [4]. Wortmannin forms a covalent bond with the ATP-binding site located on the p110 catalytic subunit, leading to the permanent inhibition of PI3K. LY294002, similar to most other inhibitors, is a synthetic molecule that competes reversibly with ATP by displacing it from the ATP-binding pocket. Despite the significant use of both compounds in in vitro investigations, their toxicity levels were deemed excessive for clinical application. Numerous exclusively targeted small compounds have been created as a result of the crystal structures of the catalytic p110 isoforms and the analysis of the structural composition of these two substances. The compounds mentioned are ATP-competitive pan-PI3K inhibitors or selective inhibitors of one or two isoforms, exhibiting action within the low nanomolar range. Several of these drugs have progressed from clinical studies to cancer therapy. Although pan-isoform inhibitors have a significant toxicity, their therapeutic effectiveness is limited results, perhaps due to the simultaneous suppression of all isoforms. Research on the varied tissue location of p110s and the symptoms resulting from isoform-specific genetic change have shown distinct biological activities for each PI3K isoform. Consequently, there has been a focus on developing inhibitors that specifically target these isoforms [30]. The subsequent discussion will focus on the effectiveness of distinct agents targeting PI3Kα and β in within the sphere of prostate cancer.

In recent decades, a number of successive generations of mTOR blockages have emerged and thoroughly examined in both preclinical and clinical settings. The chemicals include both ATP-pocket and allosteric binding agents for mTOR. The macrolide rapamycin, which is generated from bacteria, acts as an allosteric inhibitor that exhibits specificity toward mTORC1. However, with extended therapy, it might additionally restrain mTORC2. Rapamycin and its analogs, often referred to as rapalogs, including temsirolimus (CC1–779) and everolimus (RAD001), interact with FKBP12 to produce a complex that subsequently binds to mTORC1. The suppression of mTORC1 substrates, particularly p70S6K and to a minor extent 4EBP1, is shown by a reduction in phosphorylation. The drugs RAD001 and temsirolimus have received approval from both the US Food and Drug Administration (FDA) and the European Medicines Agency (EMA) [30]. Currently, phase II clinical trials in the field of oncology are underway to assess how effective ATP-competitive mTOR inhibitors like vistusertib and sapanisertib are in suppressing DNA-PK/mTOR pathway, or both mTOR-C1 and mTOR-C2 [30, 31]. In order to address the issue of rapamycin resistance, researchers are now working on the creation of an innovative category of mTOR inhibitors known as rapalinks. These inhibitors combine rapamycin with MNL0128, which is an inhibitor of mTOR by binding to DNA. Despite its significant level of interest, the safety and effectiveness of this medicine in prostate cancer therapy have not yet been assessed [32].

The majority of AKT inhibitors exhibit binding affinity toward the adenosine triphosphate (ATP) site of AKT. Nevertheless, there have also been allosteric inhibitors that imitate the allosteric control of AKT activity via the binding of PI (3,4,5) P3 to the PH domain. The chemical perifosine, an alkylphospholipid and lipophilic choline analog, has been the first substance within its class to undergo cell and animal model study. Mechanistically it involves inhibiting the AKT translocation to the cytosol membrane and following activation. Regrettably, despite encouraging outcomes seen in preclinical investigations, no clinical trial evaluating perifosine as a standalone treatment has shown substantial effectiveness across a diverse array of tumor types. Therefore, the following paragraph will focus only on pharmaceutical substances that have shown encouraging outcomes in preclinical prostate cancer models and subsequently progressed to clinical trials [33] (Fig. 8.1).

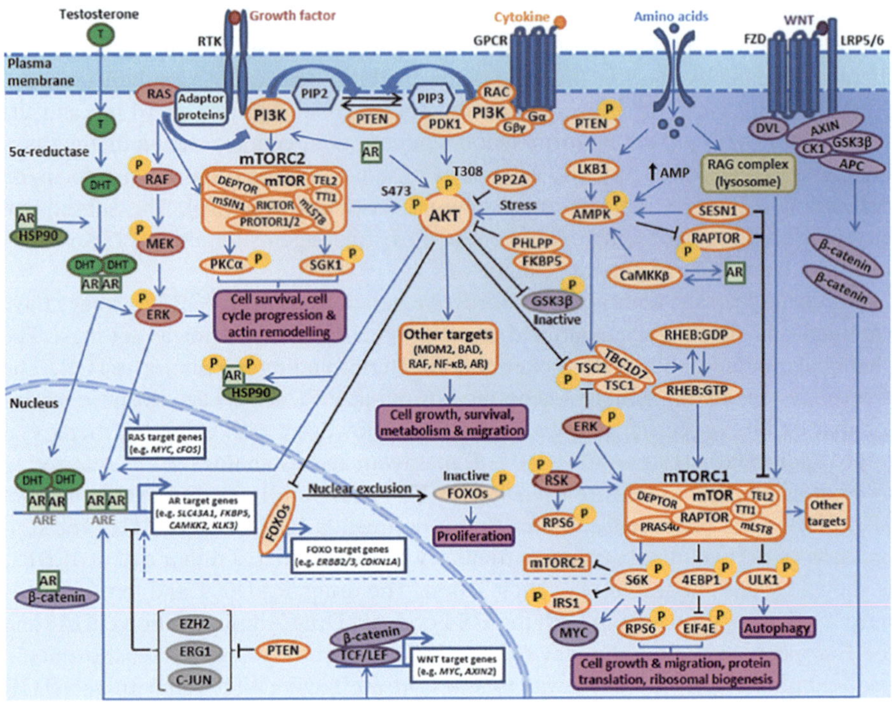

Fig. 8.1 The cross-talk between the PI3K/mTOR pathway and the AR signaling pathway [34]

8.4 The Dysregulation of PTEN/PI3K and PI3K/mTOR Pathways in the Context of Prostate Cancer Therapy

The presence of gene amplifications, deletions, insertions, and missense mutations is mostly seen in the PIK3CA gene, encoding the Class IA p110α subunit [9]. According to a study, it has been shown that PIK3CA mutations exist in roughly 4% of prostate cancer cases, while PIK3CA copy number increase or amplification is seen in approximately 66% of cases [35]. There are two significant hotspot mutations identified in this study, namely exon 9 E542K and E545K located in the helical region and exon 20 H1047R in the kinase domain [35]. Recent research has provided evidence indicating that the induction of invasive prostate cancer in cell lines may be attributed to the presence of PIK3CA H1047, thereby establishing it as a genetic driver of prostate cancer [35]. While there is currently no documentation of PIK3CB mutations, the involvement of PI3Kβ in carcinogenesis is significant due to the intricate cross-regulation across PI3K isoforms. While it is true that PI3Kα is the primary isoform found in prostate epithelial cells, investigations have shown that the loss of PTEN causes the activation of oncogenic pathways and promotes tumor development through PI3Kβ [36–38]. Consistent with the aforementioned data, it was shown in a mouse model with PTEN deficiency that PI3Kβ has a significant role in the formation of prostate tumors [39]. The aforementioned investigations have provided evidence supporting the presence of a therapeutic approach for targeting PI3K via isoform-specific inhibitors, including AZD8186, SAR260301, and GSK2636771 [36]. Nevertheless, the subsequent data did not meet the anticipated standards. The suppression of PI3Kβ led to a subsequent high level of PI3Kα activity, most likely due to the upregulation of FOXO and/or p70S6K/rpS6, which caused the rebound activity of AKT and mTOR [40]. In contrast, the administration of medicines that specifically target both isoforms of PI3K effectively disrupted subsequent signaling pathways and resulted in a decrease in tumor development. The effectiveness of the treatment was found to be restricted to mice models of prostate cancer that expressed the wild-type PTEN gene, as indicated by a previous study [40]. The aforementioned characteristic was recently subjected to additional analysis in mice with prostate-specific biallelic PTEN deletion and PIK3CA-H1047R, as compared to a control group consisting of animals with just PTEN loss [35]. These sophisticated research models facilitated the investigation of the potential impact of PTEN expression on PI3K activity by modulating the isoform-specific upstream activators, including RAS and RAC1 for PI3Kα and PI3Kβ, respectively. The study revealed that there was a persistent activation of the RAS/pERK signaling pathway in mice that had both PTEN deletion and PIK3CA H1047R mutation, as well as in animals that only had PTEN deletion. In contrast, it was shown that a significant increase in RAC1 activity was only evident in PTEN-null/wild-type PIK3CA. This finding suggests that the continuous RAC1/PI3Kβ activity may be responsible for the advancement of tumors in these particular animal models. Given the limited effectiveness of pharmaceuticals that inhibit PI3Kβ, the researchers of this study proposed a treatment approach for PTEN-deleted individuals by combining the disabling RAC using PI3Kβ inhibitors [35].

The exploration of alternative techniques includes the extensive examination of inhibiting PI3Kα/β or PI3K/mTOR. In cellular experiments, simultaneous inhibition of PI3Kβ using AZD8186 and mTOR using vistusertib effectively prevented the reactivation of signaling in PTEN-null prostate cancer cell lines. This was demonstrated by the notably low levels of phosphorylation observed in AKT and rpS6, even after prolonged exposure. Conversely, the administration of either drug as a standalone treatment was unsuccessful in controlling the reactivation process [36]. Additionally, it should be noted that the medication combination had comparable outcomes in prostate tumor xenografts. However, it is worth mentioning that the in vivo reduction of rpS6 phosphorylation was not as successful [36].

Furthermore, it has been reported that BKM120, an orally administered pan PI3K reversible inhibitor, as well as the dual PI3K/mTOR inhibitors PP242 (mTOR allosteric) and NVP-BEZ235 (ATP-competitive), exhibit anticancer effects in both cellular and animal model investigations [41]. These findings provide confirmation that the upregulation of the PI3K pathway is implicated not only in the initiation but also in the advancement of the disease [42]. Specifically, when examining PTEN-null mice models of high-grade prostatic intraepithelial neoplasia, it was observed that the administration of either BKM120 or BEZ235 for a duration of up to 8 weeks led to a remarkable decrease in tumor proliferation and a promotion in rate of apoptosis. Additionally, the aforementioned treatment led to the reversal of the phenotype mentioned above. These findings provide support for applying PI3K-targeted treatment in clinical settings. To assess the impact of PI3K and/or mTOR inhibition, the extended dephosphorylation of both rpS6 and AKT has been observed. The effectiveness of BEZ235 was further evaluated in a more advanced model of PTEN-null CRPC. Surprisingly, the sensitivity of this model to BEZ235 was found to be lower than anticipated. According to the authors, the proposed explanation is that the simultaneous overactivation of androgen receptor, MAPK, and PI3K signaling pathways resulted in resistance to treatment [43]. However, the combination of BEZ235 with AZD6224 (a MAPK inhibitor) was shown to efficiently overcome resistance, suggesting that individuals with PTEN-deleted prostate cancers may get therapeutic benefits from PI3K signaling inhibitors [43].

Unfortunately, the previous administration of BKM120 or BEZ235 as monotherapy to patients has been constrained by significant toxicity. Moreover, in the monotherapy by BKM120, unintended consequences result from its interaction with tubulin. The substitution of BKM120 with the new dual PI3K/mTOR inhibitor PQR 309 has been suggested for nonsolid tumors [44]. During the preclinical phase of research. The investigational drug PQR 309 has shown encouraging outcomes in clinical trials and is now undergoing phase II testing for the treatment of lymphoma. However, there is currently a lack of published evidence about its effectiveness in prostate cancer. The investigation explored the administration of BKM120 in combination with abiraterone acetate and prednisone. Abiraterone acetate is a strong inhibitor against androgen synthesis that hampers AR transcription mediated by AR. Abiraterone acetate is currently utilized in the treatment of advanced CRPC. This investigation was prompted by the mutual regulation observed between AR and PI3K signaling, as described earlier [45]. Despite the encouraging first findings, the study was halted due to the delayed accrual of participants (NCT01741753).

The efficacy of combining abiraterone with BEZ 235 was evaluated in an experimental rat model of androgen-dependent prostate cancer. The findings of the study indicated that the administration of this particular medication combination in rats resulted in the impairment of the inflammatory response and the prevention of tumor development from the premalignant stage to the malignant one [46]. Furthermore, the effectiveness of the drug BEZ235 combined with abiraterone acetate has been evaluated in a phase 1b clinical study including patients with CRPC. The study exhibited suboptimal tolerability of the combination, perhaps due to an overabundance of pathway blockage resulting in adverse effects both on the intended target and unintended targets [47]. A further investigation was conducted on male individuals afflicted with CRPC, whereby the efficacy of both BEZ235 and BKM120 was examined [48]. The present investigation was unsuccessful in achieving the desired outcomes, mostly attributed to the little effectiveness seen despite the presence of significant levels of toxicity. The efficacy of BKM120, either alone or combined with enzalutamide, which is a second generation of androgen receptor inhibitors, was shown to be unsatisfactory in a phase II clinical trial including patients with a similar phenotype, mostly owing to issues related to poor tolerance [49]. A recent preclinical investigation examined the impact of X480 (a dual PI3K/

mTOR inhibitor) on the promotion of bone metastases, activation of osteoclasts, and function of osteoblasts both in cell lines and in xenograft models of prostate cancer bone metastases. It is worth noting that the inhibition of PI3K/mTOR led to a declination in tumor development in both primary and bone metastatic locations, as well as a substantial increase in survival rates with prostate cancer [50].

8.5 Perspectives and Conclusion

The PI3K/AKT/mTOR signaling has been widely acknowledged as one of the primary pathways in tumor progression, playing a crucial role in cancer cell proliferation, growth, migration, and survival. Extensive research has been devoted to developing specific inhibitors through the design and implementation of preclinical and clinical studies. However, the increasing complexity of this pathway continues to present challenges in effectively targeting it for therapeutic purposes. Despite the existence of many powerful and selective drugs, the progress in targeting PI3K signaling therapeutically for cancer has been disheartening, with the majority of compounds failing to advance beyond phase II trials. Over the last decade, preclinical investigations have elucidated the underlying factors contributing to this lack of success, therefore offering a justification for the development of future pharmaceutical agents. The PI3K/AKT/mTOR pathway is commonly depicted as a sequential series of events in which each component transmits the signal to downstream factors. However, recent evidence has revealed that this pathway exhibits extensive network divergence and significant intercommunication with other signaling cycles. Consequently, the inhibitory effects of drugs on this pathway can be overridden, leading to the restoration of active signaling through various mechanisms. These factors encompass a range of mechanisms, including, but not limited to, the increased expression of RTKs [51, 52], signaling redundancies, excessive inhibition, loss of function deletions of PTEN, activating point mutations in PI3K including the PIK3CA H1047RK, and interruption of inhibitory feedback loops that restrict the effectiveness of treatments like the AKT activation triggered by rapamycin [53].

Consequently, it is unsurprising that the clinical efficacy of medications that specifically target PI3K signaling as a standalone treatment for prostate cancer has so far shown poor results. In spite of the existence of several active-site inhibitors or allosteric inhibitors, as well as dual kinase and pan- or isoform-specific inhibitors, the number of medicines authorized by the FDA and EMA remains limited, with none specifically indicated for prostate cancer treatment. On the other hand, the use of additional substances in combination shows more potential as a strategy. However, caution must be exercised when adding medications that have comparable bad effects, as this might result in heightened toxicity. An example of this is the interaction between mTOR and PI3K inhibitors with traditional chemotherapy. Nevertheless, promising results have been observed in a phase Ib/II clinical trial evaluating the efficacy of GDC-0068 (ipatasertib), an ATP-competitive AKT inhibitor, in combination with abiraterone acetate for the treatment of metastatic CRPC [54]. CRCP patients under consideration exhibit a state of constitutive activation in the PI3K/AKT/mTOR and AR signaling pathways, which is closely linked to a very worse prognosis. Despite the generally favorable outcomes seen in this trial, it is noteworthy that patients with PTEN loss exhibited a notable deceleration in disease progression and a higher level of treatment tolerance. These encouraging findings have prompted the initiation of a subsequent randomized phase III research focused on PTEN-null CRPC. While the outcomes of the aforementioned phase III clinical trial are currently unavailable, the potential combination of GDC-0068/ipatasertib with abiraterone acetate has the potential to be a significant study in the treatment of PTEN-null CRPC patients. Furthermore, it may have implications for the treatment of prostate cancer patients with a similar genetic profile during the early stages of their disease. Hence, it is essential to comprehensively analyze the genetic background and signaling circuitry in order to effectively devise therapeutic interventions for prostate cancer.

References

1. Yang J, Nie J, Ma X, Wei Y, Peng Y, Wei X. Targeting PI3K in cancer: mechanisms and advances in clinical trials. Mol Cancer. 2019;18(1):26.
2. Manning BD, Toker A. AKT/PKB signaling: navigating the network. Cell. 2017;169(3):381–405.
3. Hoxhaj G, Manning BD. The PI3K-AKT network at the interface of oncogenic signalling and cancer metabolism. Nat Rev Cancer. 2020;20(2):74–88.
4. Manning BD, Cantley LC. AKT/PKB signaling: navigating downstream. Cell. 2007;129(7):1261–74.
5. Wong KK, Engelman JA, Cantley LC. Targeting the PI3K signaling pathway in cancer. Curr Opin Genet Dev. 2010;20(1):87–90.
6. Park S, Kim YS, Kim DY, So I, Jeon JH. PI3K pathway in prostate cancer: all resistant roads lead to PI3K. Biochim Biophys Acta Rev Cancer. 2018;1870(2):198–206.
7. Feng Q, He B. Androgen receptor signaling in the development of castration-resistant prostate cancer. Front Oncol. 2019;9:858.
8. Chappell WH, Candido S, Abrams SL, Akula SM, Steelman LS, Martelli AM, et al. Influences of TP53 and the anti-aging DDR1 receptor in controlling Raf/MEK/ERK and PI3K/Akt expression and chemotherapeutic drug sensitivity in prostate cancer cell lines. Aging (Albany NY). 2020;12(11):10194–210.
9. Samuels Y, Wang Z, Bardelli A, Silliman N, Ptak J, Szabo S, et al. High frequency of mutations of the PIK3CA gene in human cancers. Science. 2004;304(5670):554.
10. Geering B, Cutillas PR, Nock G, Gharbi SI, Vanhaesebroeck B. Class IA phosphoinositide 3-kinases are obligate p85-p110 heterodimers. Proc Natl Acad Sci USA. 2007;104(19):7809–14.
11. Backer JM. The regulation and function of Class III PI3Ks: novel roles for Vps34. Biochem J. 2008;410(1):1–17.
12. Gewinner C, Wang ZC, Richardson A, Teruya-Feldstein J, Etemadmoghadam D, Bowtell D, et al. Evidence that inositol polyphosphate 4-phosphatase type II is a tumor suppressor that inhibits PI3K signaling. Cancer Cell. 2009;16(2):115–25.
13. Levine DA, Bogomolniy F, Yee CJ, Lash A, Barakat RR, Borgen PI, et al. Frequent mutation of the PIK3CA gene in ovarian and breast cancers. Clin Cancer Res. 2005;11(8):2875–8.

14. Gao X, Wang Y, Ribeiro CF, Manokaran C, Chang H, Von T, et al. Blocking PI3K p110β attenuates development of PTEN-deficient castration-resistant prostate cancer. Mol Cancer Res. 2022;20(5):673–85.
15. Jia S, Liu Z, Zhang S, Liu P, Zhang L, Lee SH, et al. Essential roles of PI(3)K-p110beta in cell growth, metabolism and tumorigenesis. Nature. 2008;454(7205):776–9.
16. Zhao JJ, Liu Z, Wang L, Shin E, Loda MF, Roberts TM. The oncogenic properties of mutant p110alpha and p110beta phosphatidylinositol 3-kinases in human mammary epithelial cells. Proc Natl Acad Sci USA. 2005;102(51):18443–8.
17. Conciatori F, Bazzichetto C, Falcone I, Ciuffreda L, Ferretti G, Vari S, et al. PTEN function at the interface between cancer and tumor microenvironment: implications for response to immunotherapy. Int J Mol Sci. 2020;21(15):5337.
18. Bunney TD, Katan M. Phosphoinositide signalling in cancer: beyond PI3K and PTEN. Nat Rev Cancer. 2010;10(5):342–52.
19. Knowles MA, Platt FM, Ross RL, Hurst CD. Phosphatidylinositol 3-kinase (PI3K) pathway activation in bladder cancer. Cancer Metastasis Rev. 2009;28(3–4):305–16.
20. Hinz N, Jücker M. Distinct functions of AKT isoforms in breast cancer: a comprehensive review. Cell Commun Signal. 2019;17(1):154.
21. Stahl JM, Sharma A, Cheung M, Zimmerman M, Cheng JQ, Bosenberg MW, et al. Deregulated Akt3 activity promotes development of malignant melanoma. Cancer Res. 2004;64(19):7002–10.
22. Kim J, Guan KL. mTOR as a central hub of nutrient signalling and cell growth. Nat Cell Biol. 2019;21(1):63–71.
23. Yan X, Li W, Yang L, Dong W, Chen W, Mao Y, et al. MiR-135a protects vascular endothelial cells against ventilator-induced lung injury by inhibiting PHLPP2 to activate PI3K/Akt pathway. Cell Physiol Biochem. 2018;48(3):1245–58.
24. Sarbassov DD, Ali SM, Kim DH, Guertin DA, Latek RR, Erdjument-Bromage H, et al. Rictor, a novel binding partner of mTOR, defines a rapamycin-insensitive and raptor-independent pathway that regulates the cytoskeleton. Curr Biol. 2004;14(14):1296–302.
25. Yellen P, Saqcena M, Salloum D, Feng J, Preda A, Xu L, et al. High-dose rapamycin induces apoptosis in human cancer cells by dissociating mTOR complex 1 and suppressing phosphorylation of 4E-BP1. Cell Cycle. 2011;10(22):3948–56.
26. Carver BS, Chapinski C, Wongvipat J, Hieronymus H, Chen Y, Chandarlapaty S, et al. Reciprocal feedback regulation of PI3K and androgen receptor signaling in PTEN-deficient prostate cancer. Cancer Cell. 2011;19(5):575–86.
27. Goldstein AS, Zong Y, Witte ON. A two-step toward personalized therapies for prostate cancer. Sci Transl Med. 2011;3(72):72ps7.
28. Vivanco I, Sawyers CL. The phosphatidylinositol 3-kinase AKT pathway in human cancer. Nat Rev Cancer. 2002;2(7):489–501.
29. Bitting RL, Armstrong AJ. Targeting the PI3K/Akt/mTOR pathway in castration-resistant prostate cancer. Endocr Relat Cancer. 2013;20(3):R83–99.
30. Hillmann P, Fabbro D. PI3K/mTOR pathway inhibition: opportunities in oncology and rare genetic diseases. Int J Mol Sci. 2019;20(22):5792.
31. Tsuji T, Sapinoso LM, Tran T, Gaffney B, Wong L, Sankar S, et al. CC-115, a dual inhibitor of mTOR kinase and DNA-PK, blocks DNA damage repair pathways and selectively inhibits ATM-deficient cell growth in vitro. Oncotarget. 2017;8(43):74688–702.
32. Jhanwar-Uniyal M, Wainwright JV, Mohan AL, Tobias ME, Murali R, Gandhi CD, et al. Diverse signaling mechanisms of mTOR complexes: mTORC1 and mTORC2 in forming a formidable relationship. Adv Biol Regul. 2019;72:51–62.
33. Braglia L, Zavatti M, Vinceti M, Martelli AM, Marmiroli S. Deregulated PTEN/PI3K/AKT/mTOR signaling in prostate cancer: still a potential druggable target? Biochim Biophys Acta Mol Cell Res. 2020;1867(9):118731.
34. Shorning BY, Dass MS, Smalley MJ, Pearson HB. The PI3K-AKT-mTOR pathway and prostate cancer: at the crossroads of AR, MAPK, and WNT signaling. Int J Mol Sci. 2020;21(12):4507.

35. Pearson HB, Li J, Meniel VS, Fennell CM, Waring P, Montgomery KG, et al. Identification of Pik3ca mutation as a genetic driver of prostate cancer that cooperates with Pten loss to accelerate progression and castration-resistant growth. Cancer Discov. 2018;8(6):764–79.
36. Lynch JT, Polanska UM, Hancox U, Delpuech O, Maynard J, Trigwell C, et al. Combined inhibition of PI3Kβ and mTOR inhibits growth of PTEN-null tumors. Mol Cancer Ther. 2018;17(11):2309–19.
37. Wee S, Wiederschain D, Maira SM, Loo A, Miller C, deBeaumont R, et al. PTEN-deficient cancers depend on PIK3CB. Proc Natl Acad Sci USA. 2008;105(35):13057–62.
38. Ni J, Liu Q, Xie S, Carlson C, Von T, Vogel K, et al. Functional characterization of an isoform-selective inhibitor of PI3K-p110β as a potential anticancer agent. Cancer Discov. 2012;2(5):425–33.
39. Jia L, Yu W, Wang P, Sanders BG, Kline K. In vivo and in vitro studies of anticancer actions of alpha-TEA for human prostate cancer cells. Prostate. 2008;68(8):849–60.
40. Schwartz S, Wongvipat J, Trigwell CB, Hancox U, Carver BS, Rodrik-Outmezguine V, et al. Feedback suppression of PI3Kα signaling in PTEN-mutated tumors is relieved by selective inhibition of PI3Kβ. Cancer Cell. 2015;27(1):109–22.
41. Ren H, Zhao L, Li Y, Yue P, Deng X, Owonikoko TK, et al. The PI3 kinase inhibitor NVP-BKM120 induces GSK3/FBXW7-dependent Mcl-1 degradation, contributing to induction of apoptosis and enhancement of TRAIL-induced apoptosis. Cancer Lett. 2013;338(2):229–38.
42. Park HS, Hong SK, Oh MM, Yoon CY, Jeong SJ, Byun SS, et al. Synergistic antitumor effect of NVP-BEZ235 and sunitinib on docetaxel-resistant human castration-resistant prostate cancer cells. Anticancer Res. 2014;34(7):3457–68.
43. Jia S, Gao X, Lee SH, Maira SM, Wu X, Stack EC, et al. Opposing effects of androgen deprivation and targeted therapy on prostate cancer prevention. Cancer Discov. 2013;3(1):44–51.
44. Bohnacker T, Prota AE, Beaufils F, Burke JE, Melone A, Inglis AJ, et al. Deconvolution of Buparlisib's mechanism of action defines specific PI3K and tubulin inhibitors for therapeutic intervention. Nat Commun. 2017;8:14683.
45. Fan L, Dong B, Chi C, Wang Y, Gong Y, Sha J, et al. Abiraterone acetate for chemotherapy-naive metastatic castration-resistant prostate cancer: a single-centre prospective study of efficacy, safety, and prognostic factors. BMC Urol. 2018;18(1):110.
46. Gonçalves BF, de Campos SGP, Fávaro WJ, Brandt JZ, Pinho CF, Justulin LA, et al. Combinatorial effect of abiraterone acetate and NVP-BEZ235 on prostate tumor progression in rats. Horm Cancer. 2018;9(3):175–87.
47. Wei XX, Hsieh AC, Kim W, Friedlander T, Lin AM, Louttit M, et al. A phase I study of abiraterone acetate combined with BEZ235, a dual PI3K/mTOR inhibitor, in metastatic castration resistant prostate cancer. Oncologist. 2017;22(5):503–e43.
48. Yeh YA, Yang S, Constantinescu M, Chaudoir C, Tanner A, Henry M, et al. Prostatic adenocarcinoma with novel NTRK3 gene fusion: a case report. Am J Clin Exp Urol. 2019;7(5):341–5.
49. Armstrong AJ, Halabi S, Healy P, Alumkal JJ, Winters C, Kephart J, et al. Phase II trial of the PI3 kinase inhibitor buparlisib (BKM-120) with or without enzalutamide in men with metastatic castration resistant prostate cancer. Eur J Cancer. 2017;81:228–36.
50. Mancini A, Colapietro A, Pompili S, Del Fattore A, Delle Monache S, Biordi LA, et al. Dual PI3 K/mTOR inhibition reduces prostate cancer bone engraftment altering tumor-induced bone remodeling. Tumour Biol. 2018;40(4):1010428318771773.
51. Serra V, Scaltriti M, Prudkin L, Eichhorn PJ, Ibrahim YH, Chandarlapaty S, et al. PI3K inhibition results in enhanced HER signaling and acquired ERK dependency in HER2-overexpressing breast cancer. Oncogene. 2011;30(22):2547–57.
52. Rodon J, Dienstmann R, Serra V, Tabernero J. Development of PI3K inhibitors: lessons learned from early clinical trials. Nat Rev Clin Oncol. 2013;10(3):143–53.
53. Chandarlapaty S. Negative feedback and adaptive resistance to the targeted therapy of cancer. Cancer Discov. 2012;2(4):311–9.
54. Hongo H, Kosaka T, Nakatsuka S, Oya M. A long-term survivor of metastatic neuroendocrine prostate cancer treated with multimodal therapy: genetic consideration from next-generation sequencing. Int Cancer Conf J. 2021;10(3):174–80.

Chapter 9
Prostate Cancer and Noncoding RNAs: A Focus on miRNAs, lncRNAs, and circRNAs

Ahmad Nazari, Parisa Osati, Siavash Seifollahy Fakhr, Mahnaz Akhound-Attar, Nazanin Pazhouhesh Far, Morteza Rajabi, Mahshid Seyed Karimi, Nasim Ebrahimi, Mostafa Haji-Fatahaliha, and Amir Reza Aref

Abstract Noncoding RNAs (ncRNAs) are a class of regulatory transcripts that play important functions in the pathogenesis of several cancer types, including prostate cancer (PCa). Within the framework of prostate cancer, non-coding RNAs have

The original version of the chapter has been revised. A correction to this chapter can be found at https://doi.org/10.1007/978-981-97-4612-5_15

A. Nazari
Tehran University of Medical Science, Tehran, Iran

P. Osati
Department of Chemical Engineering, Fouman Faculty of Engineering, College of Engineering, University of Tehran, Tehran, Iran

S. S. Fakhr
Department of Biotechnology, Faculty of Applied Ecology, Agricultural Science and Biotechnology, Campus Hamar, Inland Norway University of Applied Sciences, Hamar, Norway

M. Akhound-Attar
Department of Biology, Faculty of Sciences, Yazd University, Yazd, Iran

N. P. Far
Department of Microbiology, Faculty of Advanced Science and Technology, Tehran Medical Science, Islamic Azad University, Tehran, Iran

M. Rajabi
Department of Genetics, Faculty of Basic Science, Central Tehran Branch, Islamic Azad University, Tehran, Iran

M. Seyed Karimi
Department of Surgery and Anesthesiology, Shariati Hospital, Tehran University of Medical Sciences, Tehran, Iran

N. Ebrahimi (✉)
Division of Genetics, Department of Cell and Molecular Biology and Microbiology, Faculty of Biological Science and Technology, University of Isfahan, Isfahan, Iran

G. Sethi et al. (eds.), *Prostate Cancer: Molecular Events and Therapeutic Modalities*, https://doi.org/10.1007/978-981-97-4612-5_9

the capacity to function as either oncogenic or tumor-suppressive agents. ncRNAs have the potential to participate in the prostate cancer progression by influencing the signaling of the androgen receptor (AR), the degradation process of AR via ubiquitin-proteasome pathways, or other critical signaling pathways. This chapter provides a detailed review of the involvement of ncRNAs in the evolutionary processes of PCa, with a particular emphasis on their significance in the development of innovative biomarker profiles and targets for cancer treatment.

Keywords Androgen receptor (AR) · Double-stranded RNAs (dsRNAs) · RNA interference (RNAi) · Prostate cancer · CRISPR-Cas9

9.1 Introduction

The first investigations into carcinogenesis mostly focused on genes that encode proteins, since proteins are regarded as fundamental components of molecular biology [1]. The discovery of several noncoding RNA (ncRNAs) species has been facilitated by advancements in transcriptional sequencing methods. Furthermore, extensive evidence has shown the involvement of several noncoding RNAs in various essential cellular processes and pathological conditions, particularly in cancer [2]. ncRNAs may be classified into some distinct categories considering their sequence length. The first category comprises short noncoding RNAs (sncRNAs), which are featured by their size being fewer than 200 nucleotides (nt). Examples of sncRNAs include microRNAs (miRNAs) and Piwi-interacting RNAs (piRNAs). The second group consists of long noncoding RNAs (lncRNAs), which include circular RNAs (circRNAs) and pseudogenes [2, 3]. miRNAs and lncRNAs have garnered significant interest among the many types of ncRNAs [4–6].

miRNAs as a category of short ncRNAs are typically composed of 18–22 nt. These molecules have a pivotal function in the regulation of several developmental and physiological processes. Extensive research conducted over the last 20 years has provided substantial evidence supporting the involvement of miRNAs in numerous health conditions [7–9]. A considerable count of miRNAs has been found in more advanced eukaryotes, and research has shown that they exhibit a high degree of conservation across different species. Their primary role is to negatively control the expression of coding and noncoding genes at the post-transcriptional stage [7]. The discovery of lin-4 miRNA occurred in 1993, marking the first identification of a microRNA. The coming to light of the regulatory role of the short

M. Haji-Fatahaliha
Department of Immunology, Faculty of Medicine, Tabriz University of Medical Sciences, Tabriz, Iran

A. R. Aref (✉)
Mass General Cancer Center, Department of Surgery, Massachusetts General Hospital, Harvard Medical School, Boston, MA, USA

Broad Institute of MIT and Harvard, Harvard Medical School, Cambridge, MA, USA
e-mail: aaref@mgh.harvard.edu

non-protein-coding RNA lin-4 in the transcription of the lin-4 gene via its 3′-UTR (untranslated region) was reported separately by two research teams [9, 10]. In a subsequent study conducted by Fire and colleagues, the elucidation of the RNA interference (RNAi) process in the worm *Caenorhabditis elegans* was revealed. This was achieved by the observation of the impact of double-stranded RNAs (dsRNAs) on the RNAi activation mechanism and subsequent suppressing messenger RNAs (mRNAs) [11]. Based on the data gathered subsequent to the identification of this mechanism and the subsequent discovery of let-7, the first mammalian miRNA, it is now postulated that RNA interference (RNAi) is present in all animal species [12, 13].

The early indication of the involvement of miRNAs in tumorigenesis was presented by Croce and his collaborators, who discovered a tumor-suppressive sequence located at chromosome 13q14 [14]. The research conducted has shown a high frequency of deletions in the area indicated above among individuals diagnosed with chronic lymphocytic leukemia. Additionally, it has been observed that this sequence encodes two distinct miRNA genes, namely miR-16a and miR-15a. The miRNA genes in question exhibit deletions or experience transcriptional downregulation in blood-related tumors, such as chronic lymphocytic leukemia [14]. Subsequent investigations have provided additional evidence indicating that both miR-15a and miR-16a serve as tumor-suppressive miRNAs by promoting cell death via the repression of an anti-apoptotic protein known as B-cell lymphoma 2 (Bcl-2). Notably, Bcl-2 is found to be excessively expressed in blood-related tumors [15, 16]. These data were reaffirmed by experimental studies, which demonstrated that the removal of a cluster of tumors suppressive miRNAs in animal models replicated the phenotypes associated with B-cell malignancies seen in humans. This finding offers compelling support for the tumor-suppressor roles of these miRNAs [17, 18]. The in vitro and in vivo functional validation of miRNAs has contributed to a deeper understanding of pathophysiological and physiological mechanisms in both regular growth and pathological conditions in humans [19–21]. The aforementioned research has shown a novel method of post-transcriptional regulation that exhibits significant dysregulation in cancerous cells [22, 23]. The dysregulation of miRNAs in a spectrum of disorders, including infectious afflictions, cardiovascular diseases, and different types of human cancer, including prostate cancer (PCa), has been demonstrated using advanced high-throughput techniques like single-cell analysis, next-generation sequencing (NGS), and expression microarrays along with clustered regularly interspaced short palindromic repeats (CRISPR) approaches [24–28]. The prognostic, diagnostic, or theragnostic consequences of improperly expressed miRNAs may be determined using their expression profiles [29]. The comprehensive analysis of the miRNome at the genomic level enabled the precise differentiation of various cancer types and the identification of the tissue from which poorly differentiated cancers originated [25, 30].

In contrast to miRNAs and other tiny ncRNAs, which typically consist of less than 200 ribonucleotides, lncRNAs exhibit more heterogeneity in terms of length, spanning from 200 to several thousand ribonucleotides [31, 32]. In contemporary times, there is a growing acknowledgment that lncRNAs exhibit a higher degree of regulation and are more precisely confined to certain cellular contexts as compared to messenger RNAs (mRNAs) [33]. Despite little overall sequence similarity, these elements exhibit frequent and evolutionarily conserved activities, secondary structures, and microhomology areas [34]. There is a growing body of data that supports the participation of lncRNAs in the control of transcription and translation processes, as well as their association with many human disorders [35]. Notably, lncRNAs have undergone thorough investigation within the realm of cancer [36].

This chapter aims to explain the distinctive attributes and significant implications of ncRNAs, including miRNA, lncRNA, and circRNA, in relation to prostate cancer progression and its related mechanism in therapy resistance. The noncoding RNAs mentioned have the capacity to serve as therapeutic targets in the treatment of medication resistance in prostate cancer (Fig. 9.1).

9.2 miRNAs in Prostate Cancer

The evidence has clearly demonstrated that any disruption in the expression level of miRNAs, including the upregulation of oncogenic miRNAs and the downregulation of tumor-suppressive miRNAs, can be associated with the initiation and progression of prostate tumors [38]. Multiple studies have confirmed the correlation between dysregulation in miRNA expression and the onset and development of metastatic phenotype in prostate cancer. These miRNAs regulate key processes including epithelial-to-mesenchymal transition (EMT), tumor proliferation, AR signaling, metastasis, and apoptosis [39].

9.3 miRNAs and Prostate Cancer Progression and Invasion

One of the miRNAs that has been investigated and shows promise is miR-18a, which is a member of the miR-17–92 cluster. It is increased in PCa and acts as a promoter of tumor growth [40, 41]. The miR-18a-5p overexpression induces the prostate cancer cell growth via targeting solute carrier family 40 member 1 (SLC40A1), which is an iron transporter [42]. Furthermore, miR-18a-5p has the ability to decrease the transcription of a pro-apoptotic protein known as serine/threonine kinase 4 (STK4), leading to an elevation in phosphorylated-protein kinase b (AKT) levels and ultimately promoting the survival of tumor cells [43]. Additionally, it has been shown that the miR-221/miR-222 oncogenic cluster is present at elevated levels in prostate cancer. A suggested mechanism of miR-221/miR-222 action includes the reduction of p27kip1 expression, which then impacts the transcription of many genes contributed to the progression of cell cycle and cell proliferation, including cyclin D1, cyclin A, and S-phase kinase-associated protein 2 (Skp2) [44]. Additionally, it has been shown that miR-122 has a role as a tumor-suppressor microRNA in the prostate cancer progression. The downregulation of this entity has been associated with overexpression of ROCK2 protein [45]. In a separate investigation, it was revealed that reduced

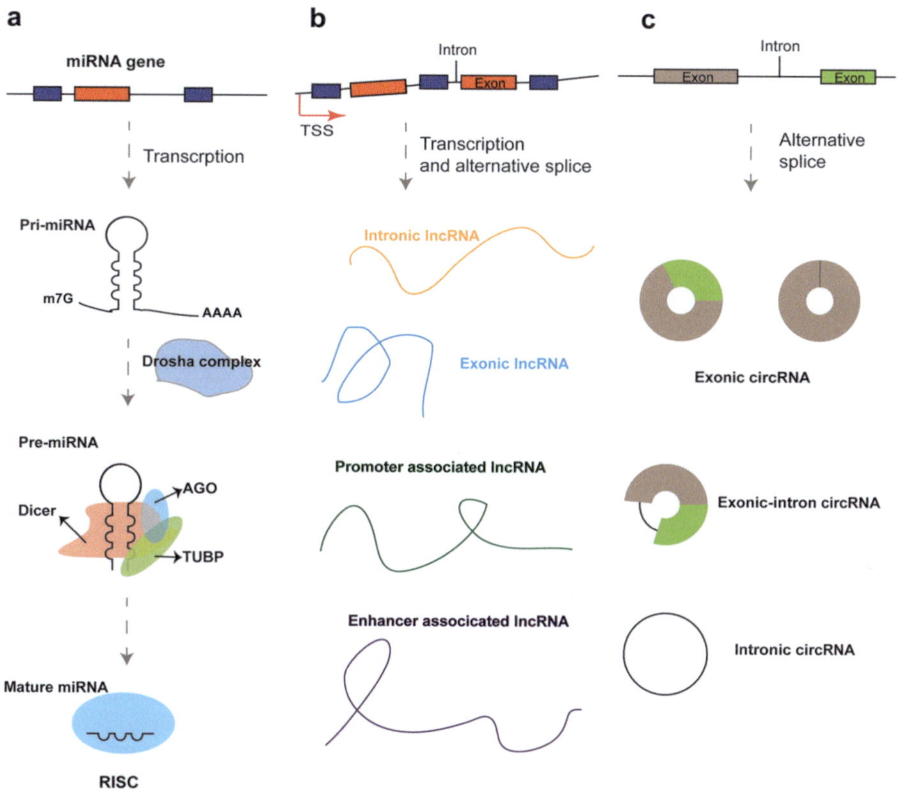

Fig. 9.1 The biogenesis of several noncoding RNAs. The regulation of miRNA transcription is controlled by RNA polymerase II. **a**) The primary microRNAs (pri-miRNAs) undergo a series of sequential cleavage events to generate mature microRNAs (miRNAs) due to their transcriptional origin. Ultimately, fully developed microRNAs (miRNAs) are integrated into the Argonaute protein, resulting in the formation of the miRNA-induced silencing complex (RISC). **b**) Based on the information provided by diverse origin transcription sites, lncRNAs may be categorized into many distinct categories, including intronic lncRNAs, exonic lncRNAs, promoter-associated lncRNAs, and enhancer-associated lncRNAs. **c**) The majority of circRNAs originate from precursor mRNA (pre-mRNA). CircRNAs are categorized into many categories based on their distinct compositions [37]

transcription of miR-122 was concomitant with heightened proliferation, suppressed apoptosis, and enhanced resistance of prostate cancer to docetaxel. This effect was presumably mediated via the regulation of pyruvate kinase M2 (PKM2) enzyme expression [46]. Furthermore, it has been shown that the absence of the tumor-suppressor cluster (miR-16-1 and -15a) has a significant impact on the prostate cancer cell's growth and survival. This effect is achieved via the regulation of many genes, including CDK6, cyclin D1, cyclin E1, and BCL2 [47]. miR-204-5p has been extensively studied as a tumor suppressor that exerts its influence on the formation of PCa prostate cancer by regulating the levels of BCL2, Meis Homeobox 1 (MEIS1), and Homeobox A10 (HOXA10) expression [48, 49].

In addition, it is noteworthy that a tumor-suppressive family of miRNAs, known as miR-200, plays a pivotal role in EMT regulation. The family comprises miR-200a/b/c, -141, and -429. Research was conducted to examine the impact of miR-200c-3p on the invasiveness of prostate cancer cells. The findings revealed a considerable downregulation of miR-200c-3p in human prostate cancer cell lines, such as PC3 and DU145, in comparison to the normal prostatic epithelial cell line (RWPE1). The inhibitory effects of miR-200c-3p on cell motility, cell migration, and cell invasion have been suggested to occur via its targeting of zinc finger E-box binding homeobox 2 (ZEB2), which acts as a repressor of E-cadherin and a promoter of EMT [50]. The inhibition of miR-200b in prostate cancer has been shown to downregulate epithelial-mesenchymal transition, hinder growth, and impede metastasis via a route mediated by ZEB1, which is comparable to previous findings [51]. In a study, it was observed that the downregulation of miR-141-3p plays a role in the metastasis and invasiveness of prostate cancer by activating the nuclear factor kappa b (NF-κB) signaling pathway [52]. Moreover, miR-141-3p enrichment enhances the stemness features in prostate cancer stem cells (PCSCs) by inhibiting a group of genes associated with promoting metastasis, such as Ras homologous (Rho) GTPases, EZH2, and CD44 [53]. Furthermore, the reduced expression of miR-204 5p was linked with disease progression and metastasis, in addition to its established function in regulating cell proliferation and cell death through the apoptosis pathway. Wa and colleagues demonstrated that miR-204-5p exerts inhibitory effects on invasion, migration, and bone metastasis. These effects are achieved through the suppression of NF-κB signaling, which is accomplished by targeting three key proteins at the same time: tumor necrosis factor receptor-associated factor 1 (TRAF1), TGF-β activated kinase 1 (MAP3K7) binding protein 3 (TAB3), and mitogen-activated protein kinase kinase kinase 3 (MAP3K3) [54]. Furthermore, many studies have provided insights into the significant incorporation of the miR-34a tumor suppressor in the invasiveness of prostate cancer, with a noticeable decrease in its expression reported in prostate tumors [55]. The study conducted by Liang and coworkers demonstrated the inhibitory impact of miR-34a on the Wnt signaling pathway, leading to the suppression of migration and invasion associated with EMT in prostate tumors [56]. Liu's team showed that miR-34a has a role in the development of resistance to paclitaxel-based chemotherapy in prostate cancer cells. This resistance is achieved by the direct inhibition of the JAG1/Notch1 axis [57]. Furthermore, Yan and coworkers (2015) provided evidence for the engagement of miR-34a in the regulation of PCSCs and the process of metastasis by its direct repression of CD44 expression. In addition, a comprehensive analysis was conducted in a recent study to thoroughly examine the participation of many microRNAs, such as miR-185, miR-148, and miR-145 in the regulation of the phenotype of PCSCs and their contribution to the invasive and metastatic properties of prostate cancer [58, 59].

Zhiping and colleagues showed that miR-181a expression was significantly elevated in metastatic prostate tumors in comparison to native prostate cancers. The miR-181a upregulation has been seen to have a role in the acquisition of the EMT phenotype. This is achieved by the increased levels of E-cadherin and other epithelial markers, in contrast to elevated levels of vimentin, N-cadherin, and Snail expression, which are mesenchymal indicators. The upregulation of miR-181 has been shown to facilitate the mobility of prostate cancer cells via the direct targeting of TGF-β induced factor 2 protein (TGIF2) [60]. Additionally, it has been shown that it involves in prostate cancer cells resistance to docetaxel and cabazitaxel. This resistance is partially attributed to its ability to modulate p53 phosphorylation and apoptosis [61]. The miR-93 expression level is seen to be increased in prostate cancer, since it is a constituent of the miR-106b-25 cluster. The involvement of this factor in the course of diseases is characterized by its ability to upregulate the expression levels of LATS2, ITGB8, and TGFβR2. Additionally, it has been shown that miR-93 has a substantial correlation with many clinical indicators in prostate cancer, including TNM stage, Gleason score, bone metastases, and lymph node involvement [62, 63].

9.4 lncRNAs Engagement in Prostate Cancer Progression

9.4.1 Oncogenic lncRNAs

The application of quantitative real-time PCR has revealed the upregulation of multiple lncRNAs in prostate cancer tissues when compared to adjacent non-cancerous tissues or samples of benign prostate hyperplasia (BPH). This observation suggests that lncRNA transcripts have an oncogenic role in the advancement of prostate cancer. The study of lncRNAs in this area has mostly focused on small nucleolar RNA host genes (SNHGs). Several carcinogenic lncRNAs, including nuclear paraspeckle assembly transcript 1 (NEAT1), taurine up-regulated gene 1 (TUG1), plasmacytoma variant translocation 1 (PVT1), metastasis associated lung adenocarcinoma transcript 1 (MALAT1), differentiation antagonizing non-protein coding rna (DANCR), and colon cancer associated transcript 1 (CCAT1), have been revealed to function as oncogenes in prostate cancer, similar to their roles in other types of cancer. For example, DANCR can develop taxol resistance in this particular kind of tumor by influencing the miR-33b-5p/LDHA axis [64]. The expression of lncRNA has shown an upregulation in blood samples obtained from individuals diagnosed with prostate cancer, concomitant with a decrease in miR-214-5p. Significantly, there exists an association between the DANCR expression and other clinical parameters such as T stage, Gleason score, and prostate-specific antigen (PSA) level in the aforementioned patient population. The expression of DANCR has been shown to have diagnostic significance in prostate cancer, as well as the ability to predict poor prognosis in patients with this form of disease. The enhancement of cell growth and cell migration, prevention of apoptosis, and induction of TGF-β signaling may be achieved by the increased levels of DANCR or the inhibition of miR-214-5p expression, as shown by previous research [65]. DANCR has been shown to have the ability to target miR-185-5p, therefore facilitating the upregulation of LIM and SH3 protein 1, which in turn promotes the progression of prostate tumors through the PI3K/FAK/GSK3b /AKT/snail axis [66].

The process of epigenetic suppression of the androgen receptor (AR) corepressor contributes crucially to the activation of the AR. The regulation of ARLNC1 is likewise influenced by androgens, leading to an increase in androgen receptor mRNA stability via its binding to the 3′-UTR. Consistent with this observation, the inhibition of ARLNC1 results in the downregulation of androgen receptor expression and the repression of AR signaling, ultimately leading to the reduction of prostate cancer development. ARLNC1 plays a significant role in maintaining a positive feedback loop that triggers and sustains androgen receptor activation throughout the advancement of prostate cancer [67]. Furthermore, a number of lncRNAs that are particular to CRPC and controlled by the AR have a significant role in the upregulation of androgen receptors and their variation. The expression levels of long non-coding RNAs controlled by androgen receptors are shown to be significantly higher in tissues of CRPC. The results of the experiment indicate that the reduction of CRPC tumor development and inhibition of androgen receptor and androgen receptor variant expression may be achieved by the knockdown of (prkag2 antisense RNA 1) PRKAG2-AS1 and hoxc cluster antisense RNA 1 (HOXC)-AS1 in these cells. The functional role of PRKAG2-AS1 involves the regulation of the intracellular distribution of the splicing factor u2 small nuclear rna auxiliary factor 2 (U2AF2). The splicing component in U2AF2 has an important role in the AR splicing system [68].

Hox transcript antisense RNA (HOTAIR), a lncRNA, is well recognized as an androgen receptor-repressed molecule. Its expression is seen to increase during androgen deprivation therapy (ADT) and in the context of CRPC. In a mechanistic manner, the lncRNA known as HOTAIR forms a binding relationship with the AR protein, resulting in the inhibition of its connections with the E3 ubiquitin ligase mouse double minute 2 (MDM2). Consequently, this inhibition suppresses the process of androgen receptor ubiquitination and subsequent destruction. Consequently, the HOTAIR molecule stimulates androgen-independent activation of AR and facilitates the transcriptional program regulated by AR in the absence of androgen [69]. Recent research has shown that NEAT1 facilitates the promotion of cancerous development in prostate tissue by modulating the epigenetic modifications in the promoters of target genes, hence stimulating their transcription [70]. Additionally, it has been shown that prostate cancer gene expression marker 1 (PCGEM1) and prostate cancer associated non-coding RNA 1 (PRNCR1) exhibit binding affinity toward AR and facilitate the process of selective looping, whereby AR-bound enhancers are brought into close proximity with target gene promoters [71]. In a similar vein, it has been shown that the suppressor-of-cytokine-2-antisense RNA 1 (SOCS2-AS1) gene interacts with the androgen receptor to facilitate co-factor interaction [72].

Chen and colleagues in their study aimed to examine the involvement of lncRNA plasmacytoma variant translocation 1 (PVT1) in the pathogenesis of prostate tumor progression [73]. The findings of the study reveal that the PVT1 levels are markedly increased in both prostate cancer tissues and cells. The expression of PVT1 is mechanistically upregulated by the process of METTL3-mediated N6-methyladenosine (m6A) alterations. Increased levels of PVT1 contribute to the promotion of heightened invasion, migration, and proliferation capabilities in prostate cancer cells, while a reduction in PVT1 levels leads to contrasting outcomes. Interestingly, miR-27b-3p has been recognized as a regulator of both PVT1 and bloom syndrome protein (BLM). PVT1 functions by sequestering miR-27b-3p, so indirectly facilitating the development of BLM. The research findings also demonstrate that increased levels of BLM have a mitigating effect on the negative outcomes of PVT1 knockdown, namely in relation to the migration, proliferation, and invasion of prostate cancer cells. The cumulative findings of this study indicate that PVT1 has a role in promoting the aggressiveness of prostate cancer by influencing the miR-27b-3p/BLM axis. These results provide valuable insights into prospective targets for the development of treatment methods for prostate cancer [73].

9.4.2 *Tumor-Suppressive lncRNAs*

Several other lncRNAs have been identified as exerting tumor-suppressive effects in the context of prostate cancer. For example, it has been shown that the gene LINC00893 may impede the advancement of this particular kind of cancer by regulating the miR-3173-5p/SOCS3/JAK2/STAT3 axis [74]. In a similar vein, the impact of LINC01679 on miR-3150a-3p is implicated in the suppression of prostate cancer advancement via modulating the SLC17A9 transcription [75]. MIR22HG is an additional lncRNA that functions as a tumor suppressor by serving as a decoy for miR-9-3p [76]. The involvement of RP1-59D14.5 in prostate tumorigenesis is attributed to its tumor-suppressor function, which is facilitated by the trigger of the Hippo signaling pathway and augmentation of autophagy [77]. Furthermore, previous studies have shown that MAGI2-AS3 is a miR-424-5p sponge, leading to the inhibition of STAT3 signaling and the subsequent suppression of proliferation in prostate cancer cells [78]. NEAT1-interacting transcriptional repressor (NXTAR) is an additional lncRNA that regulates the AR expression and influences enzalutamide resistance [79]. Indeed, the quantity of discerned tumor-suppressive lncRNAs in the context of prostate cancer is much lower in comparison to the abundance of oncogenic lncRNAs.

9.4.3 *Circular RNAs in Prostate Cancer*

Circular RNAs, also known as circRNAs, are a category of ncRNA molecules that possess a covalently closed structure, lacking both 3′ and 5′ ends. The widely used technique for the discovery of novel circRNAs is high-throughput RNA-sequencing (RNA-seq), which involves the detection of spliced reads including the back-splicing junctions. After their formation, circRNAs exhibit a remarkable level of stability owing to their unique circular conformation. Hence, the use of circRNAs as potential biomarkers in various bodily tissues, blood samples, or urine specimens has been suggested by Wen's team study. The precise cellular activities of the majority of circRNAs remain elusive [80]. In recent years, research on specific circRNAs has revealed their potential to act as miRNA sponges, interact with RNA-binding proteins to influence their function, regulate alternative splicing and transcription, and even undergo translation to generate new bioactive peptides [81, 82]. CircRNAs exhibit abnormal expression patterns in several types of malignant tumors, including renal cell carcinoma [83], breast [84], and prostate tumors [85]. The dysregulation of circRNAs has been reported in several dimensions of malignant tumor growth, such as tumor development, metastasis, immunosuppression, and drug resistance [86]. According to Zhang et al. (2019), research conducted on patient-derived xenograft (PDX) mice models shows that the administration of intratumor injections of siRNA specifically targeting oncogenic circRNA has significant potential as a treatment strategy for gastric cancer therapy [87]. Furthermore, it has been shown that circRNAs have potential as reliable indicators for predicting the prognosis or diagnosing malignant tumors, as evidenced by studies conducted by recent studies [88, 89]. Both dysregulated and functional circRNAs have significant contributions in several dimensions of prostate cancer, such as metastasis, cell cycle, tumor proliferation, invasion, migration, radiosensitivity, and treatment resistance. Certain circRNAs have the capacity to function as valuable biomarkers for both prognostic and diagnostic purposes.

CircRNAs have a significant role in the EMT regulation. Yan and coworkers (2020) conducted an RNA-seq analysis to identify circRNAs associated with EMT in cells stimulated by interferon-gamma (IFN-γ). Their findings revealed that hsa_circ_0001165 and hsa_circ_0001085 have a regulatory function in the EMT process during prostate tumorigenesis [90]. Feng and colleagues (2019), showed that circ0005276 molecules facilitated cellular proliferation and EMT via interacting with FUS [91]. The study conducted by Han and coworkers revealed the downregulation of circSMAD2 in prostate cancer tissues. The suppression of the defective EMT process may be achieved by the restoration of circSMAD2, which in turn inhibits miR-9 [92]. According to Yang et al., it was said that the regulation of EMT by p53 occurs via the circAMOTL1L/miR-193a-5p/Pcdha regulatory axis [93]. According to the findings of Li et al., it was proposed that circ-0016068 can enhance the EMT in prostate cancer cells via the regulation of the miR-330 3p/BMI-1 axis [94]. Shen et al. showed that circFoxo3 has inhibitory effects on the cell motility and invasiveness of prostate cancer cells by modulating the expression of Foxo3 and EMT [95]. Furthermore, apart from their role in EMT, circRNAs can regulate the metastatic process of prostate cancer through other mechanisms. In their study, Xu and coworkers discovered that circRNA-51,217 acts as a sponge for miRNA-646, resulting in the activation of the TGFb1/p-Smad2/3 signaling and subsequent promotion of prostate cancer cell invasion [96]. According to the findings of Weng et al., it has been proposed that the circular RNA_LARP4 has the ability to impede cell migration and invasion by upregulating the FOXO3A [97]. The study conducted by Si-Tu and colleagues revealed that circ-102,004 exhibited an oncogenic function by facilitating the metastasis-related processes in cells of prostate cancer [98]. The upregulation of circ-102,004 modulates the signaling pathways of Hedgehog, c-JUN N-terminal kinase (JNK), and extracellular signal-regulated kinase (ERK)

[98]. It has been shown that circSOBP effectively suppressed the amoeboid migration and metastasis of prostate cancer cells. This inhibitory effect was mediated via the involvement of the miR-141 3p/MYPT1/p-MLC2 axis [99].

Moreover, recent evidence has shown the engagement of circRNAs in the processes of cell cycle regulation, cell proliferation, and cell death in prostate tumors. For example, Shan et al. documented that the suppression of circFMN2 resulted in the inhibition of tumor development in vivo and the reduction of proliferation in prostate cancer cells [100]. This effect was achieved by the cell cycle checkpoint activation and apoptosis, which was mediated through the regulation of the miR-1238/LHX2 axis [100]. In their study, Mao et al. found a significant association between circPDHX and many clinical factors in prostate cancer, including overall survival, pathological T, stage, and Gleason score. Furthermore, their findings demonstrated that circPDHX had a role in promoting cell growth in laboratory settings and tumor progression in animal models [101]. According to Liu et al., it was proposed that the expression of circHIPK3 was increased in prostate cancer and that it facilitated the transition from the G2 to the M phase by serving as a miR-338-3p sponge [102]. According to Deng et al., the inhibition of circ_0088233 resulted in a decrease in cellular proliferation and led to G1 phase arrest and cell death by specifically inhibiting hsa-miR-185-3p [103]. The suppression of circ_0057553 was shown to impede cellular viability and promote apoptosis [104]. In addition, it was proposed that the inhibition of tumor development in animal models and cell cycle progression in tumor cells might be achieved by the suppression of circABCC4, which targets the miR-1182-FOXP4 regulatory axis [105].

CircRNAs have been shown to be important for the development of treatment resistance in several types of cancer. Recent research has examined the involvement of circRNAs in CRPC. In their study, Cao et al. (2019) applied RNA-seq techniques to detect a total of 13 circRNAs originating from the androgen receptor gene. This analysis was conducted on a diverse set of samples, including 47 metastatic CRPC samples, cell models, and patient-derived xenografts (PDXs), with the additional utilization of RNase R RNA sequencing. The upregulation of the four most prevalent circRNAs is seen throughout the growth of castration-resistant PDXs, and these circRNAs may be identified in the plasma of patients diagnosed with prostate cancer [106]. The circRNAs produced from AR have the potential to function as CRPC biomarkers. In their study, Greene and colleagues discovered that circRNAs exhibited a higher frequency of downregulation in prostate cancer cells that were resistant to enzalutamide. This finding was obtained by the use of a high-throughput circRNA microarray [107]. Hsa_circ_0004870, a circRNA that was shown to be decreased, has been implicated in potentially facilitating the progression of enzalutamide resistance in prostate cancer. Wu and coworkers (2019) showed that the circRNA17 expression was much lower in enzalutamide-resistant cell lines derived from CRPC C4–2 cells, in comparison to the parental sensitive cells. This study proposes that circRNA17 may regulate the sensitivity of cells to enzalutamide by means of the miR-181c-5p/ARv7 axis [108]. Xiang et al. (2019) indicated that circUCK2 expression was reduced in cells that had developed resistance to enzalutamide. The potential therapeutic efficacy of targeting these circRNAs might be important in the development of novel treatment strategies for CRPC [109].

Docetaxel is the first chemotherapeutic medication that has been substantiated to effectively extend the life duration of individuals diagnosed with metastatic CRPC. The findings of the STAMPEDE study support the recommendation for the first administration of docetaxel in individuals diagnosed with metastatic hormone-naive prostate cancer. Recent research has shown that circRNAs have a role in the susceptibility of prostate cancer to docetaxel. Shen et al. (2020) proposed that the downregulation of circFoxo3 contributed to an increase in chemoresistance to docetaxel in prostate cancer patients. The siRNAs utilized to deplete circFoxo3 resulted in the promotion of docetaxel resistance in mice xenografts. Conversely, the administration of circFoxo3 led to an extension in the survival of animals with tumors and an augmentation in the sensitivity to docetaxel [94]. According to the findings of Gao et al. (2020), it was demonstrated that the hsa_circ_0000735 expression was increased in prostate cancer tissues that were resistant to docetaxel treatment. Moreover, this upregulation was found to be associated with a worse overall survival outcome. The downregulation of hsa_circ_0000735 resulted in increased responsiveness of prostate cancer cells to docetaxel treatment and reduced cell viability in an in vivo setting. Furthermore, the suppression of hsa_circ_0000735 was shown to enhance the sensitivity to docetaxel and inhibit tumor development in vivo [110]. A study conducted by Zhang's team demonstrated that the exosomal circ-XIAP molecule had an important role in the docetaxel resistance development in prostate cancer by modulating the miR-1182/TPD52 axis [111].

9.4.4 Discussion and Potential of ncRNAs in Prostate Cancer Diagnosis and Treatment

Numerous ncRNAs have a pivotal role in the prostate cancer progression through influencing and regulating androgen receptor signaling, the degradation process of androgen receptors via ubiquitin-proteasome mechanisms, or other critical signaling pathways. Certain biomarkers, such as lncRNA-PCA3, have a high degree of specificity toward prostate cancer, making them suitable for diagnostic purposes. Various tumors have differential expression levels of certain genes, which may either be overexpressed or under-expressed. These genes have the potential to serve as therapeutic targets for a diverse array of human malignancies. The disparities in the expression of certain ncRNAs between CRPC and cases that respond to androgen deprivation therapy suggest that these transcripts participate crucially in determining patients' response to this therapy approach. Moreover, these transcripts can be considered as potential targets for addressing resistance to this therapy.

While a considerable number of ncRNAs unique to prostate cancer or related to prostate cancer have been identified, only a limited number of these ncRNAs have been validated in separate groups of patients or authorized for clinical use. One of the significant advancements in the domain of lncRNA investigation is perhaps the endorsement of urine lncRNA-PCA3 as an indicator for the identification of prostate cancer by the FDA [112]. PCA3 has significant potential as a biomarker for prostate cancer diagnosis by urine testing, demonstrating a more effective performance when compared to prostate-specific antigen (PSA) in the urinary identification of this condition. Additional research is required to identify other lncRNA biomarkers that are suitable for this particular kind of cancer. LncRNAs profiles have the potential to be used for the identification of prostate cancer patients who may get therapeutic benefits from radiation. For example, it has been shown that UCA1 has a role in modulating the susceptibility of prostate cancer cell lines to radiation, suggesting its potential as a biomarker for anticipating the effectiveness of radiotherapy in this patient population. The impact of UCA1 on radiosensitivity is mediated via its influence on the course of the cell cycle [113]. The significance of ncRNAs in regulating cellular processes such as cell metastasis, invasiveness, and proliferation has positioned them as promising targets for therapeutic interventions in prostate cancer. The findings from animal research have shown considerable potential, especially in relation to some non-coding RNAs that are controlled by androgen receptors. It is worth noting that non-coding RNAs also have a role in the development of drug resistance in prostate cancer cells, making them suitable candidates for therapeutic intervention [114]. As an example, the upregulation of HORAS5 has the potential to induce taxane resistance in CRPC cells by upregulating BCL2A1. The silencing of HORAS5 has been shown to decrease the cabazitaxel resistance of prostate cancer cells, hence improving the effectiveness of chemotherapy [115].

The involvement of signaling pathways in prostate cancer including STAT3, p53, PI3K/AKT/mTOR, TGF-β, Wnt/β-catenin, FAK/AKT/β-catenin, FAK/PI3K/AKT/GSK3b/Snail, NF-κB, FOXO, and Ras/ERK signaling pathways, has been extensively covered in previous chapters. These signaling pathways, which are subject to modulation by ncRNAs, are also relevant regarding prostate cancer. Furthermore, numerous diverse ncRNAs exhibit intercommunication with one another. For example, it has been shown that some lncRNAs or circRNAs function as molecular decoys, effectively sequestering miRNAs and therefore modulating the expression of target miRNAs.

While the expression profile of ncRNAs has been extensively evaluated in tumoral tissues of individuals diagnosed with prostate cancer, there has been a relatively limited focus on the investigation of their levels in serum or urine samples. Given the accessibility of these resources for non-invasive diagnostic tests, it is recommended that future research concentrate on these biological fluids in order to enhance the early identification of prostate cancer using non-invasive means. Collectively, ncRNAs have a considerable role in the tumorigenesis of prostate cancer in many ways. The aforementioned transcripts have the potential to act as viable subjects for targeted therapy in the context of this particular malignancy.

References

1. Wong CM, Tsang FH, Ng IO. Non-coding RNAs in hepatocellular carcinoma: molecular functions and pathological implications. Nat Rev Gastroenterol Hepatol. 2018;15(3):137–51.
2. Slack FJ, Chinnaiyan AM. The role of non-coding RNAs in oncology. Cell. 2019;179(5):1033–55.
3. Zhang Y, Yang M, Yang S, Hong F. Role of noncoding RNAs and untranslated regions in cancer: a review. Medicine (Baltimore). 2022;101(33):e30045.
4. Geisler S, Coller J. RNA in unexpected places: long non-coding RNA functions in diverse cellular contexts. Nat Rev Mol Cell Biol. 2013;14(11):699–712.
5. Beermann J, Piccoli MT, Viereck J, Thum T. Non-coding RNAs in development and disease: background, mechanisms, and therapeutic approaches. Physiol Rev. 2016;96(4):1297–325.
6. Cipolla GA, de Oliveira JC, Salviano-Silva A, Lobo-Alves SC, Lemos DS, Oliveira LC, et al. Long non-coding RNAs in multifactorial diseases: another layer of complexity. Noncoding. RNA. 2018;4:2.
7. Tong AW, Nemunaitis J. Modulation of miRNA activity in human cancer: a new paradigm for cancer gene therapy? Cancer Gene Ther. 2008;15(6):341–55.
8. Almeida MI, Reis RM, Calin GA. MicroRNA history: discovery, recent applications, and next frontiers. Mutat Res. 2011;717(1–2):1–8.
9. Wightman B, Ha I, Ruvkun G. Posttranscriptional regulation of the heterochronic gene lin-14 by lin-4 mediates temporal pattern formation in C. elegans. Cell. 1993;75(5):855–62.
10. Lee RC, Feinbaum RL, Ambros V. The C. elegans heterochronic gene lin-4 encodes small RNAs with antisense complementarity to lin-14. Cell. 1993;75(5):843–54.
11. Fire A, Xu S, Montgomery MK, Kostas SA, Driver SE, Mello CC. Potent and specific genetic interference by double-stranded RNA in Caenorhabditis elegans. Nature. 1998;391(6669):806–11.
12. Reinhart BJ, Slack FJ, Basson M, Pasquinelli AE, Bettinger JC, Rougvie AE, et al. The 21-nucleotide let-7 RNA regulates developmental timing in Caenorhabditis elegans. Nature. 2000;403(6772):901–6.
13. Song E, Lee SK, Wang J, Ince N, Ouyang N, Min J, et al. RNA interference targeting Fas protects mice from fulminant hepatitis. Nat Med. 2003;9(3):347–51.
14. Calin GA, Dumitru CD, Shimizu M, Bichi R, Zupo S, Noch E, et al. Frequent deletions and down-regulation of micro-RNA genes miR15 and miR16 at 13q14 in chronic lymphocytic leukemia. Proc Natl Acad Sci USA. 2002;99(24):15524–9.
15. Cimmino A, Calin GA, Fabbri M, Iorio MV, Ferracin M, Shimizu M, et al. miR-15 and miR-16 induce apoptosis by targeting BCL2. Proc Natl Acad Sci USA. 2005;102(39):13944–9.
16. Calin GA, Cimmino A, Fabbri M, Ferracin M, Wojcik SE, Shimizu M, et al. MiR-15a and miR-16-1 cluster functions in human leukemia. Proc Natl Acad Sci USA. 2008;105(13):5166–71.
17. Klein U, Lia M, Crespo M, Siegel R, Shen Q, Mo T, et al. The DLEU2/miR-15a/16-1 cluster controls B cell proliferation and its deletion leads to chronic lymphocytic leukemia. Cancer Cell. 2010;17(1):28–40.
18. Otmani K, Lewalle P. Tumor suppressor miRNA in cancer cells and the tumor microenvironment: mechanism of deregulation and clinical implications. Front Oncol. 2021;11:708765.
19. Roush S, Slack FJ. The let-7 family of microRNAs. Trends Cell Biol. 2008;18(10):505–16.
20. Tili E, Michaille JJ, Croce CM. MicroRNAs play a central role in molecular dysfunctions linking inflammation with cancer. Immunol Rev. 2013;253(1):167–84.
21. Gurha P. MicroRNAs in cardiovascular disease. Curr Opin Cardiol. 2016;31(3):249–54.
22. Esquela-Kerscher A, Slack FJ. Oncomirs—microRNAs with a role in cancer. Nat Rev Cancer. 2006;6(4):259–69.

23. García-Cárdenas JM, Guerrero S, López-Cortés A, Armendáriz-Castillo I, Guevara-Ramírez P, Pérez-Villa A, et al. Post-transcriptional regulation of colorectal cancer: a focus on RNA-binding proteins. Front Mol Biosci. 2019;6:65.
24. Esteller M. Non-coding RNAs in human disease. Nat Rev Genet. 2011;12(12):861–74.
25. Iorio MV, Croce CM. MicroRNA dysregulation in cancer: diagnostics, monitoring and therapeutics. A comprehensive review. EMBO Mol Med. 2012;4(3):143–59.
26. Lu J, Getz G, Miska EA, Alvarez-Saavedra E, Lamb J, Peck D, et al. MicroRNA expression profiles classify human cancers. Nature. 2005;435(7043):834–8.
27. Strobel EJ, Yu AM, Lucks JB. High-throughput determination of RNA structures. Nat Rev Genet. 2018;19(10):615–34.
28. Yang J, Meng X, Pan J, Jiang N, Zhou C, Wu Z, et al. CRISPR/Cas9-mediated noncoding RNA editing in human cancers. RNA Biol. 2018;15(1):35–43.
29. Croce CM. Causes and consequences of microRNA dysregulation in cancer. Nat Rev Genet. 2009;10(10):704–14.
30. Volinia S, Calin GA, Liu CG, Ambs S, Cimmino A, Petrocca F, et al. A microRNA expression signature of human solid tumors defines cancer gene targets. Proc Natl Acad Sci USA. 2006;103(7):2257–61.
31. Mattick JS. The genetic signatures of noncoding RNAs. PLoS Genet. 2009;5(4):e1000459.
32. Wang Y, Fu Y, Lu Y, Chen S, Zhang J, Liu B, et al. Unravelling the complexity of lncRNAs in autophagy to improve potential cancer therapy. Biochim Biophys Acta Rev Cancer. 2023;1878(5):188932.
33. Cabili MN, Trapnell C, Goff L, Koziol M, Tazon-Vega B, Regev A, et al. Integrative annotation of human large intergenic noncoding RNAs reveals global properties and specific subclasses. Genes Dev. 2011;25(18):1915–27.
34. Hezroni H, Koppstein D, Schwartz MG, Avrutin A, Bartel DP, Ulitsky I. Principles of long noncoding RNA evolution derived from direct comparison of transcriptomes in 17 species. Cell Rep. 2015;11(7):1110–22.
35. Chen G, Wang Z, Wang D, Qiu C, Liu M, Chen X, et al. LncRNADisease: a database for long-non-coding RNA-associated diseases. Nucleic Acids Res. 2013;41(Database issue):D983-6.
36. Schmitt AM, Chang HY. Long noncoding RNAs in cancer pathways. Cancer Cell. 2016;29(4):452–63.
37. Ding L, Wang R, Shen D, Cheng S, Wang H, Lu Z, et al. Role of noncoding RNA in drug resistance of prostate cancer. Cell Death Dis. 2021;12(6):590.
38. Zhang B, Pan X, Cobb GP, Anderson TA. microRNAs as oncogenes and tumor suppressors. Dev Biol. 2007;302(1):1–12.
39. Moustafa AA, Kim H, Albeltagy RS, El-Habit OH, Abdel-Mageed AB. MicroRNAs in prostate cancer: from function to biomarker discovery. Exp Biol Med (Maywood). 2018;243(10):817–25.
40. Al-Kafaji G, Al-Naieb ZT, Bakhiet M. Increased oncogenic microRNA-18a expression in the peripheral blood of patients with prostate cancer: a potential novel non-invasive biomarker. Oncol Lett. 2016;11(2):1201–6.
41. Song CJ, Chen H, Chen LZ, Ru GM, Guo JJ, Ding QN. The potential of microRNAs as human prostate cancer biomarkers: a meta-analysis of related studies. J Cell Biochem. 2018;119(3):2763–86.
42. Liang B, Zhou C, Cui S, Lu H, Xu R, Xue D, et al. Upregulation of miR-18a-5p promotes the proliferation of prostate cancer via inhibiting the expression of SLC40A1. Pathol Res Pract. 2021;224:153448.
43. Hsu TI, Hsu CH, Lee KH, Lin JT, Chen CS, Chang KC, et al. MicroRNA-18a is elevated in prostate cancer and promotes tumorigenesis through suppressing STK4 in vitro and in vivo. Oncogenesis. 2014;3(4):e99-e.
44. Mercatelli N, Coppola V, Bonci D, Miele F, Costantini A, Guadagnoli M, et al. The inhibition of the highly expressed miR-221 and miR-222 impairs the growth of prostate carcinoma xenografts in mice. PLoS One. 2008;3(12):e4029.

45. Liu H, Hou T, Ju W, Xing Y, Zhang X, Yang J. MicroRNA-122 downregulates Rho-associated protein kinase 2 expression and inhibits the proliferation of prostate carcinoma cells. Mol Med Rep. 2019;19(5):3882–8.
46. Zhu Z, Tang G, Yan J. MicroRNA-122 regulates docetaxel resistance of prostate cancer cells by regulating PKM2. Exp Ther Med. 2020;20(6):247.
47. Bonci D, De Maria R. miR-15/miR-16 loss, miR-21 upregulation, or deregulation of their target genes predicts poor prognosis in prostate cancer patients. Mol Cell Oncol. 2016;3(4):e1109744.
48. Lin YC, Lin JF, Tsai TF, Chou KY, Chen HE, Hwang TI. Tumor suppressor miRNA-204-5p promotes apoptosis by targeting BCL2 in prostate cancer cells. Asian J Surg. 2017;40(5):396–406.
49. Yang F, Bian Z, Xu P, Sun S, Huang Z. MicroRNA-204-5p: A pivotal tumor suppressor. Cancer Med. 2023;12(3):3185–200.
50. Zhang J, Zhang H, Qin Y, Chen C, Yang J, Song N, et al. MicroRNA-200c-3p/ZEB2 loop plays a crucial role in the tumor progression of prostate carcinoma. Ann Transl Med. 2019;7(7):141.
51. Williams LV, Veliceasa D, Vinokour E, Volpert OV. miR-200b inhibits prostate cancer EMT, growth and metastasis. PLoS One. 2013;8(12):e83991.
52. Huang S, Wa Q, Pan J, Peng X, Ren D, Huang Y, et al. Downregulation of miR-141-3p promotes bone metastasis via activating NF-κB signaling in prostate cancer. J Exp Clin Cancer Res. 2017;36(1):173.
53. Liu C, Liu R, Zhang D, Deng Q, Liu B, Chao H-P, et al. MicroRNA-141 suppresses prostate cancer stem cells and metastasis by targeting a cohort of pro-metastasis genes. Nat Commun. 2017;8(1):14270.
54. Wa Q, Huang S, Pan J, Tang Y, He S, Fu X, et al. miR-204-5p represses bone metastasis via inactivating NF-κB signaling in prostate cancer. Mol Ther Nucleic Acids. 2019;18:567–79.
55. Lodygin D, Tarasov V, Epanchintsev A, Berking C, Knyazeva T, Körner H, et al. Inactivation of miR-34a by aberrant CpG methylation in multiple types of cancer. Cell Cycle. 2008;7(16):2591–600.
56. Liang J, Li Y, Daniels G, Sfanos K, De Marzo A, Wei J, et al. LEF1 targeting EMT in prostate cancer invasion is regulated by miR-34a. Mol Cancer Res. 2015;13(4):681–8.
57. Liu X, Luo X, Wu Y, Xia D, Chen W, Fang Z, et al. MicroRNA-34a attenuates paclitaxel resistance in prostate cancer cells via direct suppression of JAG1/Notch1 Axis. Cell Physiol Biochem. 2018;50(1):261–76.
58. Coradduzza D, Cruciani S, Arru C, Garroni G, Pashchenko A, Jedea M, et al. Role of miRNA-145, 148, and 185 and stem cells in prostate cancer. Int J Mol Sci. 2022;23:3.
59. Yan X, Tang B, Chen B, Shan Y, Yang H. Replication study: the microRNA miR-34a inhibits prostate cancer stem cells and metastasis by directly repressing CD44. elife. 2019:8.
60. Zhiping C, Shijun T, Linhui W, Yapei W, Lianxi Q, Qiang D. MiR-181a promotes epithelial to mesenchymal transition of prostate cancer cells by targeting TGIF2. Eur Rev Med Pharmacol Sci. 2017;21(21):4835–43.
61. Armstrong CM, Liu C, Lou W, Lombard AP, Evans CP, Gao AC. MicroRNA-181a promotes docetaxel resistance in prostate cancer cells. Prostate. 2017;77(9):1020–8.
62. Wang C, Tian S, Zhang D, Deng J, Cai H, Shi C, et al. Increased expression of microRNA-93 correlates with progression and prognosis of prostate cancer. Medicine (Baltimore). 2020;99(22):e18432.
63. Liu JJ, Zhang X, Wu XH. miR-93 promotes the growth and invasion of prostate cancer by upregulating its target genes TGFBR2, ITGB8, and LATS2. Mol Ther Oncolytics. 2018;11:14–9.
64. Wang YY, Chen C. lncRNA-DANCR promotes Taxol resistance of prostate cancer cells through modulating the miR-33b-5p-LDHA Axis. Dis Markers. 2022;2022:9516774.

65. Deng H, Zhu B, Dong Z, Jiang H, Zhao X, Wu S. miR-214-5p targeted by LncRNA DANCR mediates TGF-β signaling pathway to accelerate proliferation, migration and inhibit apoptosis of prostate cancer cells. Am J Transl Res. 2021;13(4):2224–40.
66. Sun W, Zu S, Shao G, Wang W, Gong F. Long non-coding DANCR targets miR-185-5p to upregulate LIM and SH3 protein 1 promoting prostate cancer via the FAK/PI3K/AKT/GSK3β/snail pathway. J Gene Med. 2021;23(7):e3344.
67. Zhang Y, Pitchiaya S, Cieślik M, Niknafs YS, Tien JC, Hosono Y, et al. Analysis of the androgen receptor-regulated lncRNA landscape identifies a role for ARLNC1 in prostate cancer progression. Nat Genet. 2018;50(6):814–24.
68. Kamada S, Takeiwa T, Ikeda K, Horie-Inoue K, Inoue S. Long non-coding RNAs involved in metabolic alterations in breast and prostate cancers. Front Oncol. 2020;10:593200.
69. Zhang A, Zhao JC, Kim J, Fong KW, Yang YA, Chakravarti D, et al. LncRNA HOTAIR enhances the androgen-receptor-mediated transcriptional program and drives castration-resistant prostate cancer. Cell Rep. 2015;13(1):209–21.
70. Chakravarty D, Sboner A, Nair SS, Giannopoulou E, Li R, Hennig S, et al. The oestrogen receptor alpha-regulated lncRNA NEAT1 is a critical modulator of prostate cancer. Nat Commun. 2014;5:5383.
71. Yang L, Lin C, Jin C, Yang JC, Tanasa B, Li W, et al. lncRNA-dependent mechanisms of androgen-receptor-regulated gene activation programs. Nature. 2013;500(7464):598–602.
72. Misawa A, Takayama K, Urano T, Inoue S. Androgen-induced Long noncoding RNA (lncRNA) SOCS2-AS1 promotes cell growth and inhibits apoptosis in prostate cancer cells. J Biol Chem. 2016;291(34):17861–80.
73. Chen B, Liu C, Long H, Bai G, Zhu Y, Xu H. N(6)-methyladenosine-induced long non-coding RNA PVT1 regulates the miR-27b-3p/BLM axis to promote prostate cancer progression. Int J Oncol. 2023;62:1.
74. Yu C, Fan Y, Zhang Y, Liu L, Guo G. LINC00893 inhibits the progression of prostate cancer through miR-3173-5p/SOCS3/JAK2/STAT3 pathway. Cancer Cell Int. 2022;22(1):228.
75. Mi YY, Sun CY, Zhang LF, Wang J, Shao HB, Qin F, et al. Long non-coding RNAs LINC01679 as a competitive endogenous RNAs inhibits the development and progression of prostate cancer via regulating the miR-3150a-3p/SLC17A9 Axis. Front Cell Dev Biol. 2021;9:737812.
76. Zhang W, Shi C, Xu Q, Chen X, Zhu H, Zheng B. Long non-coding RNA MIR22HG suppresses cell proliferation and promotes apoptosis in prostate cancer cells by sponging microRNA-9-3p. Bioengineered. 2022;13(5):13108–17.
77. Jiang S, Li Z, Dou R, Lin Z, Zhang J, Zhang W, et al. Construction and validation of a novel cuproptosis-related long noncoding RNA signature for predicting the outcome of prostate cancer. Front Genet. 2022;13:976850.
78. Wei X, Hou Y, Zhang Y, Zhang H, Sun Z, Meng X, et al. Long non-coding RNA MAGI2-AS3 inactivates STAT3 pathway to inhibit prostate cancer cell proliferation via acting as a microRNA-424-5p sponge. J Cancer. 2022;13(1):343–53.
79. Ghildiyal R, Sawant M, Renganathan A, Mahajan K, Kim EH, Luo J, et al. Loss of long non-coding RNA NXTAR in prostate cancer augments androgen receptor expression and enzalutamide resistance. Cancer Res. 2022;82(1):155–68.
80. Wen G, Zhou T, Gu W. The potential of using blood circular RNA as liquid biopsy biomarker for human diseases. Protein Cell. 2021;12(12):911–46.
81. Kristensen LS, Andersen MS, Stagsted LVW, Ebbesen KK, Hansen TB, Kjems J. The biogenesis, biology and characterization of circular RNAs. Nat Rev Genet. 2019;20(11):675–91.
82. Xiao MS, Ai Y, Wilusz JE. Biogenesis and functions of circular RNAs come into focus. Trends Cell Biol. 2020;30(3):226–40.
83. Wang Y, Zhang Y, Wang P, Fu X, Lin W. Circular RNAs in renal cell carcinoma: implications for tumorigenesis, diagnosis, and therapy. Mol Cancer. 2020;19(1):149.
84. Jahani S, Nazeri E, Majidzadeh AK, Jahani M, Esmaeili R. Circular RNA; a new biomarker for breast cancer: a systematic review. J Cell Physiol. 2020;235(7–8):5501–10.

85. Chao F, Wang S, Zhang C, Han D, Ma Z, Chen G. Circular RNA circSMARCA5 is a prognostic biomarker in patients with malignant tumor: a meta-analysis. BMC Cancer. 2021;21(1):600.
86. Chao F, Wang S, Zhang C, Han D, Xu G, Chen G. The emerging role of circular RNAs in prostate cancer: a systematic review. Front Cell Dev Biol. 2021;9:681163.
87. Zhang X, Wang S, Wang H, Cao J, Huang X, Chen Z, et al. Circular RNA circNRIP1 acts as a microRNA-149-5p sponge to promote gastric cancer progression via the AKT1/mTOR pathway. Mol Cancer. 2019;18(1):20.
88. Wang M, Yang Y, Xu J, Bai W, Ren X, Wu H. CircRNAs as biomarkers of cancer: a meta-analysis. BMC Cancer. 2018;18(1):303.
89. Rajappa A, Banerjee S, Sharma V, Khandelia P. Circular RNAs: emerging role in cancer diagnostics and therapeutics. Front Mol Biosci. 2020;7:577938.
90. Yan Z, Xiao Y, Chen Y, Luo G. Screening and identification of epithelial-to-mesenchymal transition-related circRNA and miRNA in prostate cancer. Pathol Res Pract. 2020;216(2):152784.
91. Feng Q, He B. Androgen receptor signaling in the development of castration-resistant prostate cancer. Front Oncol. 2019;9:858.
92. Retracted: circSMAD2 governs migration and epithelial-mesenchymal transition by inhibiting microRNA-9. J Cell Biochem. 2021;122(9):1253.
93. Yang Z, Qu CB, Zhang Y, Zhang WF, Wang DD, Gao CC, et al. Dysregulation of p53-RBM25-mediated circAMOTL1L biogenesis contributes to prostate cancer progression through the circAMOTL1L-miR-193a-5p-Pcdha pathway. Oncogene. 2019;38(14):2516–32.
94. Li Q, Wang W, Zhang M, Sun W, Shi W, Li F. Circular RNA circ-0016068 promotes the growth, migration, and invasion of prostate cancer cells by regulating the miR-330-3p/BMI-1 Axis as a competing endogenous RNA. Front Cell Dev Biol. 2020;8:827.
95. Shen Z, Zhou L, Zhang C, Xu J. Reduction of circular RNA Foxo3 promotes prostate cancer progression and chemoresistance to docetaxel. Cancer Lett. 2020;468:88–101.
96. Xu H, Sun Y, You B, Huang CP, Ye D, Chang C. Androgen receptor reverses the oncometabolite R-2-hydroxyglutarate-induced prostate cancer cell invasion via suppressing the circRNA-51217/miRNA-646/TGFβ1/p-Smad2/3 signaling. Cancer Lett. 2020;472:151–64.
97. Weng XD, Yan T, Liu CL. Circular RNA_LARP4 inhibits cell migration and invasion of prostate cancer by targeting FOXO3A. Eur Rev Med Pharmacol Sci. 2020;24(10):5303–9.
98. Si-Tu J, Cai Y, Feng T, Yang D, Yuan S, Yang X, et al. Upregulated circular RNA circ-102004 that promotes cell proliferation in prostate cancer. Int J Biol Macromol. 2019;122:1235–43.
99. Chao F, Song Z, Wang S, Ma Z, Zhuo Z, Meng T, et al. Novel circular RNA circSOBP governs amoeboid migration through the regulation of the miR-141-3p/MYPT1/p-MLC2 axis in prostate cancer. Clin Transl Med. 2021;11(3):e360.
100. Shan G, Shao B, Liu Q, Zeng Y, Fu C, Chen A, et al. circFMN2 sponges miR-1238 to promote the expression of LIM-Homeobox gene 2 in prostate cancer cells. Mol Ther Nucleic Acids. 2020;21:133–46.
101. Mao Y, Li W, Hua B, Gu X, Pan W, Chen Q, et al. Circular RNA_PDHX promotes the proliferation and invasion of prostate cancer by sponging MiR-378a-3p. Front Cell Dev Biol. 2020;8:602707.
102. Liu F, Fan Y, Ou L, Li T, Fan J, Duan L, et al. CircHIPK3 facilitates the G2/M transition in prostate cancer cells by sponging miR-338-3p. Onco Targets Ther. 2020;13:4545–58.
103. Deng ZH, Yu GS, Deng KL, Feng ZH, Huang Q, Pan B, et al. Hsa_circ_0088233 alleviates proliferation, migration, and invasion of prostate cancer by targeting hsa-miR-185-3p. Front Cell Dev Biol. 2020;8:528155.
104. Zhang Y, Shi Z, Li Z, Wang X, Zheng P, Li H. Circ_0057553/miR-515-5p regulates prostate cancer cell proliferation, apoptosis, migration, invasion and aerobic glycolysis by targeting YES1. Onco Targets Ther. 2020;13:11289–99.

105. Huang C, Deng H, Wang Y, Jiang H, Xu R, Zhu X, et al. Circular RNA circABCC4 as the ceRNA of miR-1182 facilitates prostate cancer progression by promoting FOXP4 expression. J Cell Mol Med. 2019;23(9):6112–9.
106. Cao S, Ma T, Ungerleider N, Roberts C, Kobelski M, Jin L, et al. Circular RNAs add diversity to androgen receptor isoform repertoire in castration-resistant prostate cancer. Oncogene. 2019;38(45):7060–72.
107. Greene J, Baird AM, Casey O, Brady L, Blackshields G, Lim M, et al. Circular RNAs are differentially expressed in prostate cancer and are potentially associated with resistance to enzalutamide. Sci Rep. 2019;9(1):10739.
108. Wu G, Sun Y, Xiang Z, Wang K, Liu B, Xiao G, et al. Preclinical study using circular RNA 17 and micro RNA 181c-5p to suppress the enzalutamide-resistant prostate cancer progression. Cell Death Dis. 2019;10(2):37.
109. Xiang Z, Xu C, Wu G, Liu B, Wu D. CircRNA-UCK2 increased TET1 inhibits proliferation and invasion of prostate cancer cells via sponge MiRNA-767-5p. Open Med (Wars). 2019;14:833–42.
110. Gao Y, Liu J, Huan J, Che F. Downregulation of circular RNA hsa_circ_0000735 boosts prostate cancer sensitivity to docetaxel via sponging miR-7. Cancer Cell Int. 2020;20:334.
111. Zhang H, Li M, Zhang J, Shen Y, Gui Q. Exosomal Circ-XIAP promotes docetaxel resistance in prostate cancer by regulating miR-1182/TPD52 Axis. Drug Des Devel Ther. 2021;15:1835–49.
112. Hua JT, Chen S, He HH. Landscape of noncoding RNA in prostate cancer. Trends Genet. 2019;35(11):840–51.
113. Fotouhi Ghiam A, Taeb S, Huang X, Huang V, Ray J, Scarcello S, et al. Long non-coding RNA urothelial carcinoma associated 1 (UCA1) mediates radiation response in prostate cancer. Oncotarget. 2017;8(3):4668–89.
114. Mirzaei S, Paskeh MDA, Okina E, Gholami MH, Hushmandi K, Hashemi M, et al. Molecular landscape of LncRNAs in prostate cancer: a focus on pathways and therapeutic targets for intervention. J Exp Clin Cancer Res. 2022;41(1):214.
115. Pucci P, Venalainen E, Alborelli I, Quagliata L, Hawkes C, Mather R, et al. LncRNA HORAS5 promotes taxane resistance in castration-resistant prostate cancer via a BCL2A1-dependent mechanism. Epigenomics. 2020;12(13):1123–38.

Chapter 10
Prostate Cancer and Tumor Microenvironment

Ahmad Nazari, Parisa Osati, Nazanin Pazhouhesh Far, Al-Hasnawi Rasool Riyadh Abdulwahid, Ferdos Faghihkhorasani, Nasim Ebrahimi, Mostafa Haji-Fatahaliha, and Amir Reza Aref

Abstract Prostate cancer (PCa) is the most frequently detected malignancy among males on a global scale. Notwithstanding their initial susceptibility to androgen restriction, individuals afflicted with advanced disease inevitably acquire refusal to treatment and may succumb to metastatic castration-resistant prostate cancer (mCRPC). One of the primary difficulties encountered in the therapy of PCa is the presence of clinical heterogeneity, which poses a significant difficulty due to its unpredictable nature and the limitations of currently available biomarkers in accurately predicting its occurrence. There exists a substantial unmet need to establish precise molecular biomarkers for PCa that can effectively contribute to the diagno-

A. Nazari
Tehran University of Medical Science, Tehran, Iran

P. Osati
Department of Chemical Engineering, Fouman Faculty of Engineering, College of Engineering, University of Tehran, Tehran, Iran

N. P. Far
Department of Microbiology, Faculty of Advanced Science and Technology, Tehran Medical Science, Islamic Azad University, Tehran, Iran

A.-H. R. R. Abdulwahid · F. Faghihkhorasani
Medical Campus, Xi'an Jiaotong University, Xi'an, Shaanxi Province, China

N. Ebrahimi (✉)
Division of Genetics, Department of Cell and Molecular Biology and Microbiology, Faculty of Biological Science and Technology, University of Isfahan, Isfahan, Iran

M. Haji-Fatahaliha
Department of Immunology, Faculty of Medicine, Tabriz University of Medical Sciences, Tabriz, Iran

A. R. Aref (✉)
Mass General Cancer Center, Department of Surgery, Massachusetts General Hospital, Harvard Medical School, Boston, MA, USA

Broad Institute of MIT and Harvard, Harvard Medical School, Cambridge, MA, USA
e mail: aaref@mgh.harvard.edu

G. Sethi et al. (eds.), *Prostate Cancer: Molecular Events and Therapeutic Modalities*, https://doi.org/10.1007/978-981-97-4612-5_10

sis process and differentiate patients who would benefit from intensive therapy from people who would be better off avoiding excessive treatment. The etiology of PCa extends beyond the cancerous epithelial cells and encompasses the intricate interplay between these cells and the surrounding tumor microenvironment. The interaction between stroma and epithelial cells in prostate cancer has been demonstrated to have a significant impact on the advancement of the illness and its spread to other parts of the body. Several important indicators of reactive stroma have been found, including markers for stem/progenitor cells, inflammatory mediators originating from stromal cells, connective tissue growth factors, regulators of angiogenesis, wingless homologs (Wnts), and integrins. In this chapter, we present a summary of the intercommunication between stromal and epithelial cells in PCa, with a specific emphasis on the molecular biomarkers associated with the tumor microenvironment. We explore the significance of these biomarkers in the areas of diagnosis, prognosis, and the advancement of therapeutic strategies.

Keywords Androgen deprivation therapy (ADT) · Cancer-associated fibroblasts (CAFs) · Tumor microenvironment (TME) · TME heterogeneity · Androgen receptor (AR)

10.1 Introduction

Prostate cancer (PCa) is the most prevalent neoplasm impacting the male population and ranks as the second primary contributor to mortality associated with cancer in males on a global scale [1]. Tumors that exhibit a low pathological grade and are localized inside the prostate upon diagnosis often have a high likelihood of being successfully treated. Conversely, tumors characterized by progressive "International Society of Urological Pathology (ISUP)" grade groups and the presence of metastasis are associated with a less favorable prognosis [2]. Indolent neoplastic tumors of the prostate gland can manifest as either asymptomatic or accompanied by lower urinary tract symptoms (LUTS). On the other hand, it is worth noting that advanced tumors can give rise to more pronounced symptoms associated with the diffusion of cancer cells across multiple organs, leading to conditions such as vertebral fractures or compression of the spinal cord [3]. The involvement of androgens in the development of PCa is significant, therefore making it imperative to employ therapy strategies that target the modulation of androgen receptor (AR) signaling pathways [4]. The conventional treatment for disseminated illness is the use of gonadal androgen deprivation therapy (ADT). Nevertheless, in spite of the primary efficacy of androgen deprivation therapy (ADT), it is inevitable that resistance to this treatment will develop, leading to the emergence of castration-resistant prostate cancer [5].

The involvement of several cell types, along with epithelial cells, immune cells, and non-immune cells, is crucial in the expansion and advancement of PCa [6]. Prostatic oncogenesis is characterized by the interplay among epithelial cells and the adjacent stroma, facilitated by a series of inherent cellular transformations and modifications in the microenvironment. The involvement of many biomarkers associated with stromal activity has been suggested in the development of PCa [7]. The tumor microenvironment (TME) is a complex and interconnected ecosystem consisting of various cell types, including fibroblasts, immune cells, mesenchymal/stromal stem cells, myofibroblasts (MFB), endothelial cells, and neural crest cells. These cells secrete a range of factors, such as extracellular matrices (ECMs), chemokines, matrix-degrading enzymes, and cytokines [8]. The complex alterations observed in the surrounding stromal agents, which are influenced by the interaction among prostatic epithelial cells and the TME, play a crucial role in determining the severity of the disease, the ability of the tumor to metastasize, and its resistance to standard therapies [8]. Given the significant impact of the tumor microenvironment on PCa, it is imperative to identify new biomarkers that can effectively assess stromal activity. This is vital for the successful therapy of the disease. This study focuses on the interaction among epithelial and stromal cells, with a particular emphasis on relevant biomarkers that indicate stromal activity. They also discuss the significance of these biomarkers in the diagnosis, prognosis, and development of therapies for various diseases.

10.2 TME Heterogeneity in PCa

Tumor heterogeneity has emerged as a significant factor contributing to adverse outcomes, such as deadly consequences, resistance to drugs, and therapeutic inefficacy. Consequently, it poses a substantial obstacle to the achievement of precision medicine objectives. Given the observed correlation between tumor heterogeneity and unfavorable prognostic outcomes, it is plausible that quantifying heterogeneity itself could serve as a valuable prognostic indicator. The prevalent understanding is that the heterogeneity of cancers in the prostate is mostly due to genetic diversity. However, recent research suggests that, besides genetic determinants, tumor heterogeneity may also arise from non-genetic variations. The stroma plays a consequential role in inhibiting the expansion of cancer in benign tissue. However, the presence of cancer cells triggers important alterations that transform the surrounding environment into one that promotes the growth of tumors. The alterations encompass fibroblast recruitment, migration of immunocytes, remodeling of the extracellular matrix, formation of tumor-specific vasculature, and the presence of an abnormal epigenetic landscape. Each of these modifications has the potential to contribute to the heterogeneity of the tumor microenvironment (TME). The local diversity of selection forces in TME, including but not limited to hypoxia, acidity, and growth factors, plays an active role in shaping the morphology of tumors. It is plausible that the unique environmental characteristics of a tumor contribute significantly to its variability. TME exhibits a dynamic nature, characterized by variations in composition over space and time, as a result of environmental pressures and the administration of anticancer treatments. The ongoing communication between the adjacent microenvironment and tumor cells plays a crucial role in tumor initiation, phenotypic alterations, the advancement of cancer, and the development of resistance to therapeutic interventions.

The consensus in the scientific community is that the development of tumors is influenced not only by genetic changes and epigenetic modifications within cancer cells but also by TME.

The tumor microenvironment consists of various cell types, including fibroblasts, pericytes, immunocytes, and endotheliocytes. These cells have the ability to interact with cancer cells in a dynamic manner. The typical characterization of the impact of microenvironmental factors on cancer cells involves the examination of several regions. Tumorigenesis, in turn, is influenced by the heterogeneity of hypoxia, acidity, and cytokines within the tumor environment. In addition, cancer-associated fibroblasts (CAFs) are a prominent component within tumor microenvironment, playing a consequential role in promoting the malignant characteristics of cancer cells across various aspects. CAFs consist of diverse clusters that perform many tasks, including promoting tumor growth, facilitating the angiogenic process and remodeling of the stromal environment, contributing to drug resistance, and facilitating tumor spread. The clusters of the CAF exhibit either suppressive or stimulating actions on tumors. The observed variability can be attributed to various processes, including the dynamic interplay among stromal cells and tumor cells, the extracellular matrix, and the secretion of cytokines and growth hormones into TME.

The heterogeneity of cancer-associated fibroblasts is believed to be, at least in part, a result of their diverse origins. Cancer-associated fibroblasts are often believed to arise from resident fibroblasts due to the presence of transforming growth factor-beta (TGF-β), which is secreted by stromal cells and cancer cells. The topic of discussion is the pathway involving hypoxia-inducible factor (HIF)-1α. The production of transforming growth factor-beta (TGF-β) and C-X-C motif chemokine ligand 12 (CXCL-12) by CAFs plays an influential role in maintaining the myofibroblast phenotype and facilitating the interaction among the surrounding stromal cells and tumor cells. There is evidence indicating that cancer-associated fibroblasts may also originate from an epithelial-mesenchymal transition or endothelial-mesenchymal, which is facilitated by transforming growth factor-beta or suppressor of mothers against decapentaplegic homolog (SMAD) signaling. Additional types of fully developed cells, such as pericytes or inflammatory cells found in the supportive tissue, may also undergo a process called transdifferentiation to become CAFs. This transformation is facilitated by the influence of TGF-β, which regulates the activation of a cellular transition known as mesenchymal-to-mesenchymal transition. An alternative viewpoint posits that mesenchymal stromal cells generated from bone marrow have the potential to undergo differentiation into CAFs. The process of recruiting mesenchymal stromal cells and inducing their transformation into CAFs is accelerated by the secretion of TGF-β and CXCL-12 by cancer cells. Finally, it has been shown that cancer stem cells (CSCs) are identified as a significant source of CAFs. The process by which cancer stem cells undergo a transition into stromal cells provides a novel perspective that elucidates the phenomenon of tumor heterogeneity. In general, the presence of different sources contributes to the diversity of CAFs.

10.3 TME Heterogeneity in NEPC

Current scholarly investigations have been mostly directed toward comprehending the intricate terrain of castration-resistant prostate cancer (CRPC). Bluemn and coworkers (2017) conducted a comprehensive investigation involving phenotypic and genomic analyses of rapid autopsy CRPC tumors obtained from the University of Washington [9]. Their findings revealed that although most treatment-resistant CRPCs maintain androgen receptor (AR) signaling, there was a notable rise in the occurrence of double-negative prostate cancer (DNPC) and small-cell or neuroendocrine prostate cancer (NEPC) over a period of 20 years. The study revealed that the cells were experiencing adaptive changes in response to therapeutic pressure, resulting in a reduced need for AR for proliferation. Additionally, these cells were observed to undergo transdifferentiation, leading to the development of separate phenotypes with unique molecular characteristics [9].

Numerous research studies have been dedicated to investigating the mechanisms underlying the emergence and development of NEPC, with a particular emphasis on transdifferentiation processes. Additionally, considerable attention has been given to comprehending the intricate epigenomic and genomic aspects of this disease. Simultaneously, research endeavors are directed toward understanding the dynamic interaction among tumor cells and the surrounding tumor microenvironment. TME, which encompasses a complex interplay of fibroblasts, immune cells, the extracellular matrix, and blood vessels, is believed to contribute to the extension of prostate cancer and its metastasis to distant sites [10]. It is worth mentioning that within the context of NEPC, the administration of hormonal-based therapies, which include androgen deprivation therapy (ADT), has the potential to influence the interactions occurring within the tumor microenvironment. CAFs, a specific subtype of activated fibroblasts implicated in the secretion of factors and cellular plasticity associated with metastasis and tumor development [11], have been shown to initiate the proliferation of primary PC tumors and facilitate their metastatic dissemination in xenograft mouse models [12]. The association between epigenetic modifications occurring in cancer-associated fibroblasts and the process of NEPC reprogramming has been postulated. The study conducted by Mishra et al. (2018) employed a comprehensive examination of methylation patterns throughout the entire genome in fibroblasts obtained from prostate cancer tissue [13]. The findings of this investigation revealed the presence of epigenetic silencing of RASAL3, a known inhibitor of the Ras signaling pathway. The process of silencing, which is initiated through the administration of ADT, triggers a series of interconnected reactions encompassing activation of Ras, the macropinocytosis initiation, and the production of glutamine. The observed effects indicate that stromal glutamine plays a role in facilitating neuroendocrine differentiation through the provision of energy to prostate epithelial cells. Notably, increased levels of glutamine were observed in patients undergoing ADT, as reported by Mishra and coworkers (2018), further recommending its involvement in the neuroendocrine distinction procedure [13]. Enriquez et al. (2021) discovered an additional potential method by which stromal cells can exert their influence on NEPC [14]. This mechanism is believed to be activated as a response to castration resistance in the context of ADT and androgen receptor signaling inhibitor (ARSI) treatment. The initiation of castration circumstances resulted in the overexpression of GRP78, which led to the downregulation of SPARC, an extracellular matrix protein, in the adjacent stroma, mediated by microRNA (miR29-b). The downregulation of SPARC resulted in the induction of interleukin-6 (IL-6), a cytokine known for its role in facilitating a neuroendocrine milieu. The authors of the study conducted an experiment to investigate the potential of GRP78 as a therapeutic target for NEPC. They administered a powerful inhibitor of GRP78, isoliquiritigenin, to castrated mice with tumors and observed a reduction in neuroendocrine differentiation [14].

There is additional heterogeneity observed within the fibroblast populations found in CRPC, wherein a specific fraction of fibroblasts expresses CD105, a membrane glycoprotein that has been associated with epithelial-mesenchymal transition [15]. The population of cells expressing CD105 had an impact on the expression of secreted frizzled-related protein 1 (SFRP1), a regulator of NEPC development. This effect was shown in cell line models, where treatment with SFRP1 resulted in heightened expression of genes associated with neuroendocrine function [15]. Furthermore, it was observed that the administration of enzalutamide resulted in a significant augmentation of CD105 cell surface expression on both fibroblasts and epithelial cells, as reported by Kato and coworkers in 2019. This finding further supports the notion that androgen deprivation therapy (ADT) stimulates TME, promoting the expansion of a neuroendocrine phenotype [15].

Familial adenomatous polyposis (FAP) serves as a crucial mediator in the context of cancer-associated fibroblasts, exhibiting potential as a prognostic marker and displaying an association with unfavorable clinical outcomes. The study investigated by Lai and coworkers (2012) showed a correlation between the silencing of FAP in ovarian cancer models and a reduction in cancer-associated fibroblasts [16]. This finding suggests that fibroblast activation protein plays a crucial role in regulating this specific cell type. Through an evaluation of PC tumors accessible via the public database cBioPortal, Vlachostergios et al. (2022) determined a significant correlation between FAP and poorer overall survival in CRPC. Moreover, the study revealed that heightened expression of FAP was linked to elevated neuroendocrine pathway scores and diminished AR pathway scores, thereby providing additional evidence of the interplay between FAP and the tumor microenvironment [17]. Further investigation of fibroblast activation protein by immunohistochemistry revealed an augmented expression profile as the illness progressed from primary to metastatic CRPC. Significantly, it is worth noting that imaging techniques focused on FAP, such as [68Ga] Ga-FAPI-04 positron emission tomography/computed tomography (PET/CT), have exhibited notable levels of positive impact in CRPC. Consequently, these modalities hold potential as a theragnostic approach for patients with NEPC in the future [18].

The varied connections discovered between the fibroblasts and stroma within the tumor microenvironment and PC cells provide additional insight into the numerous cell signaling pathways that have a role in the development of neuroendocrine prostate cancer. Furthermore, it is evident that current anti-androgen treatments contribute to the development of a neuroendocrine-rich setting, implying that modifying conventional therapeutic strategies could be advantageous.

10.4 Prostate Cancer TME

When examining the tapestry of the tumor microenvironment (TME), it is considerable to analyze the overall impact of immune cells on the development of cancer, as well as strategies to alter the functional balance of these resident populations in order to restore anti-tumor immune responses. The intricate nature of the immunosuppressive cell populations found in PCa and the influence of the tumor microenvironment in facilitating cancer progression highlight the numerous elements that must be taken into account while devising innovative immunotherapeutic strategies. The existing clinical studies on immunotherapy in prostate cancer have been subject to thorough examination in previous literature [19]. Nevertheless, the relatively low tumor mutational burden observed in PCa and the limited efficacy of existing immune checkpoint blockade (ICB) treatments indicate the necessity of stratifying PCa patients for future therapeutic interventions. Hence, the integration of immunogenomic categorization has the potential to facilitate the identification of suitable individuals for personalized combination therapies.

The immune microenvironment has the potential to influence the biological progression of PCa via the process of N6 methyl adenosine (m6A) methylation [20]. The objective of this work was to examine the interplay between m6A methylation and the immunological milieu, as well as to identify possible biomarkers that could enhance the efficacy of immunotherapy. Initially, based on the analysis of 11 differentially expressed m6A genes in normal and tumor samples, patients with PCa were classified into two immune microenvironment subtypes, namely immune signature 1 (IMS1) and IMS2. This classification was made by extracting m6A gene profiles from the TCGA database. The IMS2 condition was found to exhibit an immunological "cold" phenotype, which was associated with poorer prognoses. Through the analysis of protein-protein interaction networks, heterogeneous nuclear ribonucleoprotein C (HNRNPC) was discovered as the biomarker for IMS2. Moreover, by employing bioinformatics analysis and conducting in vitro studies, the researchers discovered that individuals with elevated levels of HNRNPC exhibited a tumor microenvironment characterized by immune suppression, as seen by a greater presence of regulatory T (Treg) cells. In conclusion, the researchers conducted a co-culture experiment using transfected PCa cells and peripheral blood mononuclear cells (PBMC). Through their investigation, they confirmed that HNRNPC hinders tumor immunity by increasing the activation of regulatory T (Treg) cells and suppressing the activity of effector CD8 T cells. In summary, a "cold" immunological phenotype was observed in PCa, and it was determined that HNRNPC has a role in modulating the activation of regulatory T cells (Treg cells).

Targeting HNRNPC as a means to activate the immune microenvironment could potentially serve as a viable treatment approach for advanced prostate cancer [20].

10.5 Stromal Compartment in Prostate Cancer

The prostatic stromal milieu encompasses several anatomical and physiological elements that are relevant to the proper functioning of the gland. The genesis and progression of PCa are influenced by changes in several stromal elements. The phenomenon of epithelial neoplastic change in the prostate gland is intricately linked to its surrounding environment. In addition to the influence of microenvironmental variables, molecular changes occurring inside the cells themselves are known to exert a substantial impact on this process. The progression and spread of prostate tumors are dependent on the complex interaction between malignant cells and the components of the surrounding stroma [21]. Fibroblasts have a crucial role in the composition of the prostatic stroma. Epithelial cells are preserved in their structural integrity through continuous remodeling and dynamic interactions with various components inside the organ [22]. Fibroblasts have a role in the production of ECM by secreting collagen type I and type III. They also facilitate tissue regeneration by orchestrating the controlled creation of granulation tissue and subsequent transformation into myofibroblasts (MFB). During the process of prostatic neoplastic transformation, the stromal smooth muscle cells undergo replacement by a distinct type of fibroblasts known as CAF. The presence of cancer stroma has been found to stimulate the upregulation of fibroblast-specific markers, including vimentin, fibroblast-specific protein (FSP), and alpha-smooth muscle actin (α-SMA), while concurrently downregulating the expression of desmin [8]. CAFs are significant contributors to the process of angiogenesis and the modification of ECM components. These effects are mediated by various factors, including interleukin-6 (IL-6), fibroblast growth factor (FGF), transforming growth factor beta (TGF-β), hypoxia inducible factor 1 alpha (HIF-1α), growth differentiation factor 15 (GDF15), vascular endothelial growth factor (VEGF), and hepatocyte growth factor (HGF) [23, 24]. According to Sahai et al. (2020), the interaction between tumor cells and Cancer-associated fibroblasts results in the development of an unregulated "reactive stroma," which promotes the proliferation and aggressiveness of cancer cells and influences their response to treatment [25].

The development of prostate tumors is undeniably reliant, to some degree, on the stimulation of angiogenesis. The development of blood vessels has a vital role in promoting the survival and proliferation of cancer cells [26, 27]. Within the context of normal prostatic tissue, a state of equilibrium is observed in the interplay among smooth muscle cells, pericytes, and endothelial cells. Nevertheless, the vasculature of tumors is distinguished by the abnormal development of juvenile blood vessels that are permeable and do not possess pericyte coverage [28]. The process of angiogenesis, which involves the formation of new blood vessels, is facilitated by the interaction among tumor cells and stromal endothelial cells. This interaction leads to the activation of an "angiogenic switch" by upregulating the expression of pro-angiogenic proteins, including vascular endothelial growth factor [28]. The study conducted by Zhao et al. (2018) provided evidence supporting the notion that endothelial cells play a significant role in the tumor microenvironment by promoting metastatic activity through the suppression of androgen receptor (AR) expression and transcriptional activity [29]. Consequently, the researchers suggested that inhibiting endothelial cells could potentially impede the progression of PCa.

Immune cells are often present within a state of normalcy in the prostatic tissue of individuals who are in good health, and they serve a defensive function by guarding against the invasion of infections [30]. Histological investigations have revealed a correlation between high-grade PCa and heightened infiltration of stromal immune cells, with variations in cellular composition based on the stage of the tumor [31]. The progress of a chronic inflammatory state within the prostate can be influenced by ongoing stresses, including a high-fat diet, direct infection, estrogens, and urinary reflux [32]. In the context of ongoing inflammation, the stromal compartment experiences an inflow of various immune cells, including macrophages, natural killer (NK) cells, $CD3^+$ T cells, macrophages, $CD20^+$ B cells, and mast cells [6]. Inflammatory cells are known to generate substantial quantities of cytokines and chemokines, including but not limited to tumor necrosis factor (TNF), interleukin-6 (IL-6), interleukin-8 (IL-8), vascular endothelial growth factor (VEGF), and nuclear factor kappa B (NF-κB). These proteins, along with others, are involved in the adjustment of angiogenesis, cellular proliferation, and inflammation. Worthington et al. (2012) assert that they facilitate the progression toward a malignant phenotype in PCa [33]. The involvement of inflammation in prostate cancer has facilitated the exploration of new anti-inflammatory medications for the prevention and potential treatment of PCa [34].

The concept of "tight interlocking" refers to a close and interconnected relationship between different elements or components. The extracellular matrix (ECM) that envelops prostate epithelial cells consists of many non-collagenous proteins and collagenous fibers, including osteocalcin, fibronectin, osteonectin, cadherin, vitronectin, and bone sialoprotein [35]. ECM serves as a structural support system that facilitates the maintenance of cellular homeostasis within various organ systems. As the neoplastic process occurs and metastatic progression takes place, there is an alteration in the expression of several extracellular constituents, resulting in upregulation, downregulation, or loss. The expression of collagen type VII is observed to decrease, while the manufacturing of bone sialoproteins is observed to increase in association with advanced prostate cancer [36, 37]. The dependency of metastatic development on the disruption of the ECM barrier is apparent. In order for invasion and metastasis to take place, malignant cells are required to generate a variety of proteases and protein-degrading enzymes [38]. Matrix metalloproteinases (MMPs) are a class of peptidases that require zinc for their enzymatic activity. These enzymes have a broad range of binding affinities toward ECM proteins, including collagens, fibronectins, and laminin [39]. The expression of MMPs, including MMP-1, MMP-2, MMP-7, MMP-9, and MT1-MMP, becomes more evident in the stroma and bloodstream as PCa progresses. This suggests that these molecules may have predictive value, as shown by Gong et al. (2014) [40]. However, despite their theoretical potential in targeting PCa, MMP-inhibiting medicines such as batimastat and marimastat could not demonstrate efficacy in phase III clinical studies [41].

10.6 The Microenvironment of PCA and the Markers Associated with Cancer Stem/Progenitor Cells

The initial discovery of prostate stem cells was documented in the 1980s by English and coworkers (1987) [42]. Subsequently, there has been a growing acceptance among the scientific community about the possibility that prostate cancer (PCa) may originate from cancer stem cells (CSCs). There has been an increasing surge of scientific inquiry focused on the characterization of these stem cells [43, 44]. The distinctive capacity for plasticity, self-renewal, pluripotency, and the ability to restore complete tumor heterogeneity have ushered in a new era of therapeutics and diagnostics. Consequently, there is now a critical need to comprehensively comprehend the methods for detecting prostate cancer stem cells and identifying their potential markers [45–47]. The resistance of prostate CSCs to therapeutic interventions, including radiotherapy, can be attributed to various intricate mechanisms. These mechanisms contain the presence of a hypoxic microenvironment, enhanced DNA repair capabilities, epithelial-to-mesenchymal transition processes [48], increased intracellular scavenging of activation of anti-apoptotic signaling pathways, autophagy, and reactive oxygen species [49]. It is crucial to acknowledge that prostate cancer stem cells represent a small proportion of the overall tumor mass, primarily localized in the proximal areas of the prostatic ducts. The stem cells are situated within specialized habitats that possess intricate microenvironments that are strongly intertwined with the surrounding host cells. The prevailing consensus in the scientific community is that prostate cancer stem cells are primarily found in the basal cell compartment. However, there is continuous debate and extensive research about the presence of these cells in the luminal compartment [50]. The significant decline in the survival rates of individuals with recurring or metastatic tumors served as a primary catalyst for the exploration of CSCs in the context of prostate cancer.

Harris and colleagues (2017) have shown that the formation and progression of PCa are influenced by a wide range of CSC indicators [51]. These markers not only contribute to therapy resistance and the ability of cancer cells to colonize and proliferate in distant sites but also play a significant role in the overall pathogenesis of PCa. The extracellular markers associated with CSCs in PCa, although not particularly exclusive to this particular cancer type, include CD166/ALCAM, CD117/c-kit, CXCR4, α6 integrin, CD133, Trop2, CD44, α2β1 integrin, E-cadherin, cytokeratin 5, EpCAM, ABCG2, PSA, and AR variant 7 [52]. The intracellular indicators that have been identified include ALDH1, TG2, and EZH2. It is vital to acknowledge the conventional stemness markers, including Nanog, OCT3/4, c-MYC, SOX2, and KLF4, as stated by Harris and Kerr (2017) [51]. After discussing the aforementioned indicators, it is necessary to emphasize the latest developments in the identification of prostate CSCs. In a recent study, Hu and coworkers discovered a strong correlation between the expression of basic transcription factor 3 (BTF3) and the presence of stemness characteristics. The reduction in metastatic potential and self-renewal capacities was observed in cases of basic transcription factor 3 deletion, whereas an increase in these characteristics was observed in cases of BTF3 overexpression. The proposed method is centered on the hypothesis that BTF3 has the ability to enhance the stability of BMI1, a critical regulator of self-renewal in prostate CSCs. The researchers additionally provided evidence to support the notion that BTF3 has the potential to serve as a strong predictor of an unfavorable prognosis. Consequently, it can be utilized as a means to categorize patients based on their risk levels [53]. Mawaribuchi and colleagues showed that the recombinant lectin rBC2LCN exhibits potential as a cancer stem cell marker in prostate cancer. The fraction of PC-3 rBC2LCN-positive cells displayed characteristics commonly associated with CSCs, including reduced proliferation, increased cell motility, the ability to develop independently of anchorage, and resistance to therapy [54].

Simeckova and colleagues conducted an evaluation of the expression of Skp2, a crucial element of the SCF E3 ubiquitin ligase, which is commonly observed to be upregulated in PCa and other neoplastic conditions. The findings of the study indicated that Skp2 exhibited a significant upregulation in PCa cells that possessed characteristics like stem cells and mesenchymal cells, as opposed to epithelial cells. It is important to mention that a shift from an epithelial to a non-epithelial/mesenchymal phenotype has been earlier demonstrated to be associated with the observed invasiveness in cancer stemness [55].

The expression of the stemness trait was diminished in cells exhibiting a suppressed Skp2 gene. Furthermore, the downregulation of Skp2 resulted in a decrease in the subpopulation of $CD44^{+}/CD24^{-}$ prostate cancer stem cell (PCSC), providing additional evidence for the significant role of Skp2 in maintaining the stem-like properties of PCa [55]. Through the utilization of lineage retracing, Yoo and coworkers successfully recognized a specific subpopulation of $Bmi1^{+}$ $Sox2^{+}$ CRPC cells that may serve as a plausible origin for the recurrence of disease in an in vivo setting [56]. The results of this study may provide support for the strategic focus on particular subgroups responsible for the observed effects, with the aim of developing targeted treatment interventions [56]. Federer-Gsponer et al. (2020) demonstrated the presence of a stemness-associated marker pattern in both hormone naïve and castration-resistant samples, suggesting a potential association with castration resistance [57]. An intriguing discovery was made regarding a distinct pattern of mutual exclusivity observed in the expression of ALDH1A1 and ALDH1A3. It is important to highlight that this particular trend was identified within publicly available datasets at the transcriptome level. Hence, it is imperative to do additional research in order to unravel this pattern and gain a more comprehensive comprehension of the distinct impact of these markers.

Another type of marker that is important pertains to stromal markers. For example, Mahal and coworkers demonstrated the significance of these markers by a comprehensive examination of radical prostatectomy samples at the genomic level [58]. After conducting an analysis that involved examining the correlation between expression scores and classical stromal genes, as well as other important stromal markers such as Transgelin (TAGLN), Caveolin-1 (CAV1), and Vimentin (VIM), along with CD3 and CD4 markers and basal activity, the investigator reached the conclusion that the highest 10% of stromal expression was linked to elevated genomic risk scores (Decipher ≥0.6), Gleason 9 to 10 disease, an increased likelihood of metastasis (hazard ratio, 2.35; 95% CI, 1.37–4.02; $p = 0.001$), and high Cancer of the Prostate Risk Assessment-Postsurgical (CAPRA-S) scores. Furthermore, it was observed that an elevated stromal infiltration score was linked to a decrease in the expression of DNA repair genes and an increase in radiation sensitivity genomic scores, as reported by Mahal et al. (2020) [56]. Yasumizu et al. directed their attention toward the mucin 1 C-terminal subunit (MUC1-C) protein, which exhibits significant expression levels in castration-resistant neoplasms and neuroendocrine prostate cancer. The overexpression of MUC1-C in androgen-dependent prostate cancer cells inhibits the functionality of both p53 signaling pathways and the androgen receptor [59]. Conversely, it also results in the upregulation of OCT4, KLF4, MYC, and SOX2 (together referred to as the Yamanaka factors), promoting an augmented state of pluripotency. Hence, from a therapeutic perspective, it is plausible to consider MUC1-C as a potential target for combating the stemness of prostate cancer [59].

The present advancements primarily center around liquid biopsies as a minimally invasive approach for characterizing CSCs. However, a potential breakthrough in marker identification could involve transitioning from utilizing prostate cancer cell lines to patient-derived tumors. This shift would offer a more comprehensive comprehension of metastatic mechanisms and treatment resistance processes. The utilization of patient-derived organoids, which possess the ability to accurately mimic the molecular, biochemical, and structural characteristics of the original tumor, has the potential to enhance ongoing research endeavors and address the challenges associated with sustaining an in vitro luminal phenotype [60].

Bone metastasis is a frequently observed occurrence in PCa and necessitates significant therapeutic intervention. When PCa spreads to the bone, the resulting milieu can trigger changes in the epigenome and remodeling of cancer cells with stem cell-like properties. This process enhances the ability of cancer cells to adapt to the bone microenvironment, ultimately leading to the development of secondary tumor metastasis [61]. The research team has earlier discovered that the RNA binding motif 3 (RBM3) has an impact on the stem cell-like characteristics of prostate cancer by disrupting the process of alternative splicing of CD44. The current understanding of the ability of RBM3, a stress-response protein, to counteract the microenvironmental changes associated with PCa bone metastases is still lacking. Through the process of co-culturing PCa cells with osteoblasts, researchers were able to create a model that mimics the bone metastasis of PCa. This model allowed them to observe that RBM3, a specific protein, increases the level of

N6-methyladenosine (m6A) methylation on the messenger RNA (mRNA) of catenin beta 1 (CTNNB1). This increase in methylation was found to be dependent on the presence of methyltransferase 3 (METTL3), which is a catalytic subunit of the N6-adenosine-methyltransferase complex. As a result, this alteration leads to a reduction in the stability of CTNNB1 mRNA, subsequently causing the inactivation of wingless homolog (Wnt) signaling. Consequently, this inhibits the remodeling of prostate cancer cells by osteoblasts, so affecting their stemness. Therefore, the current investigation has the potential to enhance knowledge regarding the inhibitory function of RBM3, specifically in relation to bone metastases of prostate cancer [61].

10.7 Conclusion

The involvement of a reactive tumor stroma has been demonstrated to have a pivotal impact on both the start and progression of tumors. Indeed, it is widely recognized that prostate cancer stem cells (CSCs) have the potential to undergo a process of recruitment, leading to their differentiation into myofibroblasts or carcinoma-associated fibroblasts. Several crucial regulators of this recruiting and conversion procedure have been found. The intricate and multifaceted interplay between the carcinoma and the stroma is precisely regulated by the aforementioned parameters. It is important to consider that the reactive stroma can develop early, potentially even during preneoplastic stages. Additionally, the lack of success in clinical trials involving inhibitors of angiogenesis and other processes related to the prostate microenvironment in cancer underscores the need for further investigation. Researchers should actively search for clinically significant targets before the stromal components exert their complete cancer-promoting influence [62]. Circulating plasma and urine biomarkers hold significant value and have the potential to contribute to the diagnosis, selection of treatment, and evaluation of response in the context of PCa in the foreseeable future. Furthermore, it is imperative to recognize that there are valuable insights to be gained from the limitations encountered in past trials of anti-angiogenic drugs. Consequently, it is crucial that scientific endeavors are focused on avenues that circumvent errors that have been previously made. Furthermore, it is imperative to address the unfulfilled requirement of completely harnessing the capabilities of biomarkers beyond prostate-specific antigen (PSA), as the issues of excessive diagnosis and treatment of patients are of paramount concern. Two other biomarkers that have received approval from the US Food and Drug Administration (FDA) are the prostate health index (PHI) and the prostate cancer antigen 3 (PCA3). While the PHI is known for its affordability, the non-invasive 4Kscore blood test has also demonstrated the ability to predict clinically significant prostate cancer. Consequently, this has the potential to reduce the number of unnecessary biopsies. Additional urine liquid biopsy tests, such as Select MdX and Exosome Dx, have demonstrated significant potential. However, it is imperative to conduct further investigations in order to create comprehensive clinical integration.

Further investigation is necessary to achieve a comprehensive consensus on a specific marker, as suggested by Becerra et al. (2020) [63]. The process of changing the neoplastic environment is a critical factor in driving tumor invasiveness. The efficacy of this process relies significantly on the extent of extracellular matrix penetration, the reorganization of fibrillar components, and the interaction between cancer and stroma.

References

1. Siegel RL, Miller KD, Fuchs HE, Jemal A. Cancer statistics, 2021. CA Cancer J Clin. 2021;71(1):7–33.
2. Martin NE, Mucci LA, Loda M, Depinho RA. Prognostic determinants in prostate cancer. Cancer J (Sudbury, Mass). 2011;17(6):429–37.
3. Merriel SWD, Funston G, Hamilton W. Prostate cancer in primary care. Adv Ther. 2018;35(9):1285–94.
4. Schrecengost R, Knudsen KE. Molecular pathogenesis and progression of prostate cancer. Semin Oncol. 2013;40(3):244–58.
5. Polotti CF, Kim CJ, Chuchvara N, Polotti AB, Singer EA, Elsamra S. Androgen deprivation therapy for the treatment of prostate cancer: a focus on pharmacokinetics. Expert Opin Drug Metab Toxicol. 2017;13(12):1265–73.
6. Shiao SL, Chu GC, Chung LW. Regulation of prostate cancer progression by the tumor microenvironment. Cancer Lett. 2016;380(1):340–8.
7. Filella X, Fernández-Galan E, Fernández Bonifacio R, Foj L. Emerging biomarkers in the diagnosis of prostate cancer. Pharmgenomics Pers Med. 2018;11:83–94.
8. Hägglöf C, Bergh A. The stroma-a key regulator in prostate function and malignancy. Cancers. 2012;4(2):531–48.
9. Bluemn EG, Coleman IM, Lucas JM, Coleman RT, Hernandez-Lopez S, Tharakan R, et al. Androgen receptor pathway-independent prostate cancer is sustained through FGF signaling. Cancer Cell. 2017;32(4):474–89. e6
10. Andersen S, Richardsen E, Moi L, Donnem T, Nordby Y, Ness N, et al. Fibroblast miR-210 overexpression is independently associated with clinical failure in prostate cancer - a multicenter (in situ hybridization) study. Sci Rep. 2016;6:36573.
11. Ping Q, Yan R, Cheng X, Wang W, Zhong Y, Hou Z, et al. Cancer-associated fibroblasts: overview, progress, challenges, and directions. Cancer Gene Ther. 2021;28(9):984–99.
12. Linxweiler J, Hajili T, Körbel C, Berchem C, Zeuschner P, Müller A, et al. Cancer-associated fibroblasts stimulate primary tumor growth and metastatic spread in an orthotopic prostate cancer xenograft model. Sci Rep. 2020;10(1):12575.
13. Mishra R, Haldar S, Placencio V, Madhav A, Rohena-Rivera K, Agarwal P, et al. Stromal epigenetic alterations drive metabolic and neuroendocrine prostate cancer reprogramming. J Clin Invest. 2018;128(10):4472–84.
14. Enriquez C, Cancila V, Ferri R, Sulsenti R, Fischetti I, Milani M, et al. Castration-induced downregulation of SPARC in stromal cells drives neuroendocrine differentiation of prostate cancer. Cancer Res. 2021;81(16):4257–74.
15. Kato M, Placencio-Hickok VR, Madhav A, Haldar S, Tripathi M, Billet S, et al. Heterogeneous cancer-associated fibroblast population potentiates neuroendocrine differentiation and castrate resistance in a CD105-dependent manner. Oncogene. 2019;38(5):716–30.
16. Lai D, Ma L, Wang F. Fibroblast activation protein regulates tumor-associated fibroblasts and epithelial ovarian cancer cells. Int J Oncol. 2012;41(2):541–50.

17. Vlachostergios PJ, Karathanasis A, Tzortzis V. Expression of fibroblast activation protein is enriched in neuroendocrine prostate cancer and predicts worse survival. Genes. 2022;13:1.
18. Kesch C, Yirga L, Dendl K, Handke A, Darr C, Krafft U, et al. High fibroblast-activation-protein expression in castration-resistant prostate cancer supports the use of FAPI-molecular theranostics. Eur J Nucl Med Mol Imaging. 2021;49(1):385–9.
19. Fay EK, Graff JN. Immunotherapy in prostate cancer. Cancers. 2020;12:7.
20. Cheng Y, Li L, Wei X, Xu F, Huang X, Qi F, et al. HNRNPC suppresses tumor immune microenvironment by activating Treg cells promoting the progression of prostate cancer. Cancer Sci. 2023;114(5):1830–45.
21. Torrealba N, Rodríguez-Berriguete G, Fraile B, Olmedilla G, Martínez-Onsurbe P, Guil-Cid M, et al. Expression of several cytokines in prostate cancer: correlation with clinical variables of patients. Relationship with biochemical progression of the malignance. Cytokine. 2017;89:105–15.
22. Gabbiani G. The myofibroblast in wound healing and fibrocontractive diseases. J Pathol. 2003;200(4):500–3.
23. Ishii K, Mizokami A, Tsunoda T, Iguchi K, Kato M, Hori Y, et al. Heterogenous induction of carcinoma-associated fibroblast-like differentiation in normal human prostatic fibroblasts by co-culturing with prostate cancer cells. J Cell Biochem. 2011;112(12):3604–11.
24. Levesque C, Nelson PS. Cellular constituents of the prostate stroma: key contributors to prostate cancer progression and therapy resistance. Cold Spring Harb Perspect Med. 2018;8:8.
25. Sahai E, Astsaturov I, Cukierman E, DeNardo DG, Egeblad M, Evans RM, et al. A framework for advancing our understanding of cancer-associated fibroblasts. Nat Rev Cancer. 2020;20(3):174–86.
26. Melegh Z, Oltean S. Targeting angiogenesis in prostate cancer. Int J Mol Sci. 2019;20:11.
27. Bates M, Kovalenko B, Wilson EL, Moscatelli D. Endothelial cells support the growth of prostate tissue in vivo. Prostate. 2008;68(8):893–901.
28. Bergers G, Benjamin LE. Tumorigenesis and the angiogenic switch. Nat Rev Cancer. 2003;3(6):401–10.
29. Zhao R, Bei X, Yang B, Wang X, Jiang C, Shi F, et al. Endothelial cells promote metastasis of prostate cancer by enhancing autophagy. J Exp Clin Cancer Res CR. 2018;37(1):221.
30. Hussein MR, Al-Assiri M, Musalam AO. Phenotypic characterization of the infiltrating immune cells in normal prostate, benign nodular prostatic hyperplasia and prostatic adenocarcinoma. Exp Mol Pathol. 2009;86(2):108–13.
31. Gurel B, Lucia MS, Thompson IM Jr, Goodman PJ, Tangen CM, Kristal AR, et al. Chronic inflammation in benign prostate tissue is associated with high-grade prostate cancer in the placebo arm of the prostate cancer prevention trial. Cancer Epidemiol Biomarkers Prev. 2014;23(5):847–56.
32. De Marzo AM, Platz EA, Sutcliffe S, Xu J, Grönberg H, Drake CG, et al. Inflammation in prostate carcinogenesis. Nat Rev Cancer. 2007;7(4):256–69.
33. Worthington JJ, Fenton TM, Czajkowska BI, Klementowicz JE, Travis MA. Regulation of TGFβ in the immune system: an emerging role for integrins and dendritic cells. Immunobiology. 2012;217(12):1259–65.
34. Stark T, Livas L, Kyprianou N. Inflammation in prostate cancer progression and therapeutic targeting. Transl Androl Urol. 2015;4(4):455–63.
35. Kiefer JA, Farach-Carson MC. Type I collagen-mediated proliferation of PC3 prostate carcinoma cell line: implications for enhanced growth in the bone microenvironment. Matrix Biol. 2001;20(7):429–37.
36. Nagle RB, Hao J, Knox JD, Dalkin BL, Clark V, Cress AE. Expression of hemidesmosomal and extracellular matrix proteins by normal and malignant human prostate tissue. Am J Pathol. 1995;146(6):1498–507.
37. Bussemakers MJ, Van Bokhoven A, Tomita K, Jansen CF, Schalken JA. Complex cadherin expression in human prostate cancer cells. Int J Cancer. 2000;85(3):446–50.

38. Stamenkovic I. Matrix metalloproteinases in tumor invasion and metastasis. Semin Cancer Biol. 2000;10(6):415–33.
39. Cooper CR, Chay CH, Gendernalik JD, Lee HL, Bhatia J, Taichman RS, et al. Stromal factors involved in prostate carcinoma metastasis to bone. Cancer. 2003;97(3 Suppl):739–47.
40. Gong Y, Chippada-Venkata UD, Oh WK. Roles of matrix metalloproteinases and their natural inhibitors in prostate cancer progression. Cancers. 2014;6(3):1298–327.
41. Coussens LM, Fingleton B, Matrisian LM. Matrix metalloproteinase inhibitors and cancer: trials and tribulations. Science (New York, NY). 2002;295(5564):2387–92.
42. English HF, Santen RJ, Isaacs JT. Response of glandular versus basal rat ventral prostatic epithelial cells to androgen withdrawal and replacement. Prostate. 1987;11(3):229–42.
43. Abou-Kheir WG, Hynes PG, Martin PL, Pierce R, Kelly K. Characterizing the contribution of stem/progenitor cells to tumorigenesis in the Pten-/-TP53-/- prostate cancer model. Stem Cells (Dayton, Ohio). 2010;28(12):2129–40.
44. Leão R, Domingos C, Figueiredo A, Hamilton R, Tabori U, Castelo-Branco P. Cancer stem cells in prostate cancer: implications for targeted therapy. Urol Int. 2017;99(2):125–36.
45. Moltzahn F, Thalmann GN. Cancer stem cells in prostate cancer. Transl Androl Urol. 2013;2(3):242.
46. Bahmad HF, Cheaito K, Chalhoub RM, Hadadeh O, Monzer A, Ballout F, et al. Sphere-formation assay: three-dimensional in vitro culturing of prostate cancer stem/progenitor sphere-forming cells. Front Oncol. 2018;8:347.
47. Bahmad HF, Elajami MK, Daouk R, Jalloul H, Darwish B, Chalhoub RM, et al. Stem cells: in sickness and in health. Curr Stem Cell Res Ther. 2021;16(3):262–76.
48. Cheaito KA, Bahmad HF, Hadadeh O, Saleh E, Dagher C, Hammoud MS, et al. EMT markers in locally-advanced prostate cancer: predicting recurrence? Front Oncol. 2019;9:131.
49. Tsao T, Beretov J, Ni J, Bai X, Bucci J, Graham P, et al. Cancer stem cells in prostate cancer radioresistance. Cancer Lett. 2019;465:94–104.
50. Xin L. Cells of origin for prostate cancer. Adv Exp Med Biol. 2019;1210:67–86.
51. Harris KS, Kerr BA. Prostate cancer stem cell markers drive progression, therapeutic resistance, and bone metastasis. Stem Cells Int. 2017;2017:8629234.
52. Di Stefano C, Grazioli P, Fontanella RA, De Cesaris P, D'Amore A, Regno M, et al. Stem-like and highly invasive prostate cancer cells expressing CD44v8-10 marker originate from CD44-negative cells. Oncotarget. 2018;9(56):30905–18.
53. Hu J, Sun F, Chen W, Zhang J, Zhang T, Qi M, et al. BTF3 sustains cancer stem-like phenotype of prostate cancer via stabilization of BMI1. J Exp Clin Cancer Res. 2019;38:1–15.
54. Mawaribuchi S, Onuma Y, Aiki Y, Kuriyama Y, Mutoh M, Fujii G, et al. The rBC2LCN-positive subpopulation of PC-3 cells exhibits cancer stem-like properties. Biochem Biophys Res Commun. 2019;515(1):176–82.
55. Šimečková Š, Kahounová Z, Fedr R, Remšík J, Slabáková E, Suchánková T, et al. High Skp2 expression is associated with a mesenchymal phenotype and increased tumorigenic potential of prostate cancer cells. Sci Rep. 2019;9(1):5695.
56. Yoo YA, Vatapalli R, Lysy B, Mok H, Desouki MM, Abdulkadir SA. The role of castration-resistant Bmi1+Sox2+ cells in driving recurrence in prostate cancer. J Natl Cancer Inst. 2019;111(3):311–21.
57. Federer-Gsponer JR, Müller DC, Zellweger T, Eggimann M, Marston K, Ruiz C, et al. Patterns of stemness-associated markers in the development of castration-resistant prostate cancer. Prostate. 2020;80(13):1108–17.
58. Mahal BA, Alshalalfa M, Zhao SG, Beltran H, Chen WS, Chipidza F, et al. Genomic and clinical characterization of stromal infiltration markers in prostate cancer. Cancer. 2020;126(7):1407–12.
59. Yasumizu Y, Rajabi H, Jin C, Hata T, Pitroda S, Long MD, et al. MUC1-C regulates lineage plasticity driving progression to neuroendocrine prostate cancer. Nat Commun. 2020;11(1):338.

60. Li JJ, Shen MM. Prostate stem cells and cancer stem cells. Cold Spring Harb Perspect Med. 2019;9:6.
61. Zhang S, Lv C, Niu Y, Li C, Li X, Shang Y, et al. RBM3 suppresses stemness remodeling of prostate cancer in bone microenvironment by modulating N6-methyladenosine on CTNNB1 mRNA. Cell Death Dis. 2023;14(2):91.
62. Barron DA, Rowley DR. The reactive stroma microenvironment and prostate cancer progression. Endocr Relat Cancer. 2012;19(6):R187–204.
63. Becerra MF, Atluri VS, Bhattu AS, Punnen S, editors. Serum and urine biomarkers for detecting clinically significant prostate cancer. Urologic Oncology: Seminars and Original Investigations; 2021: Elsevier.

Part IV
Treatments and Challenges

Chapter 11
Chemoresistance, Radioresistance, and Androgen Deprivation Therapy Resistance in Prostate Cancer

Samaneh Adelian, Amin Soltani, and Michael R. Hamblin

Abstract One of the primary obstacles encountered in the clinical care of individuals suffering from advanced, life-threatening prostate cancer is the development of resistance to therapeutic interventions, including androgen deprivation therapy (ADT), chemotherapy, and radiation. To overcome this resistance, it is essential to possess a comprehensive comprehension of the underlying processes that drive the tumor microenvironment. This knowledge should extend beyond the androgen receptor (AR)-signaling pathway and include other factors that contribute to treatment resistance. By doing so, novel pharmacological targets may be identified. The tumor microenvironment facilitates crucial signaling pathways that enhance the survival and invasive capabilities of cancer cells by conferring resistance to apoptosis. Specifically, the phenomenon known as epithelial-mesenchymal transition (EMT), which is regulated by transforming growth factor-β (TGF-β), grants stem cell characteristics and facilitates the development of a migratory and invasive phenotype by enabling resistance to anoikis. The potential effectiveness of the main drug DZ-50 in treating advanced metastatic castration-resistant prostate cancer (mCRPC) lies in its ability to induce a therapeutic response driven by anoikis. The capacity for differentiated prostate tumor gland epithelium to undergo cellular de-differentiation into mesenchymal cells via EMT and subsequent re-differentiation through mesenchymal-epithelial transition (MET) has a remarkable role in the evolution of cancers. One notable attribute of the EMT landscape is the downregulation of E-cadherin, resulting in the disruption of adherent junctions. This event effectively evades apoptosis, triggered by detachment from the extracellular matrix, hence facilitating the metastatic potential and resistance to chemotherapy. Researchers are

---

Samaneh Adelian and Amin Soltani contributed equally with all other contributors.

S. Adelian (✉) · A. Soltani
Cellular and Molecular Research Center, Basic Health Sciences Institute, Shahrekord University of Medical Sciences, Shahrekord, Iran

M. R. Hamblin (✉)
Laser Research Centre, Faculty of Health Science, University of Johannesburg, Doornfontein, South Africa

G. Sethi et al. (eds.), *Prostate Cancer: Molecular Events and Therapeutic Modalities*, https://doi.org/10.1007/978-981-97-4612-5_11

now investigating the potential linkages between AR and TGF-β signaling in order to develop more effective therapeutic approaches for the treatment of mCRPC. This chapter aims to explain the existing data about therapeutic resistance in individuals suffering from recurrent prostate cancer that is resistant to standard treatments.

Keywords Epithelial-mesenchymal transition (EMT) · Prostate cancer stem cells (PCSC) · Superoxide dismutase (SOD) · Prostate-specific antigen (PSA) · Androgen signaling pathway

11.1 Introduction

Lately, there has been substantial advancement in the comprehension of the molecular, cellular, and systemic mechanisms that underlie the genesis, development, heterogeneity, and metastatic dissemination of cancer. The use of sequencing technology and subsequent data processing has facilitated the discovery of a considerable number of genomic abnormalities present in tumors [1]. However, the current count of genes that have been identified as cancer-promoting genes is rather limited, with around 125 genes found so far. Among these genes, 55 are categorized as oncogenes, while the remaining 70 are classed as tumor-suppressor genes [2]. Common adult tumors typically contain typically, three to six gene mutations on average that are recognized to facilitate the development of tumors. However, the overall count of nonsynonymous mutations, which are anticipated to modify gene function, varies between 40 and 100 in the majority of solid tumors. In certain types of tumors, such as colorectal or lung cancers with microsatellite instability, this count can escalate to several hundred [2]. Hence, the genetic composition of a specific tumor is very intricate, characterized by a limited number of mutations that promote cancer development among a multitude of "passenger" mutations that accumulate during tumor advancement and branching clonal evolution. Regardless of the intricate nature of the genome, a significant proportion of the identified oncogenes or tumor-suppressor genes may be categorized into twelve distinct pathways [2]. Moreover, it has been observed that mutations that promote tumor growth are implicated in three primary biological mechanisms. First, these mutations affect cell survival, with sensitivity to mutations occurring in genes such as BRAF, MYC, PTEN, epidermal growth factor receptor (EGFR), PIK3CA, human epidermal growth factor 2 (HER2), and others. Second, they influence cell fate, with mutations in genes like KLF4, androgen receptor (AR), APC, GATA2, and NOTCH playing a significant role. Finally, these mutations alter genomic stability, with notable effects observed in genes such as BRCA2, BRCA1, ATM, TP53, and others. The analysis of genomic landscapes in tumors has great potential for the development of mechanism-based targeted medicines that are designed to disrupt certain oncogenic pathways. Numerous inhibitors targeting prevalent oncogenic pathways have undergone testing in preclinical cancer models and have already been incorporated into the treatment regimens for cancer patients. Examples of such inhibitors include anti-breakpoint cluster region-Ab1 (BCR-ABL1), anti-human epidermal growth factor 2 (HER2), and anti-epidermal growth factor receptor (EGFR) inhibitors. Additionally, there are ongoing assessments of these inhibitors in various clinical trial studies [3, 4].

Despite the specificity shown by several techniques, the practical application of the majority of individual treatments has not been excellent. These therapies have either proven to be useless or have only provided temporary effectiveness, followed by the development of resistance. Hence, it is essential to thoroughly evaluate the underlying processes that contribute to the restricted therapeutic outcomes, with the aim of customizing the treatment approach for individual cancer patients. The analysis of tumor genomes has not only revealed novel potential "cancer genes," but has also shown a significant level of heterogeneity within tumors [5]. Put simply, while examining a specific tumor, we encounter different patterns of mutations. Consequently, the effectiveness of a certain anti-cancer drug may not be consistent across the whole tumor. This phenomenon enhances the probability that a specific subset of malignant cells would exhibit resistance against a solitary therapeutic intervention [6]. Additionally, the therapeutic efficacy of a certain cell is influenced not only by the existence of the intended target but also by the presence or later emergence of mutations or genetic abnormalities, which might potentially impact the therapeutic response. Indeed, the biological characteristics of tumors are much more intricate than first perceived. Hanahan and Weinberg emphasize in their extensive and detailed analysis that the characteristics often referred to as the "hallmarks of cancer" extend beyond oncogenic changes that result in uncontrolled cell proliferation [7]. Undoubtedly, the progression and dissemination of tumors are impacted by a wide range of inherent cellular characteristics and their interactions with the surrounding milieu. Therefore, in the context of cancer treatment, a comprehensive understanding and integration of the many processes by which tumor cells adapt to targeted therapy is necessary. This knowledge is crucial for the development of a combination of medicines that may provide the most effective anti-tumor outcomes.

In this chapter, we focus on many significant and widely applicable processes behind the development of resistance to various treatment strategies in the context of prostate cancer. Additionally, we discuss the challenges associated with predicting therapeutic response and devising combination therapies.

11.2 Prostate Cancer and Chemotherapy Resistance

The phenomenon of tumor cell heterogeneity has been recognized and acknowledged for many decades. Similar to several other forms of cancer, prostate cancer exhibits heterogeneity. For instance, the majority of early stage prostate cancer cases primarily consist of cells that exhibit a positive expression of prostate-specific antigen (PSA) and androgen receptor (AR) [8]. In contrast, advanced prostate cancer is predominantly characterized by poorly differentiated or undifferentiated cells that exhibit a limited or absent expression of PSA and AR [9]. In order to comprehensively analyze the heterogeneity of tumor cells, researchers have developed xenograft models involving the transplantation of human cancer cells into mice. These models have revealed that cells within numerous human cancers exhibit a hierarchical organization, wherein only a small subset possesses the capacity to initiate and sustain tumor growth over an extended period of time. These cells exhibit numerous phenotypic and functional characteristics that are typically observed in regular stem cells. They are commonly referred to as cancer stem cells (CSCs) due to their ability to self-renew indefinitely and generate tumorigenic offspring. It has been extensively shown that CSCs play a crucial role in the initiation, progression, metastasis, and resistance to therapy of tumors [10, 11]. Despite notable advancements in the realm of prostate cancer therapy, there is a lack of comprehensive understanding of the processes that contribute to chemoresistance in prostate cancer and the development of castration-resistant prostate cancer (CRPC). Therefore, the investigation of the phenotypic and genetic characteristics, as well as the molecular regulators, of prostate cancer stem cells (PCSCs) could provide valuable knowledge regarding the identification of cells responsible for CRPC and offer an improved insight into the mechanisms that are at the foundation of chemoresistance in prostate cancer. This research could serve as a basis for the development of innovative therapeutic approaches that specifically target PCSCs [11]. The development of chemoresistance is attributed to a combination of intricate molecular processes, such as the activation of abnormal androgen receptor and/or ATP-binding cassette (ABC) family of membrane transporters, repression of tumor-suppressor gene expression, evasion of programmed cell death, intercommunication among crucial signaling pathways, and involvement of various miRNAs [12]. This section aims to provide a comprehensive overview of the many roles played by ABC subfamily G member 2 (ABCG2), AR, important signaling pathways, PCSCs, and miRNAs in the development of chemoresistance in prostate cancer. Additionally, it will explore emerging therapy approaches, with a particular focus on medicines targeting PCSCs [12].

11.3 Chemoresistant Mediated by AR Axis

AR is a kind of nuclear hormone receptor that is composed of eight exons. These exons are responsible for encoding four distinct functional domains inside the receptor: the NH2-terminal domain (NTD), DNA-binding domain (DBD), hinge region, and ligand-binding domain (LBD). The N-terminal domain is responsible for the bulk of androgen receptor transcriptional activity, whereas the ligand-binding domain binds to androgens and facilitates the transfer of AR to the nucleus [13]. DBD, which consists of two zinc fingers, plays a crucial role in the recognition and binding of DNA. On the other hand, the hinge domain is responsible for regulating the translocation of the AR into the nucleus [14, 15]. The proliferation and survival of prostate cancer cells are reliant on androgens via the AR axis. The AR has pivotal functions in maintaining the lineage of prostate tissue and is also involved in the beginning and progression of prostate cancer. These factors underlie the success of androgen deprivation therapy (ADT) [15]. Since the first discovery by Huggins and Hodges in 1941 that prostate cancer is sensitive to hormones and castration may serve as an effective treatment, continuous efforts have been dedicated to suppressing and eliminating AR signaling [16]. Regrettably, despite the considerable efficacy of surgical or chemical castration in reducing tumor burden, lowering serum PSA levels, and enhancing survival rates in the early stages of therapy, prostate cancer inevitably relapses within a median length of 12–24 months and progresses to CRPC over time [17]. In the past, PCa that did not respond to hormonal manipulation was referred to by other terms such as hormone-refractory/resistant PCa (HRPC) or endocrine-resistant PCa (ERPC). However, nowadays, the term CRPC is frequently used. The conventional description of CRPC has certain characteristics, which are as follows: (1) The serum testosterone levels following castration are found to be below 1.7 nM, which is significantly lower than the normal range of 10–35 nM. (2) The prostate-specific antigen (PSA) shows a pattern of three consecutive increases, occurring at two-week intervals, resulting in two instances where the PSA level rises by 50% compared to the lowest recorded value. (3) The discontinuation of anti-androgen therapy for a minimum duration of four weeks. (4) Despite implementing additional hormonal interventions, there is evidence of continued progression of PSA levels. (5) The presence of metastasis, indicating the spread of cancer to other parts of the body [18]. One of the primary distinguishing features of CRPC is its capacity to endure low levels of androgens. It has been shown that CRPC cells continue to depend on AR signaling, despite the fact that the circulating testosterone levels drop below 1.7 nM after castration [19]. Numerous investigations have shown that cells of CRPC have mutant AR, resulting in increased gene expression and heightened functional sensitivity. In the context of clinical settings, it has been reported that prostate cancer cases that have had androgen deprivation therapy have a higher prevalence of AR amplification, promiscuity, and splice variant isoforms in comparison to cases of primary prostate cancer that have not received any treatment [20]. Hence, there is a prevailing belief that the majority of cases of CRPC are not really hormone refractory. This refers to instances when androgen receptor transcription is abnormally reactivated, despite the presence of low levels of testosterone in the bloodstream after castration [21]. Conversely, mutations affecting the AR sequence were identified in ~45% of instances of CRPC [22]. Thus far, a multitude of genetic alterations in the AR gene have been documented, with about 91% classified as mis-sense and non-sense mutations [23]. These mutations in the AR mostly manifest in the LBD and NTD, whereas a mere 7% of mutations are seen in the DBD and a mere 2% in the hinge region. The therapeutic significance of genetic alteration in the LBD lies in their shown ability to enhance sensitivity and reduce selectivity in ligand binding. One notable point mutation, known as T877A, has been discovered as the most prevalent. This mutation enables the activation of the receptor by many anti-androgens, including progestin, estrogen, and hydroxyflutamide. Furthermore, there is a possibility of observing a withdrawal reaction in particular patients with the T877A mutation. This is evident when the anti-androgen bicalutamide is administered intermittently, resulting in a decline in prostate-specific antigen levels [24]. This finding provides additional support for the hypothesis that AR mutations may underlie the acquired androgen-like agonistic effects associated with continuous administration of anti-androgens, such as bicalutamide.

11.4 Role of PCSCs in Chemoresistance

The presence of a subset of CSCs was first shown in leukemia by Bonnet et al. in 1997 [25]. In the ensuing sequence, CSCs have been detected in other types of solid tumors, such as glioblastoma multiforme [26], breast [27], and prostate cancers [28]. Prostate cancer chemoresistance may be attributed to the involvement of many processes based on CSCs. These mechanisms include the activation of drug-efflux pumps, increased effectiveness of DNA repair, upregulation of detoxifying enzymes, and induction of quiescence. Previously, many populations of PCSCs have been documented in the literature [29]. Laffin et al. categorized bulk prostate cancer cells based on their expression levels of prostate-specific antigen [30]. These cells were obtained from in vitro cell line cultures, human prostate cancer cell line xenografts, and pure prostate cancer tissues. The categorization included separating the cells into two subpopulations: PSA-negative/low-expressing ($PSA^{-/lo}$) and PSA^{+} subpopulations. The study demonstrated that $PSA^{-/lo}$ cells met all the established criteria that define PCSCs [30]. In contrast to PSA^{+} cells, which exhibit a high proliferation rate and contribute to the growth of tumors, $PSA^{-/lo}$ cells have a comparatively low level of activity and are characterized by their notable tumorigenic and metastatic properties. The relatively low cycling rate of $PSA^{-/lo}$ cells was hypothesized to provide intrinsic resistance to chemotherapeutic drugs, which primarily target rapidly dividing PSA^{+} cells and have anti-proliferative effects [31].

Moreover, a comprehensive analysis of the entire genome's transcriptome has brought to light distinct patterns of gene expression in $PSA^{-/lo}$ cells. These cells exhibit overexpression of numerous genes participating in stress-reducing reactions, such as detoxification-related genes (metallothioneins, GSTT2), genes responsive to hypoxia (APLN, PLAU, and THBS1), components of the p53 signaling pathway (ZBTB7A and PSME3), and genes involved in sensing and repairing DNA damage (REV1, XPA, and MSH6). This suggests that $PSA^{-/lo}$ cells not only display resistance to androgen deprivation therapy and chemotherapy drugs but also exhibit resilience to other forms of stress, like radiotherapy [32]. In particular, a distinct population of cells characterized by $ALDH^{+}CD44^{+}\alpha2\beta1^{+}$ phenotype within the $PSA^{-/lo}$ cell fraction demonstrated enhanced tumorigenicity, capable of generating serially transplantable tumors in animals that were totally castrated [1239]. Furthermore, it has been shown that cells lacking cytokeratin (CK) 18 and CK19 (CK18−/CK19−) in both docetaxel-resistant prostate cancer cell lines and in primary and metastatic PCa tissue samples are able to survive treatment with docetaxel and display a chemoresistant phenotype [27]. Recent research has provided more evidence that the transcription of CD166 has a significantly elevated presence in samples of human castration-resistant prostate cancer [33]. Collectively, the aforementioned studies indicate that PCSCs, or a pool of PCSCs that may consist of several subsets of cells resistant to chemotherapy, have the potential to serve as the genesis of CRPC. Furthermore, these PCSCs are likely to contribute, to some extent, to the development of chemoresistance in prostate cancer.

11.5 Radiotherapy Resistance in Prostate Cancer

Radiation therapy, which includes external beam radiation and brachytherapy, is a frequently used curative approach for managing localized prostate cancer. Its effectiveness is similar to that of radical prostatectomy [34]. Furthermore, the combination of irradiation and androgen restriction treatment has been shown to enhance tumor susceptibility to radiation and increase disease-specific survival [35]. Radioisotopes such as lutetium-177 (Lu-177) and radium-223 (Ra-223) are applied in the management of prostate cancer when the illness recurs or metastasizes. Ra-223 is a radioactive isotope that emits alpha particles with an 11.1-day half-life. The absorption of Ra-223 in the bloodstream by bone is facilitated by the chemical resemblance of calcium to Ra-223. The presence of osteoblastic bone lesions is a common characteristic in cases of metastatic prostate cancer, resulting in the incorporation of Ra-223 into these lesions. Subsequently, the alpha particles are situated in close proximity to the therapy region. The Phase III ALSYMPCA study demonstrated a significant improvement in overall survival among male individuals diagnosed with CRPC and had a minimum of two bone metastases who underwent treatment with Ra-223 [36]. The transmembrane protein known as PSMA has an elevated expression in cases of prostate cancer [37]. Lutetium-177 (Lu-177) is a radioactive isotope that undergoes beta decay, emitting beta particles. It has a relatively short half-life of 6.65 days. Radiopharmaceutical applications often use this substance. Lu-177-PSMA-617 is a radioligand that has a reasonably focused therapeutic effect on PSMA-positive cells while minimizing damage to surrounding normal tissue in patients with high PSMA-specific scan activity. The findings of a Phase III study, which was open-label and randomized, demonstrated that Lu-177-PSMA-617 exhibited substantial improvements in both progression-free survival and overall survival for individuals with PSMA-positive radiographic scans who were diagnosed with metastatic CRPC [38].

11.6 Antioxidants and Resistance to Radiotherapy in Prostate Cancer

The production of reactive oxygen species (ROS) plays a crucial role in determining the effectiveness of radiation treatment. However, it is important to note that ROS creation may also trigger signaling pathways that contribute to the development of resistance to radiation and the subsequent recovery of tumors [39]. There are several pathways that contribute to radioresistance mechanisms, such as antiapoptotic, antioxidant, and DNA repair systems, among other factors. This encompasses the process of activating and inducing the superoxide dismutase (SOD) family. It is noteworthy that antioxidant enzymes often operate in conjunction rather than in isolation to mitigate oxidative harm. As an example, the process of SOD involves the conversion of two superoxide radicals, together with two hydrogen ions, into hydrogen peroxide and molecular oxygen. Subsequently, other enzymes, like catalase or peroxidase, facilitate the conversion of two hydrogen peroxide molecules into water and oxygen. In addition to SOD and catalase, there exist several antioxidant enzymes. Peroxiredoxins (Prx) represent a captivating and comparatively recent cohort of enzymes that effectively eliminate peroxide and peroxynitrite. Glutathione, a thiol compound present in both the cytoplasm and organelles, has the function of reducing ROS and free radicals. The role of antioxidants in radioresistance has been implicated and is now a subject of intensive study with varied degrees of attention. The association between peroxiredoxins and radioresistance is intricate. The expression of Prx 2 is notably increased in radioresistant cancers, but Prx 1, 3, 4, 5, and 6 do not exhibit such upregulation [40]. The investigation conducted on esophageal cancer cells with varying radiosensitivity showed that the radioresistant cell line exhibited maintained levels of glutathione, but the radiosensitive cell line had a reduction in glutathione levels. The authors hypothesized that this phenomenon might potentially contribute to the development of radioresistance [41]. The upregulation of catalase, particularly when localized in the mitochondria, has been shown to provide radioprotective effects [42]. In their study, Hirose et al. conducted a comparative analysis of Chinese hamster ovary cells that overexpressed SOD2 and those that did not. The researchers observed that the cells overexpressing SOD2 exhibited a much greater survival rate after exposure to gamma radiation [43].

According to research conducted by Kalen et al., it was shown that the expression of SOD2 led to a significant increase in radioresistance, with a three- to fourfold amplification effect [44]. Significantly, the molecular mechanisms that regulate the progression of castration resistance are frequently associated with the lack of success in radiation treatment as well [45]. Redox-sensitive transcription factors, including hypoxia-inducible factor 1-alpha (HIF-1α) and nuclear factor erythroid 2-related factor 2 (Nrf-2) [46], have also shown radioprotective properties. HIF-1α is seen to increase in expression levels in conditions of low oxygen availability, known as hypoxia. This upregulation of HIF-1α has been found to have a role in promoting resistance to radiation treatment by impeding programmed cell death, hindering the repair of damage caused by irradiation, and engaging in several additional pathways. The Nrf-2 protein is responsible for activating the transcription of molecules that possess antioxidant properties, as well as molecules that inhibit programmed cell death (apoptosis). The Nrf2 pathway is used by the signaling molecule mTOR to enhance the expression of glutathione as a means of increasing resistance to radiation [47]. Besides transcription factors like HIF-1α and Nrf-2, the activation of the NF-κB pathway constitutes a noteworthy mechanism contributing to radioresistance, particularly in cells of prostate cancer origin.

11.7 Role of NF-κB Pathway in Radioresistance in Prostate Cancer

Due to the significant impact of the NF-κB pathway on the modulation of radiosensitivity and radioresistance, certain therapies such as gene therapy or medication have the potential to modify this system, thereby enhancing the radiosensitivity of prostate cancer. The observed phenomenon in androgen-dependent prostate cancer suggests that the accumulation of p52 is significantly impacted by AR activation. According to research conducted by Lessard and coworkers, it was shown that the exposure of LNCaP cells to an androgen analog resulted in a higher degree of nuclear accumulation of p52. Nevertheless, the administration of the anti-androgen bicalutamide resulted in a decrease in nuclear p52 levels [48]. According to research conducted by Fan et al., it was shown that exposure of mouse epithelial cells to a radiation dose of 10 cGy resulted in the activation of RelA. Consequently, this activation led to an upregulation of the expression of SOD2. Furthermore, several hours after this first exposure, the cells exhibited greater resistance to subsequent irradiation with a dose of 2 Gy, indicating a radioprotective effect. The expression of SOD2 and cyclin B1 was reduced upon inhibition of RelA. The study observed a reduction in radioresistance in line with SOD2 knockdown [49]. Imatinib is a pharmacological agent that functions as a selective inhibitor of tyrosine kinases, particularly those associated with the ABL gene, c-kit protein, and the receptor for platelet-derived growth factor. Leukemia is often treated with this particular intervention. Following exposure to radiation, the transcription factor RelB undergoes translocation to the cellular nucleus, where it initiates the transcription of certain genes associated with the development of radioresistance. The administration of imatinib resulted in a reduction in nuclear translocation in androgen-independent PC-3 cells, thereby leading to an increase in radiosensitivity. In a study, it was shown that imatinib led to an elevation in RelB nuclear translocation in LNCaP cells, which are known to be sensitive to androgens [50].

11.8 Role of SOD2 in Radioresistance in Prostate Cancer

As previously mentioned, it is hypothesized that SOD2 has a protective role in safeguarding prostate cells under normal physiological circumstances. The efficacy of radiation treatment in eliminating cancer cells derives from its capacity to prompt the production of free radicals. As a key antioxidant enzyme, SOD2 plays a crucial role in counteracting the detrimental effects of radiotherapy. The NF-κB pathway induces the upregulation of SOD2 in response to radiation, resulting in its radioprotective and antiapoptotic effects [51]. The activation of SOD2 by RelB is a significant mechanism via which prostate cancer cells develop resistance to radiation. RelB is classified as a member of the NF-κB family and functions as a downstream mediator within the NF-κB signaling pathway. RelB and p52 are constituents of the noncanonical route; however, RelB is furthermore subject to regulation by RelA and p50 within the canonical pathway. Cytokines have the ability to trigger the activation of transcription of the SOD2 gene via the involvement of NF-κB. Indeed, the NF-κB-binding sites within the SOD2 gene are essential for its transcription [52]. It is worth noting that NF-κB has been seen to bind to an enhancer located inside an intron of the SOD2 gene [53]. The significance of NF-κB in the induction of SOD2 by cytokines has been highlighted in research conducted by Dhar et al. It was shown that NF-κB is essential for the transcription of SOD2, but it alone is not enough for this process. Additionally, the study identified nucleophosmin, a phosphoprotein located in the nucleolus, as a crucial factor required for the expression of SOD2 by NF-κB [54].

Josson et al. conducted a research that provided evidence of RelB's ability to increase SOD2 expression in PC3 cells after exposure to radiation [55]. Consequently, there was an observed augmentation in radioresistance. The verification of this statement was accomplished by the inhibition of RelB using a dominant/negative p100 or specific siRNA. This intervention led to a significant decrease in the SOD2 levels and increased radiosensitivity of prostate cancer cell lines. In a similar vein, previous studies have shown that SOD2 exhibits an increased expression in breast cancer cells as a means of adapting to irradiation. Consequently, this overexpression subsequently bestows resistance to further radiotherapy treatments [51]. Significantly, the observed radioresistance has potential therapeutic relevance. In a cohort of males who had received radiation treatment, Margalit et al. conducted research that identified connections between certain single-nucleotide polymorphisms (SNPs) within the SOD2 gene and the occurrence of fatal prostate cancer. There was no observed connection between these single SNPs and the occurrence of fatal prostate cancer among the cohort of patients who had prostatectomy. Regrettably, the findings mentioned were not reproduced in a separate cohort for validation [56].

This finding contributes to the existing body of research that suggests a positive correlation between elevated levels of superoxide dismutase (SOD) in cells and their ability to withstand the effects of radiation. Multiple studies have used the SOD2 gene both in cell culture and animal studies to impart radioresistance [57]. In a more recent investigation conducted by Zhang and colleagues, mice were administered an oral dosage of a minicircle plasmid containing the SOD2 gene. Subsequently, these animals were subjected to irradiation of 31 Gy specifically targeting the esophagus. The survival rates of the mice that were administered the SOD2 plasmid were shown to be superior when compared to the control group. In a similar vein, it was shown that mice administered the plasmid intravenously had enhanced rates of survival when subjected to whole-body irradiation of 9.75 Gy [58]. In a research conducted by Josson's team, it was shown that PC-3 cells, which are indicative of high-grade prostate cancer, exhibited greater resistance to radiation and had higher nucleus levels of RelB compared to LNCaP cells, which are representative of low-grade prostate cancer [55]. According to the research conducted by Josson et al., it was shown that the levels of SOD2 were up in both PC-3 and LNCaP cells after exposure to radiation. However, the LNCaP cells exhibited a higher presence of superoxide radicals compared to the PC-3 cells. The introduction of an exogenous SOD2 mimic resulted in an increased radioresistance of the LNCaP cells. The PC-3 cell population exhibited higher baseline levels of SOD2 and greater activity of SOD2 compared to the LNCaP cells. A comprehensive depiction emerges when the findings of this investigation are juxtaposed with the findings of the aforementioned study by Venkataraman's team, which demonstrated that PC-3 cells exhibited diminished levels of SOD2 in comparison to immortalized prostate epithelial cells. Collectively, recent investigations align with the concept that the level of SOD2 diminishes upon cancer initiation and escalates during the advancement of the ailment [59].

The potential radioprotective efficacy of SOD2 may be restricted to conditions characterized by high levels of oxygen. In a work conducted by Urano et al., the technique of cDNA transfection was used to introduce SOD2 into tumor cells. The cell lines comprised a low SOD line, a high SOD line, and two control lines. In the presence of oxygen, it was shown that both cell lines carrying superoxide dismutase (SOD) exhibited elevated levels of survival after radiation compared to the control cell lines. The SOD cell lines exhibited increased radiosensitivity compared to the control cell lines in an oxygen-deprived environment. It is noteworthy that the lack of oxygen resulted in a reduction in tumorigenicity in cell lines containing SOD2 without providing substantial radioresistance [60]. While cells possess a variety of antioxidant pathways, some systems exhibit more radioprotective properties than others. In a recent research, three mammalian cell lines were generated to exhibit overexpression of glutathione peroxidase, SOD, and SOD2. Subsequently, the aforementioned cell lines, together with a control cell line, were subjected to irradiation. The cell line that exhibited the highest level of radioprotection was the one expressing SOD2, whereas the cell line expressing glutathione peroxidase had a lower degree of radioprotection. The cells did not exhibit a substantial change in radiosensitivity as a result of the overexpression of SOD1 [61, 62].

11.9 ADT-Resistance in Prostate Cancer

The treatment regimens for prostate malignancies have seen significant advancements since Charles Huggins was given the Nobel Prize in 1966. Huggins demonstrated that hormone modulation by orchidectomy may lead to the eradication of hormone-sensitive prostate cancer [63]. The utilization of chemical castration agents is generally seen as more favorable by a majority of patients compared to surgical methods. Consequently, the pharmaceutical business has made substantial investments in the advancement of several iterations of these medications, including enzalutamide and darolutamide. These pharmaceutical compounds possess potent inhibitory properties since they selectively bind to the androgen receptor protein with varying affinities. Ongoing evaluation of their therapeutic use is being conducted. The first design of androgen response blockers was the replication of testosterone's structure, known as steroidal anti-androgens. However, contemporary nonsteroidal anti-androgens have been molecularly tuned to enhance their inhibitory effects to the greatest extent possible [64].

Enhancements in the binding affinities of medicines for the AR target and the use of structural chemistry and molecular fitting methodologies in their development have led to notable advancements in the biochemical characteristics observed during cell culture testing. Nevertheless, the average duration between the initiation of ADT and the occurrence of recurrence, as determined by the elevation of PSA levels in the bloodstream, remains about 30 years for patients who do not have metastases, but it is half that duration for patients with metastases [65]. Additionally, there exists data suggesting that cancer with initial Gleason scores of 9/10 may have a more accelerated progression to castration-resistant illness after androgen deprivation therapy compared to a placebo [66].

Following the failure of initial ADT, using bicalutamide or luteinizing hormone-releasing hormone (LHRH) antagonists, patients may receive hormone-based treatments like abiraterone which can modify the production of androgens within the tumor itself [67]. This alteration is particularly relevant in cases of CRPC. Additionally, medications such as enzalutamide and apalutamide can effectively suppress any remaining androgen responses in individuals with CRPC [68, 69]. Following the near-inevitable lack of success shown in the later androgen-based therapies [70], there is a shift toward using less targeted, replication-based chemotherapies that are more hazardous, such as taxane treatments, for the management of CRPC. There is a potential for the development of other targeted chemotherapies, including olaparib, that specifically address the subset of prostate tumors characterized by DNA damage repair deficiencies. Recent clinical studies have shown encouraging results in this regard [71]. Currently, the oncologist's options for intervention are limited to palliative measures in order to alleviate the progression of the most lethal manifestation of the illness, characterized by a weakly differentiated histology often associated with higher Gleason grades. The lesions of advanced CRPC have either a basaloid or neuroendocrine character, known as neuroendocrine prostate cancer (NEPC), and eventually have an unfavorable prognosis [72].

The use of combination therapy, which includes the administration of both taxanes and androgen signaling suppression, has shown improved survival outcomes in patients who have just been diagnosed with high-grade metastatic illness [73]. Nevertheless, it is worth noting that several alternative immunotherapies have not shown comparable potential in the treatment of prostate cancer so far, as their effectiveness has been limited to a small subset of patients [74]. This is in contrast to the significant improvements reported in small-cell lung cancer, melanoma, and certain types of leukemias [75]. However, ADT continues to be the predominant approach for the first pharmacological intervention in prostate cancer clinical care. Prostate cancer patients who undergo hormone treatment often see improvements for a duration of 1–4 years, with a few exceptions where remission may last for as long as 10 years. The future prospects of androgen deprivation therapy seem to be closely tied to the development of novel and enhanced androgen signaling inhibitors [76]. This trajectory, however, necessitates substantial financial investments from the pharmaceutical sector and imposes additional burdens on healthcare systems. Clinical studies have examined the efficacy of combination therapies and other forms of complete androgen blocking, including both continuous and intermittent approaches [77]. Nevertheless, the recurrence of cancer persists despite the seemingly improved survival rates seen in groups receiving intermittent treatment [78], suggesting that this therapeutic approach is likely not being fully used. The lack of a definitive explanation for the limited efficacy of a combination of androgen signaling inhibitors in achieving remission or cure in CRPC, despite the tumor cells' apparent need for androgens, remains unclear [79].

The presence of several alternative signaling systems in cells expressing the androgen receptor is becoming more evident. These pathways facilitate the evasion of ADT and the preservation of androgen receptor signaling in both healthy and cancerous cells. An instance of overcoming the suppression of androgen synthesis, caused by goserelin or abiraterone, may occur via intratumoral androgen production and amplification of AR expression, or by the activation of the glucocorticoid receptor and the use of glucocorticoids, as supported by references [80–82]. In the context of evolution, the escape, salvage, and/or backup signaling pathways serve as valuable mechanisms for a cell that has been impacted, allowing for the continuation of survival and proliferative signals even in the absence of the primary ligand response. The absence of testosterone signaling in a mammalian population would have profound implications for fertility and reproduction, hence exerting significant evolutionary pressure for the development of alternative salvage mechanisms.

11.10 Conclusion

In the year 2018, advancements in molecular technology and the processing of large datasets have emerged as valuable tools for comprehending the intricate nature and diverse characteristics of prostate tumors. These developments have also facilitated the formulation of approaches aimed at averting, delaying, or alleviating the migratory and invasive traits associated with prostate cancer, extending beyond the scope of androgen receptor signaling. The utilization of epithelial-mesenchymal transition (EMT) regulatory proteins as discernible phenotypic indicators of tumor progression, alongside the identification of novel therapeutic targets such as cellular mechanisms facilitated by the transforming growth factor-β (TGF-β) non-SMAD signaling family that contribute to the creation of a tumor-promoting microenvironment, holds the potential to enhance precision diagnosis and optimize combination strategies aimed at impeding the spread of metastatic tumors and overcoming therapeutic resistance. The identification and use of specific markers that emerge from microenvironment modifiers, such as neuroendocrine cells or cancer-associated fibroblasts (CAFs), might potentially provide a clinical advantage in understanding tumor development. This approach may be particularly valuable if there are therapeutic targets accessible for the stromal pathways that have been discovered. The potential therapeutic targets/platforms represented by the tumor microenvironment, which includes myofibroblasts, cancer-associated fibroblasts, neuroendocrine cells, and myeloid-derived suppressor cells (MDSCs), have received limited attention despite the presence of compelling evidence regarding their functional role in driving tumor progression toward metastasis and the development of resistance to therapeutic interventions.

References

1. Lawrence MS, Stojanov P, Polak P, Kryukov GV, Cibulskis K, Sivachenko A, et al. Mutational heterogeneity in cancer and the search for new cancer-associated genes. Nature. 2013;499(7457):214–8.
2. Vogelstein B, Papadopoulos N, Velculescu VE, Zhou S, Diaz LA Jr, Kinzler KW. Cancer genome landscapes. Science. 2013;339(6127):1546–58.
3. Gerber DE. EGFR inhibition in the treatment of non-Small cell lung cancer. Drug Dev Res. 2008;69(6):359–72.
4. Sellers WR. A blueprint for advancing genetics-based cancer therapy. Cell. 2011;147(1):26–31.
5. Navin N, Krasnitz A, Rodgers L, Cook K, Meth J, Kendall J, et al. Inferring tumor progression from genomic heterogeneity. Genome Res. 2010;20(1):68–80.
6. Mansoori B, Mohammadi A, Davudian S, Shirjang S, Baradaran B. The different mechanisms of cancer drug resistance: a brief review. Adv Pharm Bull. 2017;7(3):339–48.
7. Hanahan D, Weinberg RA. Hallmarks of cancer: the next generation. Cell. 2011;144(5):646–74.
8. Tang DG. Understanding and targeting prostate cancer cell heterogeneity and plasticity. Semin Cancer Biol. 2022;82:68–93.
9. Qin J, Liu X, Laffin B, Chen X, Choy G, Jeter CR, et al. The PSA(-/lo) prostate cancer cell population harbors self-renewing long-term tumor-propagating cells that resist castration. Cell Stem Cell. 2012;10(5):556–69.
10. Shen MM, Abate-Shen C. Molecular genetics of prostate cancer: new prospects for old challenges. Genes Dev. 2010;24(18):1967–2000.
11. Visvader JE, Lindeman GJ. Cancer stem cells: current status and evolving complexities. Cell Stem Cell. 2012;10(6):717–28.
12. Yuan X, Cai C, Chen S, Chen S, Yu Z, Balk SP. Androgen receptor functions in castration-resistant prostate cancer and mechanisms of resistance to new agents targeting the androgen axis. Oncogene. 2014;33(22):2815–25.

13. Kahn B, Collazo J, Kyprianou N. Androgen receptor as a driver of therapeutic resistance in advanced prostate cancer. Int J Biol Sci. 2014;10(6):588–95.
14. Tanner TM, Denayer S, Geverts B, Van Tilborgh N, Kerkhofs S, Helsen C, et al. A 629RKLKK633 motif in the hinge region controls the androgen receptor at multiple levels. Cell Mol Life Sci. 2010;67(11):1919–27.
15. Egan A, Dong Y, Zhang H, Qi Y, Balk SP, Sartor O. Castration-resistant prostate cancer: adaptive responses in the androgen axis. Cancer Treat Rev. 2014;40(3):426–33.
16. Huggins C, Hodges CV. Studies on prostatic cancer. I. The effect of castration, of estrogen and androgen injection on serum phosphatases in metastatic carcinoma of the prostate. CA Cancer J Clin. 1972;22(4):232–40.
17. Schrader AJ, Boegemann M, Ohlmann CH, Schnoeller TJ, Krabbe LM, Hajili T, et al. Enzalutamide in castration-resistant prostate cancer patients progressing after docetaxel and abiraterone. Eur Urol. 2014;65(1):30–6.
18. Pienta KJ, Walia G, Simons JW, Soule HR. Beyond the androgen receptor: new approaches to treating metastatic prostate cancer. Report of the 2013 Prouts neck prostate cancer meeting. Prostate. 2014;74(3):314–20.
19. Heidenreich A, Aus G, Bolla M, Joniau S, Matveev VB, Schmid HP, et al. EAU guidelines on prostate cancer. Eur Urol. 2008;53(1):68–80.
20. Sun F, Chen HG, Li W, Yang X, Wang X, Jiang R, et al. Androgen receptor splice variant AR3 promotes prostate cancer via modulating expression of autocrine/paracrine factors. J Biol Chem. 2014;289(3):1529–39.
21. Attar RM, Takimoto CH, Gottardis MM. Castration-resistant prostate cancer: locking up the molecular escape routes. Clin Cancer Res. 2009;15(10):3251–5.
22. Beltran H, Yelensky R, Frampton GM, Park K, Downing SR, MacDonald TY, et al. Targeted next-generation sequencing of advanced prostate cancer identifies potential therapeutic targets and disease heterogeneity. Eur Urol. 2013;63(5):920–6.
23. Mostaghel EA, Plymate S. New hormonal therapies for castration-resistant prostate cancer. Endocrinol Metab Clin N Am. 2011;40(3):625–42, x.
24. Schrecengost R, Knudsen KE. Molecular pathogenesis and progression of prostate cancer. Semin Oncol. 2013;40(3):244–58.
25. Bonnet D, Dick JE. Human acute myeloid leukemia is organized as a hierarchy that originates from a primitive hematopoietic cell. Nat Med. 1997;3(7):730–7.
26. Lottaz C, Beier D, Meyer K, Kumar P, Hermann A, Schwarz J, et al. Transcriptional profiles of CD133+ and CD133—glioblastoma-derived cancer stem cell lines suggest different cells of origin. Cancer Res. 2010;70(5):2030–40.
27. Domingo-Domenech J, Vidal SJ, Rodriguez-Bravo V, Castillo-Martin M, Quinn SA, Rodriguez-Barrueco R, et al. Suppression of acquired docetaxel resistance in prostate cancer through depletion of notch—and hedgehog-dependent tumor-initiating cells. Cancer Cell. 2012;22(3):373–88.
28. Al-Hajj M, Wicha MS, Benito-Hernandez A, Morrison SJ, Clarke MF. Prospective identification of tumorigenic breast cancer cells. Proc Natl Acad Sci USA. 2003;100(7):3983–8.
29. Yang T, Rycaj K, Liu ZM, Tang DG. Cancer stem cells: constantly evolving and functionally heterogeneous therapeutic targets. Cancer Res. 2014;74(11):2922–7.
30. Laffin B, Tang DG. An old player on a new playground: bmi-1 as a regulator of prostate stem cells. Cell Stem Cell. 2010;7(6):639–40.
31. Yan J, Tang D. Prostate cancer stem-like cells proliferate slowly and resist etoposide-induced cytotoxicity via enhancing DNA damage response. Exp Cell Res. 2014;328(1):132–42.
32. Chang L, Graham PH, Hao J, Ni J, Bucci J, Cozzi PJ, et al. Acquisition of epithelial-mesenchymal transition and cancer stem cell phenotypes is associated with activation of the PI3K/Akt/mTOR pathway in prostate cancer radioresistance. Cell Death Dis. 2013;4(10):e875.
33. Jiao J, Hindoyan A, Wang S, Tran LM, Goldstein AS, Lawson D, et al. Identification of CD166 as a surface marker for enriching prostate stem/progenitor and cancer initiating cells. PLoS One. 2012;7(8):e42564.

34. D'Amico AV, Whittington R, Malkowicz SB, Schultz D, Blank K, Broderick GA, et al. Biochemical outcome after radical prostatectomy, external beam radiation therapy, or interstitial radiation therapy for clinically localized prostate cancer. JAMA. 1998;280(11):969–74.
35. Bolla M, Van Tienhoven G, Warde P, Dubois JB, Mirimanoff RO, Storme G, et al. External irradiation with or without long-term androgen suppression for prostate cancer with high metastatic risk: 10-year results of an EORTC randomised study. Lancet Oncol. 2010;11(11):1066–73.
36. Parker C, Nilsson S, Heinrich D, Helle SI, O'Sullivan JM, Fosså SD, et al. Alpha emitter radium-223 and survival in metastatic prostate cancer. N Engl J Med. 2013;369(3):213–23.
37. Kiess AP, Banerjee SR, Mease RC, Rowe SP, Rao A, Foss CA, et al. Prostate-specific membrane antigen as a target for cancer imaging and therapy. Q J Nucl Med Mol Imaging. 2015;59(3):241–68.
38. Sartor O, de Bono J, Chi KN, Fizazi K, Herrmann K, Rahbar K, et al. Lutetium-177-PSMA-617 for metastatic castration-resistant prostate cancer. N Engl J Med. 2021;385(12):1091–103.
39. Fitzgerald TJ, Wang T, Goel HL, Huang J, Stein G, Lian J, et al. Prostate carcinoma and radiation therapy: therapeutic treatment resistance and strategies for targeted therapeutic intervention. Expert Rev Anticancer Ther. 2008;8(6):967–74.
40. Forshaw TE, Holmila R, Nelson KJ, Lewis JE, Kemp ML, Tsang AW, et al. Peroxiredoxins in cancer and response to radiation therapies. Antioxidants (Basel). 2019;8(1):11.
41. Lynam-Lennon N, Reynolds JV, Pidgeon GP, Lysaght J, Marignol L, Maher SG. Alterations in DNA repair efficiency are involved in the radioresistance of esophageal adenocarcinoma. Radiat Res. 2010;174(6):703–11.
42. Epperly MW, Melendez JA, Zhang X, Nie S, Pearce L, Peterson J, et al. Mitochondrial targeting of a catalase transgene product by plasmid liposomes increases radioresistance in vitro and in vivo. Radiat Res. 2009;171(5):588–95.
43. Hirose K, Longo DL, Oppenheim JJ, Matsushima K. Overexpression of mitochondrial manganese superoxide dismutase promotes the survival of tumor cells exposed to interleukin-1, tumor necrosis factor, selected anticancer drugs, and ionizing radiation. FASEB J. 1993;7(2):361–8.
44. Kalen AL, Sarsour EH, Venkataraman S, Goswami PC. Mn-superoxide dismutase overexpression enhances G2 accumulation and radioresistance in human oral squamous carcinoma cells. Antioxid Redox Signal. 2006;8(7–8):1273–81.
45. Bonkhoff H. Factors implicated in radiation therapy failure and radiosensitization of prostate cancer. Prostate Cancer. 2012;2012:593241.
46. Zhao H, Jiang H, Li Z, Zhuang Y, Liu Y, Zhou S, et al. 2-Methoxyestradiol enhances radiosensitivity in radioresistant melanoma MDA-MB-435R cells by regulating glycolysis via HIF-1α/PDK1 axis. Int J Oncol. 2017;50(5):1531–40.
47. Woo Y, Lee HJ, Jung YM, Jung YJ. mTOR-mediated antioxidant activation in solid tumor Radioresistance. J Oncol. 2019;2019:5956867.
48. Staal J, Beyaert R. Inflammation and NF-κB signaling in prostate cancer: mechanisms and clinical implications. Cells. 2018;7(9):122.
49. Fan M, Ahmed KM, Coleman MC, Spitz DR, Li JJ. Nuclear factor-kappaB and manganese superoxide dismutase mediate adaptive radioresistance in low-dose irradiated mouse skin epithelial cells. Cancer Res. 2007;67(7):3220–8.
50. Xu Y, Fang F, Sun Y, St Clair DK, St Clair WH. RelB-dependent differential radiosensitization effect of STI571 on prostate cancer cells. Mol Cancer Ther. 2010;9(4):803–12.
51. Guo G, Yan-Sanders Y, Lyn-Cook BD, Wang T, Tamae D, Ogi J, et al. Manganese superoxide dismutase-mediated gene expression in radiation-induced adaptive responses. Mol Cell Biol. 2003;23(7):2362–78.
52. Kiningham KK, Xu Y, Daosukho C, Popova B, St Clair DK. Nuclear factor kappaB-dependent mechanisms coordinate the synergistic effect of PMA and cytokines on the induction of superoxide dismutase 2. Biochem J. 2001;353(Pt 1):147–56.
53. Xu Y, Kiningham KK, Devalaraja MN, Yeh CC, Majima H, Kasarskis EJ, et al. An intronic NF-kappaB element is essential for induction of the human manganese superoxide dismutase gene by tumor necrosis factor-alpha and interleukin-1beta. DNA Cell Biol. 1999;18(9):709–22.

54. Najar MA, Rex DAB, Modi PK, Agarwal N, Dagamajalu S, Karthikkeyan G, et al. A complete map of the calcium/calmodulin-dependent protein kinase kinase 2 (CAMKK2) signaling pathway. J Cell Commun Signal. 2021;15(2):283–90.
55. Josson S, Xu Y, Fang F, Dhar SK, St Clair DK, St Clair WH. RelB regulates manganese superoxide dismutase gene and resistance to ionizing radiation of prostate cancer cells. Oncogene. 2006;25(10):1554–9.
56. Margalit DN, Jordahl KM, Werner L, Wang X, Gwo-Shu Lee M, Penney KL, et al. GermLine variation in superoxide Dismutase-2 (SOD2) and survival outcomes after radiation therapy for prostate cancer: results of a test and validation set analysis. Clin Genitourin Cancer. 2015;13(4):370–7.e1.
57. Epperly MW, Kagan VE, Sikora CA, Gretton JE, Defilippi SJ, Bar-Sagi D, et al. Manganese superoxide dismutase-plasmid/liposome (MnSOD-PL) administration protects mice from esophagitis associated with fractionated radiation. Int J Cancer. 2001;96(4):221–31.
58. Zhang X, Epperly MW, Kay MA, Chen ZY, Dixon T, Franicola D, et al. Radioprotection in vitro and in vivo by minicircle plasmid carrying the human manganese superoxide dismutase transgene. Hum Gene Ther. 2008;19(8):820–6.
59. Venkataraman S, Jiang X, Weydert C, Zhang Y, Zhang HJ, Goswami PC, et al. Manganese superoxide dismutase overexpression inhibits the growth of androgen-independent prostate cancer cells. Oncogene. 2005;24(1):77–89.
60. Urano M, Kuroda M, Reynolds R, Oberley TD, St Clair DK. Expression of manganese superoxide dismutase reduces tumor control radiation dose: gene-radiotherapy. Cancer Res. 1995;55(12):2490–3.
61. Sun J, Chen Y, Li M, Ge Z. Role of antioxidant enzymes on ionizing radiation resistance. Free Radic Biol Med. 1998;24(4):586–93.
62. Gao Z, Sarsour EH, Kalen AL, Li L, Kumar MG, Goswami PC. Late ROS accumulation and radiosensitivity in SOD1-overexpressing human glioma cells. Free Radic Biol Med. 2008;45(11):1501–9.
63. Huggins C. Endocrine control of prostatic cancer. Science. 1943;97(2529):541–4.
64. Kolyvas EA, Caldas C, Kelly K, Ahmad SS. Androgen receptor function and targeted therapeutics across breast cancer subtypes. Breast Cancer Res. 2022;24(1):79.
65. Ross RW, Xie W, Regan MM, Pomerantz M, Nakabayashi M, Daskivich TJ, et al. Efficacy of androgen deprivation therapy (ADT) in patients with advanced prostate cancer: association between Gleason score, prostate-specific antigen level, and prior ADT exposure with duration of ADT effect. Cancer. 2008;112(6):1247–53.
66. Yang DD, Mahal BA, Muralidhar V, Martin NE, Orio PF, Mouw KW, et al. Androgen deprivation therapy and overall survival for Gleason 8 versus Gleason 9-10 prostate cancer. Eur Urol. 2019;75(1):35–41.
67. Sonpavde G, Attard G, Bellmunt J, Mason MD, Malavaud B, Tombal B, et al. The role of abiraterone acetate in the management of prostate cancer: a critical analysis of the literature. Eur Urol. 2011;60(2):270–8.
68. Scher HI, Fizazi K, Saad F, Taplin ME, Sternberg CN, Miller K, et al. Increased survival with enzalutamide in prostate cancer after chemotherapy. N Engl J Med. 2012;367(13):1187–97.
69. Smith MR, Saad F, Chowdhury S, Oudard S, Hadaschik BA, Graff JN, et al. Apalutamide and overall survival in prostate cancer. Eur Urol. 2021;79(1):150–8.
70. Tannock IF, de Wit R, Berry WR, Horti J, Pluzanska A, Chi KN, et al. Docetaxel plus prednisone or mitoxantrone plus prednisone for advanced prostate cancer. N Engl J Med. 2004;351(15):1502–12.
71. de Bono J, Mateo J, Fizazi K, Saad F, Shore N, Sandhu S, et al. Olaparib for metastatic castration-resistant prostate cancer. N Engl J Med. 2020;382(22):2091–102.
72. Matei DV, Renne G, Pimentel M, Sandri MT, Zorzino L, Botteri E, et al. Neuroendocrine differentiation in castration-resistant prostate cancer: a systematic diagnostic attempt. Clin Genitourin Cancer. 2012;10(3):164–73.

73. Kyriakopoulos CE, Chen YH, Carducci MA, Liu G, Jarrard DF, Hahn NM, et al. Chemohormonal therapy in metastatic hormone-sensitive prostate cancer: long-term survival analysis of the randomized phase III E3805 CHAARTED trial. J Clin Oncol. 2018;36(11):1080–7.
74. Rescigno P, de Bono JS. Immunotherapy for lethal prostate cancer. Nat Rev Urol. 2019;16(2):69–70.
75. Drake CG, Lipson EJ, Brahmer JR. Breathing new life into immunotherapy: review of melanoma, lung and kidney cancer. Nat Rev Clin Oncol. 2014;11(1):24–37.
76. Ito Y, Sadar MD. Enzalutamide and blocking androgen receptor in advanced prostate cancer: lessons learnt from the history of drug development of antiandrogens. Res Rep Urol. 2018;10:23–32.
77. de Leval J, Boca P, Yousef E, Nicolas H, Jeukenne M, Seidel L, et al. Intermittent versus continuous total androgen blockade in the treatment of patients with advanced hormone-naive prostate cancer: results of a prospective randomized multicenter trial. Clin Prostate Cancer. 2002;1(3):163–71.
78. Abrahamsson PA. Intermittent androgen deprivation therapy in patients with prostate cancer: connecting the dots. Asian J Urol. 2017;4(4):208–22.
79. Tsao CK, Galsky MD, Small AC, Yee T, Oh WK. Targeting the androgen receptor signalling axis in castration-resistant prostate cancer (CRPC). BJU Int. 2012;110(11):1580–8.
80. Mostaghel EA, Page ST, Lin DW, Fazli L, Coleman IM, True LD, et al. Intraprostatic androgens and androgen-regulated gene expression persist after testosterone suppression: therapeutic implications for castration-resistant prostate cancer. Cancer Res. 2007;67(10):5033–41.
81. Mostaghel EA, Zhang A, Hernandez S, Marck BT, Zhang X, Tamae D, et al. Contribution of adrenal glands to Intratumor androgens and growth of castration-resistant prostate cancer. Clin Cancer Res. 2019;25(1):426–39.
82. Hirayama Y, Sadar MD. Does increased expression of glucocorticoid receptor support application of antagonists to this receptor for the treatment of castration resistant prostate cancer? AME Med J. 2018;3:3.

Chapter 12
Plant-Derived Natural Products in Treatment of Prostate Cancer

Samaneh Adelian, Amin Soltani, and Michael R. Hamblin

Abstract Prostate cancer is the prevailing form of cancer in males and ranks as the second leading cause of cancer-related death globally. The transition from advanced prostate cancer to castration-resistant prostate cancer (CRPC) is a critical factor in the morbidity and mortality associated with the illness, presenting a substantial treatment obstacle. Resistance has been linked to the activation of androgen receptors by many methods, including alternate biosynthesis routes of dehydroepiandrosterone, other compounds that activate the androgen receptor, oncogenes, and signaling pathways involved with carcinogenesis. The tumor microenvironment is of utmost importance in both the course of cancer and the development of medication resistance. Several natural compounds have shown significant promise in combating specific or multiple resistance pathways, as evidenced by research conducted in cell lines, tumor samples, and animal models. Nevertheless, the clinical studies of these substances have been compromised due to their negative pharmacological characteristics, such as inadequate water solubility, hydrophobic nature, high excretion rate, low pharmacokinetic profile, and instability. Natural products formulated in nanoparticles provide a potential solution to the current impasse by using targeted drug administration, enhancing the pharmacokinetic drug profile, and facilitating the transit of diagnostic and therapeutic agents through biologically unpassable enclosures. This chapter presents a compilation of the existing data about the application of natural products in the treatment of prostate cancer and CRPC.

Keywords Advanced-stage cancer · Drug side effects · Flavanol compounds · Antioxidants · Natural therapeutic products

Samaneh Adelian and Amin Soltani contributed equally with all other contributors.

S. Adelian · A. Soltani
Cellular and Molecular Research Center, Basic Health Sciences Institute, Shahrekord University of Medical Sciences, Shahrekord, Iran

M. R. Hamblin (✉)
Laser Research Centre, Faculty of Health Science, University of Johannesburg, Doornfontein, South Africa

G. Sethi et al. (eds.), *Prostate Cancer: Molecular Events and Therapeutic Modalities*, https://doi.org/10.1007/978-981-97-4612-5_12

12.1 Introduction

For several years, plants have been regarded as a fundamental reservoir of medicinal substances used in the treatment of various maladies. The use of plant products in medicine may be traced back to ancient times, as shown by the discovery of clay tablets inscribed with cuneiform script, originating from the Sumerian civilization in Mesopotamia during the year 2600 BC. The tablets presented in the study demonstrated the use of over one thousand botanical components in the context of medical therapy [1]. The use of botanical resources for medicinal purposes was prevalent throughout the ancient Egyptian civilization. The examination of historical documents has shown evidence of the use of over 700 medicinal compounds produced from plants in the context of medical treatments [2]. The suboptimal efficacy and significant adverse effects associated with the application of traditional anticancer treatments have prompted researchers to prioritize the exploration and advancement of novel anticancer compounds obtained from natural sources [3]. Plant-derived secondary metabolites, like flavonoids, terpenoids, alkaloids, saponins, and other natural compounds, have been identified as significant reservoirs of strong anticancer drugs [4, 5]. A significant proportion, over 60%, of efficacious anticancer medications used in clinical settings have been derived from botanical sources, aquatic creatures, and microbes. The anticancer properties of these natural compounds are facilitated by many pathways, such as the stimulation of apoptosis, regulation of the immune system, and prevention of angiogenesis [6]. This chapter provides a summary of several plant-derived anticancer drugs. A thorough analysis was presented, including the origins of these substances from natural sources, the techniques used for their extraction, their modes of action as agents against prostate cancer, their application in clinical trials, and their formulation in the pharmaceutical industry.

12.2 Curcumin

Curcumin is classified as a curcuminoid, which is a phenolic substance consisting of diferuloylmethane, along with two other components. Curcumin, a prominent bioactive compound, is abundantly present in the desiccated rhizomes of *Curcuma longa*, a member of the Zingiberaceae family, more generally referred to as turmeric [7, 8]. At first, in 1910, curcumin's chemical structure was discovered by Milobedeska et al. [9, 10] (Fig. 12.1.). This compound has a-dicarbonyl moiety, two aromatic O-methoxy phenolic groups, and a seven-carbon bridge that contains two enone moieties. According to the International Union of Pure and Applied Chemistry

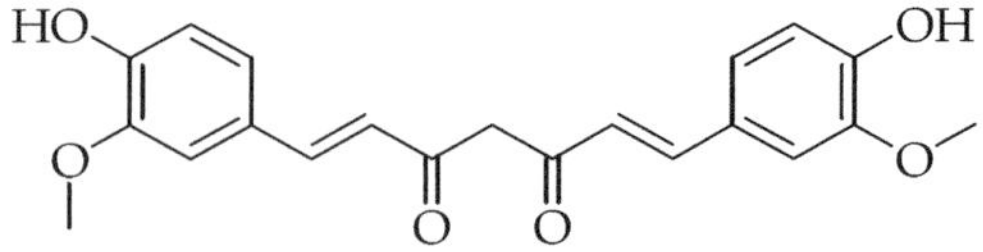

Fig. 12.1 Chemical structure of curcumin

(IUPAC) nomenclature, its designated name is (1E,6E). The compound is referred to as 1,7-bis[4-hydroxy-3-methoxyphenyl]-1,6-heptadiene-3,5,dione.

The extraction and isolation of curcumin were first accomplished by Vogel throughout the nineteenth century [10]. The extraction of curcuminoids from natural sources is often carried out using a range of standard procedures. These methods include organic solvent extraction, steam distillation, hot and cold percolation, the use of alkaline solutions [8], and the application of hydrotropes [11]. Furthermore, much research has been conducted on many sophisticated techniques, including extraction with supercritical fluid that has the notable benefit of eliminating the need for organic solvents [12]. The Soxhlet extraction method is widely recognized as the conventional benchmark technique. In comparison to more sophisticated methodologies, the Soxhlet method exhibited much greater curcumin extraction yields than enzyme-, ultrasound-, and microwave-assisted extractions [12]. The post-extraction procedures primarily include the use of chromatographic methods for the purpose of segregating the curcuminoids from other concurrently extracted volatile oils and oleoresins. These techniques are also employed to isolate curcumin from its corresponding curcuminoid molecules, such as bisdemethoxycurcumin [13]. Various organic solvents were utilized for the extraction of curcumin; nonetheless, ethanol continues to be the favored solvent [14]. Additionally, there is ongoing experimentation and utilization of food-grade solvents, like triacylglycerols [14].

The objective of the several established techniques is to reduce the quantity of organic solvents applied in extraction processes and to minimize the duration of the multi-step extraction and subsequent operations, such as the isolation of curcumin from its analogs. Furthermore, their objective is to identify a more discriminating extraction technique, characterized by a substantial output of superior quality for both nutritional and medicinal applications, which demonstrates cost-effectiveness [15].

Curcumin has been recognized for its diverse pharmacologic features, encompassing wound-healing, anti-diabetic, antioxidant, antiviral, anti-inflammatory, and antibacterial capabilities. Extensive research has been conducted to explore its potential as an anticancer and chemopreventive agent against a range of cancer types [16]. The anticancer impact of this substance is achieved by many processes, such as the reduction of cancer cell proliferation, activation of apoptosis, and suppression of metastasis in cancer cells. The processes under investigation have been examined across a diverse range of cancer types, such as colorectal, prostate, and breast cancer [17, 18]. In both prostate cancer cell lines and prostate tumor samples, it has been seen that curcumin can disrupt many cellular pathways. Some of these pathways include NF-κB, EGFR, and MAPK signaling pathways [10]. Curcumin has been shown to possess the ability to regulate autophagy and impede metastasis and angiogenesis in many types of malignancies [19]. The therapeutic use of curcumin is constrained by its instability, hydrophobic nature, low pharmacokinetic profile, and restricted water solubility, despite its possession of certain advantageous pharmacological characteristics [20]. Nanoparticles have been created as a means to enhance the transport of curcumin, hence increasing its effectiveness in cancer therapy. Nanoparticles have the capacity to safeguard pharmaceuticals against degradation, improve drug stability, provide regulated drug release, as well as enhance the pharmacokinetic properties, and reduce the toxicity profile of the medication [21]. Docetaxel (DTX) is often used as the primary therapeutic approach for the treatment of castration-resistant prostate cancer (CRPC). Over a period of time, individuals with CRPC developed a tolerance to docetaxel, which could potentially contribute to patient mortality. In a study, several pharmaceutical excipients, including Miglyol 812 and d-alpha tocopheryl polyethylene glycol succinate (TPEGS) 1000, a surfactant derived from vitamin E have been employed to create curcumin nanoparticles. The utilized surfactant in the synthesis of nanoparticles has received approval from the Food and Drug Administration (FDA) as a highly secure excipient suitable for incorporation into various formulations [22]. The inclusion of TPEGS as a surfactant is helpful due to its ability to suppress efflux via allosteric regulation of P-glycoprotein, as shown by Collnot et al. (2010). The present work included the preparation and characterization of curcumin-encapsulated nanoparticles. The nanoparticles were subjected to several analyses, including zeta potential measurement, determination of particle size, assessment of drug loading and efficiency, stability evaluation, differential scanning calorimetry analysis, and in vitro tests [23].

12.3 Epigallocatechin Gallate (EGCG)

EGCG is a naturally occurring polyphenol classified under the flavonol group [24]. The primary dietary origins of EGCG are derived from green tea (*Camellia sinensis*, Theaceae) [25] and items containing cocoa [26]. Various methods of extraction have been utilized to extract bioactive compounds from green tea [27, 28]. The extraction settings of the ultrasound-assisted technique were modified to enhance the yield of EGCG from lipid-extracted microalgae [29]. Furthermore, the use of subcritical water extraction for the EGCG extraction has been implemented by modifying the extraction parameters, leading to a yield of EGCG up to 4.66% [30]. The use of electrochemical techniques resulted in an enhancement in the extraction efficiency of epigallocatechin gallate. The use of a polymeric electrode composed of PAN/PPY, which has been enhanced with nanoparticles of TiO_2 and rGO, has been discovered to result in time savings and improved efficiency in the extraction of EGCG with high level of purity [31]. Ayyildiz and colleagues demonstrated that the use of ultrasound-assisted extraction exhibited higher efficiency in extracting EGCG compared to the hot water technique. Nevertheless, it was shown to be a viable approach for the manufacturing of green tea drinks [32]. In addition, the use of a green extracting agent such as β-cyclodextrin demonstrated enhanced extraction efficiency for EGCG and ECG when compared to conventional solvents such as water and ethanol [33].

In addition, the EGCG compound can be formed by the esterification of gallic acid and epigallocatechin [34]. Historically, green tea has been utilized in Chinese and Indian medicinal practices for its stimulant, diuretic, and astringent properties, as well as its potential to enhance cardiovascular well-being [35]. The health advantages of EGCG are shown by its ability to lower LDL cholesterol levels, limit the aberrant production of blood clots, and reduce tumor cell proliferation [36]. EGCG is identified as the most powerful agent because of its ability to reduce inflammation and its anticancer properties [37] (Fig. 12.2).

Numerous research has shown the anticancer effects of EGCG. The compound has antiproliferative, antimetastatic, and proapoptotic properties [38]. The study demonstrated that EGCG effectively inhibited the formation of prostate cancer tumors in TRAMP mice and also led to a reduction in tumor-derived blood PSA levels [39]. Similar to curcumin, many studies have provided data indicating that EGCG, a polyphenol, can hinder DNA methylation. This process has been linked to the induction of anticancer effects, demonstrating significant promise in combating prostate cancer [40, 41].

The potential of EGCG to effectively control CRPC is acknowledged; however, the issue of bioavailability remains a significant worry. In their study, Rocha et al. (2011) used a polysaccharide matrix consisting of gum arabic and maltodextrin to encapsulate EGCG. The researchers next investigated the possible anti-prostate cancer effects of this encapsulated EGCG in Du145 prostate cancer cells [42]. According to their findings, it was discovered that encapsulated EGCG exhibited not only the capacity to maintain its anti-prostate cancer properties by decreasing cell viability and inducing apoptosis but also showed improved impact in comparison to free EGCG [42]. In a study conducted by Khan's team, a formulation of chitosan nanoparticles with oral administration ability was developed. These nanoparticles were then loaded with epigallocatechin-3-gallate (EGCG) and evaluated for their potential as an antitumor agent [43]. The chitosan-EGCG nanoparticles, with a diameter of less than 200 nm, were subsequently tested in athymic nude mice that had been subcutaneously implanted with 22 Rn1 tumor xenografts. The findings of the study demonstrated that the chitosan-EGCG nanoparticles exhibited superior efficacy as an anti-prostate cancer agent in comparison to both EGCG alone and the control groups. This enhanced effectiveness was attributed to the manipulation of numerous pathways. According to Khan et al. (2014), the bioavailability problem was effectively addressed by the quicker release of EGCG in the intestinal fluid. Combination medicines have gained popularity in the management of chronic illnesses due to their potential for synergistic effects [43]. In their study, Chen et al. (2020) used a nanoparticle formulation consisting of TPGS-conjugated

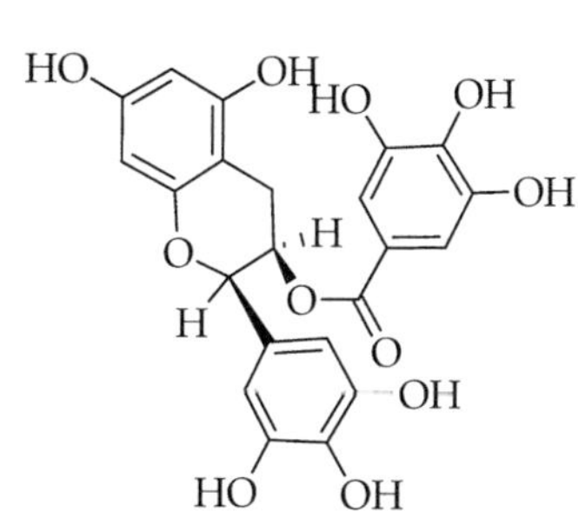

Fig. 12.2 Chemical structure of epigallocatechin-3-gallate (EGCG)

hyaluronic acid and fucoidan to encapsulate epigallocatechin gallate with low dosages of docetaxel (DTX). Among several combinations, it was observed that a ratio of EGCG to DTX at 2.00:0.20 mg/mL exhibited superior and more precise dispersion, along with notable drug loading efficiencies. The in vitro investigations revealed the uptake of these nanoparticles into prostate cancer cells, hence enhancing the specificity of the combined therapy [44]. Moreover, the in vivo investigations conducted by Chen et al. (2020) revealed a remarkable increase in M30 protein levels, which was accompanied by a reduction in tumor development, while exhibiting no discernible impact on the functioning of vital organs [44].

12.4 Emodin

Emodin is predominantly derived from the rhizomes and roots of *Rheum palmatum*, although it can also be obtained from other herbs, like *Polygonum multiflorum*, *Aloe vera*, *Polygonum cuspidatum*, and *Cassia obtusifolia* [45, 46]. Furthermore, it has been shown that this compound exhibits isolation from many fungal species, such as Aspergillus wentii [47]. Emodin, chemically referred to as 1,3,8-trihydroxy-6-methyl-anthraquinone, is a naturally occurring derivative of anthraquinone [48] (Fig. 12.3). It is recognized for its many therapeutic properties, including anticancer, anti-inflammatory, antibacterial, immunosuppressive, antiviral, and other therapeutic actions [49, 50].

In their review, Hsu and Chung (2012) discuss the molecular mechanisms associated with emodin. These mechanisms include apoptosis, upregulation of HIF-1α, cell cycle arrest, and increasing the levels of N-acetyltransferase, glutathione (GSH) S-transferase P, and glutathione detoxification enzymes. Additionally, emodin inhibits invasion, angiogenesis, migration, and the expression of p34cdc2 kinase, CKII kinase, and HER2/neu in various tumor cells [51]. According to reports, there is evidence suggesting that it may impede the process of tumor-associated angiogenesis by inhibiting the phosphorylation of ERK. Additionally, emodin has anti-metastatic and anti-proliferative properties [52]. The downregulation of survivin and β-catenin expression is seen, leading to the induction of DNA damage and inhibition of the DNA repair system [53]. Additionally, it has inhibitory effects on CKII by competing with ATP-binding sites [54]. Based on some research results, it has been shown that this substance enhances the expression of intracellular superoxide dismutases and HIF-1α, hence increasing the effectiveness of cytotoxic medications [55]. In a study conducted by Cha and colleagues, it was demonstrated that emodin

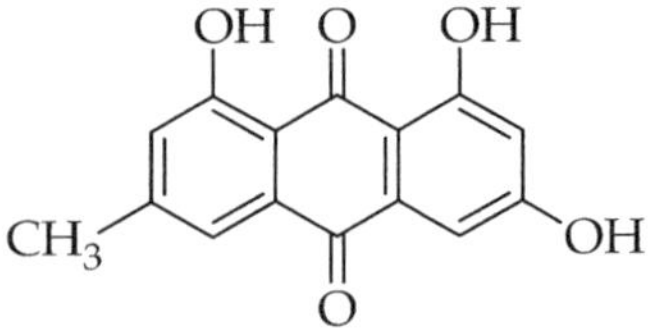

Fig. 12.3 Chemical structure of emodin

exhibited inhibitory effects on the proliferation of prostate tumor cells. This inhibition effect was attained by the decrease in AR level from heat shock protein 90 (Hsp90) and the enhancement of its cross-talk with E3 ligase MDM2. Consequently, this promoted the AR degradation mediated by proteasome in LNCaP cells [56]. Furthermore, an increase in chemosensitivity was found in DU-145 cancer cell lines (a cell line derived from multidrug-resistant prostate carcinoma) in vitro and also in tumor-bearing mice after administration of emodin and cisplatin simultaneously. The study demonstrated that the process entails the inhibition of multidrug resistance and HIF-1α in cells with high activity of HIF-1α via the mediation of ROS [57].

12.5 Thymoquinone (TQ)

Thymoquinone (TQ) is the primary bioactive phytochemical ingredient present in the volatile oil derived from *Nigella sativa* (often known as black cumin or black seed). This plant has a long history of traditional medicinal usage in several nations [58]. TQ has a range of pharmacological properties, including antihistaminic, anti-inflammatory, antibacterial, antioxidant, and immunomodulatory effects. Additionally, it has shown significant potential as an anticancer agent [59, 60] (Fig. 12.4).

The potential anticancer actions of TQ are facilitated by many methods that modulate the control of growth factors, transcription factors, cell cycle, tumor-suppressor genes, protein kinase enzymes, cell survival, apoptosis, and phase I/II enzymes [61]. Modulating the course of the cell cycle constitutes a fundamental stage in the prevention and suppression of cancer growth and advancement. The conjugation of TQ with fatty acid has potential action on several cellular mechanisms, including cell death, cell proliferation, and cell signaling pathways [61]. TQ triggers G2/M cell cycle arrest and promotes apoptosis, while also drastically reducing the expression of NF-κB in the nucleus. Furthermore, it has been shown that TQ has a significant role in enhancing the activity of PPAR-γ while simultaneously reducing the transcription of genes associated with surviving, Bcl-xL, and Bcl-2 [62]. According to the reports, it has been shown that TQ has a crucial participation in the initiation of apoptosis by downregulating the anti-apoptotic factors. Additionally, it has been observed that TQ substantially upregulates the pro-apoptotic agents [58]. The aforementioned process is facilitated by the triggering of caspases 7, 8, and 9 in a way that is dependent on the dosage. Additionally, it leads to an elevation in the PPAR-γ activity [63, 64]. TQ has been shown to elicit the breakdown of the tubulin

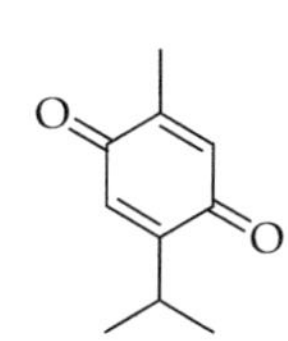

Fig. 12.4 Chemical structure of thymoquinone (TQ)

component inside cellular systems while also exhibiting inhibitory effects on telomerase enzyme activity. In addition, it induces the downregulation of both AR levels and E2F-1 that play crucial roles in the cell proliferation and cell survival of prostate cancer cells that are responsive to androgen as well as those that are not [65]. The research by Kou and colleagues indicated that thymoquinone had inhibitory effects on the metastatic characteristics and reversed EMT in prostate tumor cells. This was achieved via the negative regulation of the TGF-β/Smad2/3 signaling pathway [66]. The results of this study indicate that thymoquinone has promise as a therapeutic agent for the treatment of prostate cancer via its specific targeting of TGF-β. In addition, TQ is equipped with inhibitory effects on the active sites of cytochrome P450 enzymes that are well recognized as a crucial target in the context of prostate cancer treatment [67]. The combination of TQ with Docetaxel, at concentrations of 50 μM and 10 nM, respectively, resulted in an elevated rate of apoptosis in DU145 and C4-2B prostate cancer cells. This effect was achieved by the inhibition of the PI3K/AKT pathway and subsequent modulation of downstream signaling effectors. Additionally, it has been seen to stimulate the transcription of apoptosis inducer proteins, including BID and procaspase-3, and BAX. Conversely, it can suppress the expression of anti-apoptotic proteins like Bcl-xL [37].

Al-Trad et al. (2017) performed an in vivo investigation to investigate the potential preventive benefits of TQ against the onset of benign prostatic hyperplasia (BPH) in a group of Wistar rats. The rats were administered an oral dose of 50 mg/kg TQ daily for a duration of 14 days [68, 69]. The findings demonstrated that TQ exhibited a capacity to decrease the ratio of prostate weight to body weight, epithelial hyperplasia, serum levels of interleukin (IL)-6, TGF-β1, and VEGF-A expression in the experimental group [69]. TQ has been shown to have inhibitory impacts on prostate cancer progression at a concentration of 45 μM. This is achieved by the decrease in IL-6 production and the inhibition of phosphorylation of ERK, AKT, and STAT3 proteins in PC3 cells [70].

12.6 Genistein

Genistein, also known as 4′,5,7-trihydroxyisoflavone or 5,7-dihydroxy-3-(4-hydroxyphenyl) chromen-4-one, is an isoflavonoid compound characterized by a 15-carbon skeleton (as seen in Fig. 12.5). It falls within the category of phytoestrogens. The glycosylated or free form of this substance is often present in several dietary sources, particularly legumes. The compound has a structural resemblance

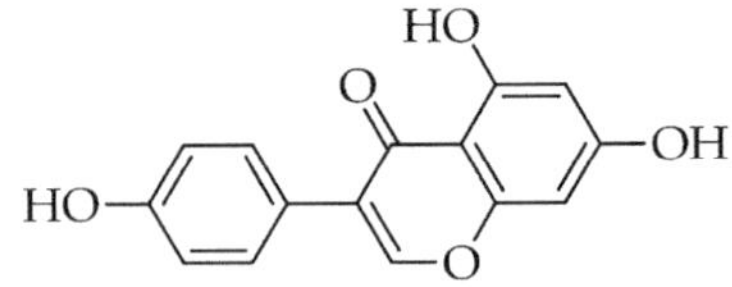

Fig. 12.5 Chemical structure of genistein

to 17β-estradiol, hence enabling its capacity to interact with and regulate the functioning of estrogen receptors [71].

The anticancer properties of genistein are manifested through various mechanisms, including apoptosis promotion, suppression of proliferation, angiogenesis inhibition, and prevention of metastasis. These effects have been demonstrated in hepatocellular cancer models of nude mice and Wistar rats, in addition to in a gastric cancer model of Wistar rats, where genistein administration resulted in reduced tumor growth and development [58]. The role of genistein in prostate cancer has been extensively studied through in vivo studies using various animal models. These models include the Lobund-Wistar rat, which is a distinctive rat model that naturally develops metastatic prostate cancer in approximately 30% of its population. Additionally, SCID mice transplanted with human prostate carcinoma cells (LNCaP, PC3, and DU-145) have also been utilized in these studies. Several in vivo investigations were conducted using normal rats to examine the potential harmful effects of genistein on the prostate, as well as its impact on the expression of androgen and estrogen receptors [72]. Furthermore, the study conducted in this research examined the effects of prostate cancer on several cell types, including VeCaP, PNT-1 and PNT-2, DU-145, PC3, and LNCaP [72]. Genistein exerts its inhibitory effects on cyclin-dependent kinases (CDKs) by the upregulation of p21. Additionally, it suppresses the cyclin D1 expression, resulting in the induction of G2/M cell cycle arrest and a reduction in tumor cell growth [73, 74]. The downregulation of matrix metalloproteinase-2 (MMP-2) expression levels in prostate cancer cell lines has been described as a result of genistein treatment. Matrix metalloproteinase (MMP) serves as the first stage in the cascade of metastasis and angiogenesis [75]. Furthermore, it should be noted that AP-1 is a cytokine involved in angiogenesis. Its activity may be suppressed by genistein, resulting in the inhibition of many targets such as MMP, Bcl-XL, cyclin D1, Bcl-2, VEGF, and uPA [76]. Furthermore, it has been shown that genistein has the ability to have an impact on the process of metastasis and trigger apoptosis in PC3 cell lines by inhibiting Akt and NF-κB cascades [77]. Additionally, it has been shown that genistein can decrease the levels of phosphorylated-Akt in LNCaP cells [78]. In a recent study, it has been observed that the boost of AR ubiquitination in LNCaP cells treated with genistein was attributed to the suppression of Hsp90 chaperones. The findings of this study provide substantial evidence in favor of the idea that genistein has the potential to serve as a chemopreventive drug for prostate cancer [79].

12.7 Parthenolide

Parthenolide is a significant metabolite that occurs naturally in medicinal plants belonging to the Asteraceae family [80]. Its prominence is particularly notable in *Tanacetum parthenium* (feverfew) [81], but it is also present in other species such as *Tanacetum vulgare* (tansy) and Tanacetum larvatum [82]. Parthenolide is mostly present in the aerial portions of plants, namely in flowers and leaves, whereas its presence in roots is little. Nevertheless, it should be noted that parthenolide, which is used for research reasons, has been obtained from *T. parthenium* leaves with a purity above 97%. The extraction of parthenolide from feverfew was conducted using traditional methods, using chloroform and petroleum ether as solvents. Subsequently, a gradient technique for high-performance liquid chromatography (HPLC) was established [58]. Several more HPLC extraction procedures were also documented. According to Zhou's team study, the extraction of parthenolide from feverfew was shown to be most effective by utilizing acetonitrile with a water content of 10% (v/v) and using bottle stirring procedures. This extraction process yielded the maximum quantity of parthenolide, with a concentration of 930 mg/100 g of raw material [83].

Parthenolide, a sesquiterpene lactone, has a methylene-γ-lactone ring and an epoxide group (Fig. 12.6), facilitating rapid interactions with biological sites [84]. Historically, parthenolide was predominantly employed for the management of migraine, fever, and rheumatoid arthritis. However, recent research has revealed that parthenolide exhibits anticancer properties in various types of tumors, such as breast, pancreatic, prostate, bladder, and leukemia [85]. The pharmacological characteristics of parthenolide are generally suboptimal due to its low solubility in water and subsequent limited bioavailability. As a result, its potential clinical application as an anticancer medication is constrained. Nonetheless, researchers have developed a range of derivatives of parthenolide to address this challenge [86].

The anticancer activity of parthenolide is elicited by many modes of action [87]. The cytotoxic activity of this compound may be attributed to its ability to disrupt DNA replication via the presence of the highly reactive methylene groups, epoxide, and lactone ring [88]. Furthermore, it facilitated the suppression of STAT3 by promoting the death receptor transcription, so activating the apoptosis pathway [89]. Moreover, the molecular mechanism behind the action of parthenolide is closely linked to its proapoptotic effects, which are mediated by the p53 activation and the enhanced generation of ROS [90]. Additionally, parthenolide leads to a decrease in cellular levels of reduced glutathione (GSH) [91]. According to the findings of Duan et al., parthenolide has the ability to selectively affect mitochondrial thioredoxin reductase, leading to the trigger of the apoptotic pathway through ROS generation [92]. In addition, it has been shown that parthenolide has inhibitory effects on microtubule production, hence impeding the growth of malignant cells [93]. Parthenolide has been shown to stimulate thrombopoiesis by inhibiting NF-κB activity, hence increasing the susceptibility of cancer cells to undergo apoptosis [94]. Moreover, it has been shown that parthenolide has the ability to hinder

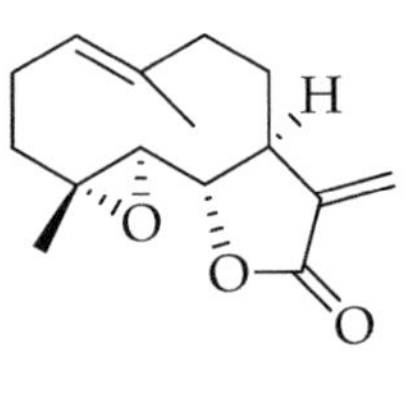

Fig. 12.6 Chemical structure of parthenolide

signaling pathways that are reliant on focal adhesion kinase. Consequently, this leads to a decrease in cell growth, survival, and movement [95]. It is noteworthy that research has shown the unique impact of parthenolide on cancer cells while exhibiting no harmful effects on normal cells [96]. The compound known as parthenolide has anticancer characteristics and has the ability to produce radiosensitivity in mouse prostate cancer cell lines. Additionally, it provides protection against radiation-induced damage in primary prostate epithelial cell lines [97].

12.8 Conclusion

Prostate cancer, a malignancy influenced by hormonal factors, is strongly linked to significant morbidity and death rates in men on a global scale. The phenomenon of castration resistance has been linked to a repertoire of over 150 chemicals that engage in interactions with androgen receptors. Therapeutic targets encompass receptors, binding compounds, and their biosynthetic pathways, which can be effectively targeted by various natural compounds. These compounds include quercetin, curcumin, eugenol, isoflavones, ericifolin, and sintokamides A to E, as well as emodin derived from the plant *Rheum palmatum*. Despite the shown anticancer efficacy of these drugs in laboratory and animal studies, their effectiveness is limited when used in clinical situations. The aforementioned limitations may be attributed to the suboptimal pharmacodynamics and pharmacokinetic qualities of the subject in question. The use of nanoparticle formulations enables the manipulation of the biodistribution and accumulation at specific target sites of natural chemicals, resulting in a precise adjustment of the equilibrium between their effectiveness and harmful effects. Without a doubt, the use of nanoformulations of natural goods is associated with higher costs in comparison to the usage of natural products in their original form. Nevertheless, these benefits are compromised by the corresponding advantages, which include enhanced precision in targeting, heightened efficacy with minimized negative outcomes, greater bioavailability, gradual release, and extended half-life provided by these substances. Furthermore, it is worth noting that the financial implications do not exhibit a proportional relationship with the societal and health-related economic burdens. The use of curcumin nanoparticles has been shown to improve its negative pharmacological characteristics, such as its limited solubility in water. The in vitro investigations have shown the potential of curcumin-encapsulated nanoparticles in the context of stability, drug loading, dispersion, and particle size. The aforementioned statement holds true for medication delivery methods in prostate cancer that are based on quercetin nanomicelles. Further research is required to evaluate the potential of nanoparticles using atraric acid, capsaicin, niphatenones A and B, betulinic acid, and sintokamide A. In future clinical investigations, nanoparticle drug design has the potential to enhance the efficacy of existing phytocompound-based anticancer medicines, such as cabazitaxel (Jevtana®). According to the investigation of Pulker and coworkers, the use of digital health apps has the potential to enhance both retrospective and prospective research methodologies, hence enabling a more thorough evaluation of natural compound-based nanoparticles [98]. The delivery of nanomedicines to patients with advanced illnesses under established regulatory frameworks may enhance research in the area. In general, there is significant promise for the application of nanomedicines derived from natural products in the treatment of prostate cancer, in particular CRPC. Nevertheless, it is imperative to validate this potential via rigorous preclinical and clinical investigations.

References

1. Atanasov AG, Waltenberger B, Pferschy-Wenzig EM, Linder T, Wawrosch C, Uhrin P, et al. Discovery and resupply of pharmacologically active plant-derived natural products: a review. Biotechnol Adv. 2015;33(8):1582–614.
2. Dias DA, Urban S, Roessner U. A historical overview of natural products in drug discovery. Meta. 2012;2(2):303–36.
3. Wright GD. Opportunities for natural products in 21(st) century antibiotic discovery. Nat Prod Rep. 2017;34(7):694–701.
4. Yin SJ, Zhang L, Zhang L, Wan J, Song W, Jiang X, et al. Metabolic responses and arginine kinase expression of juvenile cuttlefish (Sepia pharaonis) under salinity stress. Int J Biol Macromol. 2018;113:881–8.
5. Avato P, Migoni D, Argentieri M, Fanizzi FP, Tava A. Activity of Saponins from Medicago species against HeLa and MCF-7 cell lines and their capacity to potentiate cisplatin effect. Anti Cancer Agents Med Chem. 2017;17(11):1508–18.
6. Rayan A, Raiyn J, Falah M. Nature is the best source of anticancer drugs: indexing natural products for their anticancer bioactivity. PLoS One. 2017;12(11):e0187925.
7. Agarwal A, Kasinathan A, Ganesan R, Balasubramanian A, Bhaskaran J, Suresh S, et al. Curcumin induces apoptosis and cell cycle arrest via the activation of reactive oxygen species-independent mitochondrial apoptotic pathway in Smad4 and p53 mutated colon adenocarcinoma HT29 cells. Nutr Res. 2018;51:67–81.
8. Patil SS, Bhasarkar S, Rathod VK. Extraction of curcuminoids from Curcuma longa: comparative study between batch extraction and novel three phase partitioning. Prep Biochem Biotechnol. 2019;49(4):407–18.
9. Ismail NI, Othman I, Abas F, Lajis NH, Naidu R. Mechanism of apoptosis induced by curcumin in colorectal Cancer. Int J Mol Sci. 2019;20(10):2454.
10. Tomeh MA, Hadianamrei R, Zhao X. A review of curcumin and its derivatives as anticancer agents. Int J Mol Sci. 2019;20(5):1033.
11. Yue CH, Zheng LT, Guo QM, Li KP. Study on extracting and separating curcuminoids from Curcuma longa rhizome using ultrasound strengthen by microemulsion. Zhong Yao Cai. 2014;37(5):880–3.
12. Urošević M, Nikolić L, Gajić I, Nikolić V, Dinić A, Miljković V. Curcumin: biological activities and modern pharmaceutical forms. Antibiotics (Basel). 2022;11(2):135.
13. Yadav DK, Sharma K, Dutta A, Kundu A, Awasthi A, Goon A, et al. Purity evaluation of Curcuminoids in the turmeric extract obtained by accelerated solvent extraction. J AOAC Int. 2017;100(3):586–91.
14. Priyadarsini KI. The chemistry of curcumin: from extraction to therapeutic agent. Molecules. 2014;19(12):20091–112.
15. Paulucci VP, Couto RO, Teixeira CCC, Freitas LAP. Optimization of the extraction of curcumin from Curcuma longa rhizomes. Rev Bras. 2013;23(1):94–100.

16. Kunnumakkara AB, Bordoloi D, Padmavathi G, Monisha J, Roy NK, Prasad S, et al. Curcumin, the golden nutraceutical: multitargeting for multiple chronic diseases. Br J Pharmacol. 2017;174(11):1325–48.
17. Falah RR, Talib WH, Shbailat SJ. Combination of metformin and curcumin targets breast cancer in mice by angiogenesis inhibition, immune system modulation and induction of p53 independent apoptosis. Ther Adv Med Oncol. 2017;9(4):235–52.
18. Ahmed K, Zaidi SF, Cui ZG, Zhou D, Saeed SA, Inadera H. Potential proapoptotic phytochemical agents for the treatment and prevention of colorectal cancer. Oncol Lett. 2019;18(1):487–98.
19. Bar-Sela G, Epelbaum R, Schaffer M. Curcumin as an anti-cancer agent: review of the gap between basic and clinical applications. Curr Med Chem. 2010;17(3):190–7.
20. Shoba G, Joy D, Joseph T, Majeed M, Rajendran R, Srinivas PS. Influence of piperine on the pharmacokinetics of curcumin in animals and human volunteers. Planta Med. 1998;64(4):353–6.
21. Markman JL, Rekechenetskiy A, Holler E, Ljubimova JY. Nanomedicine therapeutic approaches to overcome cancer drug resistance. Adv Drug Deliv Rev. 2013;65(13–14):1866–79.
22. Tanaudommongkon I, Tanaudommongkon A, Prathipati P, Nguyen JT, Keller ET, Dong X. Curcumin nanoparticles and their cytotoxicity in docetaxel-resistant castration-resistant prostate Cancer cells. Biomedicines. 2020;8(8):253.
23. Collnot EM, Baldes C, Schaefer UF, Edgar KJ, Wempe MF, Lehr CM. Vitamin E TPGS P-glycoprotein inhibition mechanism: influence on conformational flexibility, intracellular ATP levels, and role of time and site of access. Mol Pharm. 2010;7(3):642–51.
24. Eng QY, Thanikachalam PV, Ramamurthy S. Molecular understanding of epigallocatechin gallate (EGCG) in cardiovascular and metabolic diseases. J Ethnopharmacol. 2018;210:296–310.
25. Nagle DG, Ferreira D, Zhou YD. Epigallocatechin-3-gallate (EGCG): chemical and biomedical perspectives. Phytochemistry. 2006;67(17):1849–55.
26. Rodríguez-Carrasco Y, Gaspari A, Graziani G, Santini A, Ritieni A. Fast analysis of polyphenols and alkaloids in cocoa-based products by ultra-high performance liquid chromatography and Orbitrap high resolution mass spectrometry (UHPLC-Q-Orbitrap-MS/MS). Food Res Int. 2018;111:229–36.
27. Li DC, Jiang JG. Optimization of the microwave-assisted extraction conditions of tea polyphenols from green tea. Int J Food Sci Nutr. 2010;61(8):837–45.
28. Lee LS, Lee N, Kim YH, Lee CH, Hong SP, Jeon YW, et al. Optimization of ultrasonic extraction of phenolic antioxidants from green tea using response surface methodology. Molecules. 2013;18(11):13530–45.
29. Kröger H, Donner I, Skiello G. Influence of a new virostatic compound on the induction of enzymes in rat liver. Arzneimittelforschung. 1975;25(9):1426–9.
30. Nguyen T, Duong H, Anh D, Nguyen N, Thai D, Linh D, et al. Subcritical water extraction of epigallocatechin Gallate from Camellia sinensis and optimization study using response surface methodology. Processes. 2020;8:1028.
31. Ferdosian F, Ebadi M, Zafar-Mehrabian R, Golsefidi MA, Moradi AV. Extraction of epigallocatechin Gallate from green tea and its Chracterization using polymeric electrode PAN/PPY enriched with nano particles of TiO2 and rGO. Int J Electrochem Sci. 2019;14(7):6347–65.
32. Saklar Ayyildiz S, Karadeniz B, Sagcan N, Bahar B, Us A, Alasalvar C. Optimizing the extraction parameters of epigallocatechin Gallate using conventional hot water and ultrasound assisted methods from green tea. Food Bioprod Process. 2018;111:111.
33. Wang Y, Wang K, Yan J, Zhou Q, Wang X. Recent Progress in research on mechanisms of action of natural products against Alzheimer's disease: dietary plant polyphenols. Int J Mol Sci. 2022;23(22):13886.
34. Lambert JD, Lee MJ, Lu H, Meng X, Hong JJ, Seril DN, et al. Epigallocatechin-3-gallate is absorbed but extensively glucuronidated following oral administration to mice. J Nutr. 2003;133(12):4172–7.

35. Zhao T, Li C, Wang S, Song X. Green tea (Camellia sinensis): a review of its Phytochemistry, pharmacology, and toxicology. Molecules. 2022;27(12):3909.
36. Katiyar SK, Elmets CA. Green tea polyphenolic antioxidants and skin photoprotection (review). Int J Oncol. 2001;18(6):1307–13.
37. Musial C, Kuban-Jankowska A, Gorska-Ponikowska M. Beneficial properties of green tea Catechins. Int J Mol Sci. 2020;21(5):1744.
38. Wang YQ, Lu JL, Liang YR, Li QS. Suppressive effects of EGCG on cervical cancer. Molecules. 2018;23(9):2334.
39. Chuu CP, Chen RY, Kokontis JM, Hiipakka RA, Liao S. Suppression of androgen receptor signaling and prostate specific antigen expression by (−)-epigallocatechin-3-gallate in different progression stages of LNCaP prostate cancer cells. Cancer Lett. 2009;275(1):86–92.
40. Kallifatidis G, Hoy JJ, Lokeshwar BL. Bioactive natural products for chemoprevention and treatment of castration-resistant prostate cancer. Semin Cancer Biol. 2016;40-41:160–9.
41. Wang XJ, Chen JY, Fu LQ, Yan MJ. Recent advances in natural therapeutic approaches for the treatment of cancer. J Chemother. 2020;32(2):53–65.
42. Rocha S, Generalov R, Pereira Mdo C, Peres I, Juzenas P, Coelho MA. Epigallocatechin gallate-loaded polysaccharide nanoparticles for prostate cancer chemoprevention. Nanomedicine (Lond). 2011;6(1):79–87.
43. Khan N, Bharali DJ, Adhami VM, Siddiqui IA, Cui H, Shabana SM, et al. Oral administration of naturally occurring chitosan-based nanoformulated green tea polyphenol EGCG effectively inhibits prostate cancer cell growth in a xenograft model. Carcinogenesis. 2014;35(2):415–23.
44. Chen M-L, Lai C-J, Lin Y-N, Huang C-M, Lin Y-H. Multifunctional nanoparticles for targeting the tumor microenvironment to improve synergistic drug combinations and cancer treatment effects. J Mater Chem B. 2020;8(45):10416–27.
45. Dong X, Fu J, Yin X, Cao S, Li X, Lin L, et al. Emodin: a review of its pharmacology, toxicity and pharmacokinetics. Phytother Res. 2016;30(8):1207–18.
46. Li SH, Li L, Yang RN, Liang SD. Compounds of traditional Chinese medicine and neuropathic pain. Chin J Nat Med. 2020;18(1):28–35.
47. Qiu X, Gong L, Xin X, An F. Enhancement of Emodin production by medium optimization and KH(2)PO(4) supplementation in submerged fermentation of marine-derived Aspergillus favipes HN4-13. Mar Drugs. 2021;19(8):421.
48. Tang T, Yin L, Yang J, Shan G. Emodin, an anthraquinone derivative from Rheum officinale Baill, enhances cutaneous wound healing in rats. Eur J Pharmacol. 2007;567(3):177–85.
49. Huang HC, Chu SH, Chao PD. Vasorelaxants from Chinese herbs, emodin and scoparone, possess immunosuppressive properties. Eur J Pharmacol. 1991;198(2–3):211–3.
50. Zhu S, Wang Y, Wang X, Li J, Hu F. Emodin inhibits ATP-induced IL-1β secretion, ROS production and phagocytosis attenuation in rat peritoneal macrophages via antagonizing $P2X_7$ receptor. Pharm Biol. 2014;52(1):51–7.
51. Hsu SC, Chung JG. Anticancer potential of emodin. Biomedicine (Taipei). 2012;2(3):108–16.
52. Oei AL, Sweep FC, Thomas CM, Boerman OC, Massuger LF. The use of monoclonal antibodies for the treatment of epithelial ovarian cancer (review). Int J Oncol. 2008;32(6):1145–57.
53. Vickers NJ. Animal communication: when I'm calling you, will you answer too? Curr Biol. 2017;27(14):R713–r5.
54. Yim H, Lee YH, Lee CH, Lee SK. Emodin, an anthraquinone derivative isolated from the rhizomes of Rheum palmatum, selectively inhibits the activity of casein kinase II as a competitive inhibitor. Planta Med. 1999;65(1):9–13.
55. Zhang Z, Yan J, Chang Y, ShiDu Yan S, Shi H. Hypoxia inducible factor-1 as a target for neurodegenerative diseases. Curr Med Chem. 2011;18(28):4335–43.
56. Cha TL, Qiu L, Chen CT, Wen Y, Hung MC. Emodin down-regulates androgen receptor and inhibits prostate cancer cell growth. Cancer Res. 2005;65(6):2287–95.
57. Huang XZ, Wang J, Huang C, Chen YY, Shi GY, Hu QS, et al. Emodin enhances cytotoxicity of chemotherapeutic drugs in prostate cancer cells: the mechanisms involve ROS-mediated suppression of multidrug resistance and hypoxia inducible factor-1. Cancer Biol Ther. 2008;7(3):468–75.

58. Talib WH, Daoud S, Mahmod AI, Hamed RA, Awajan D, Abuarab SF, et al. Plants as a source of anticancer agents: from bench to bedside. Molecules. 2022;27(15):4818.
59. Aslan M, Afşar E, Kırımlıoglu E, Çeker T, Yılmaz Ç. Antiproliferative effects of Thymoquinone in MCF-7 breast and HepG2 liver Cancer cells: possible role of ceramide and ER stress. Nutr Cancer. 2021;73(3):460–72.
60. Laskar AA, Khan MA, Askari F, Younus H. Thymoquinone binds and activates human salivary aldehyde dehydrogenase: potential therapy for the mitigation of aldehyde toxicity and maintenance of oral health. Int J Biol Macromol. 2017;103:99–110.
61. Tabassum S, Thakur V, Rosli N, Ichwan SJA, Mishra P, Suriyah WH. Therapeutic implications of thymoquinone and its molecular and functional mechanisms against oral and lung cancer. Gene Rep. 2022;27:101600.
62. Woo CC, Loo SY, Gee V, Yap CW, Sethi G, Kumar AP, et al. Anticancer activity of thymoquinone in breast cancer cells: possible involvement of PPAR-γ pathway. Biochem Pharmacol. 2011;82(5):464–75.
63. Ayan M, Tas U, Sogut E, Caylı S, Kaya H, Esen M, et al. Protective effect of thymoquinone against testicular torsion induced oxidative injury. Andrologia. 2016;48(2):143–51.
64. Mabrouk A, Ben CH. Thymoquinone supplementation ameliorates lead-induced testis function impairment in adult rats. Toxicol Ind Health. 2016;32(6):1114–21.
65. Talib WH, Alsalahat I, Daoud S, Abutayeh RF, Mahmod AI. Plant-derived natural products in Cancer research: extraction, mechanism of action, and drug formulation. Molecules. 2020;25(22):5319.
66. Kou B, Liu W, Zhao W, Duan P, Yang Y, Yi Q, et al. [corrigendum] Thymoquinone inhibits epithelial-mesenchymal transition in prostate cancer cells by negatively regulating the TGF-β/Smad2/3 signaling pathway. Oncol Rep. 2023;49(3):3592.
67. Fu H, He J, Mei F, Zhang Q, Hara Y, Ryota S, et al. Lung cancer inhibitory effect of epigallocatechin-3-gallate is dependent on its presence in a complex mixture (polyphenon E). Cancer Prev Res (Phila). 2009;2(6):531–7.
68. Al-Trad B, Al-Zoubi M, Qar J, Al-Batayneh K, Hussien E, Muhaidat R, et al. Inhibitory effect of Thymoquinone on testosterone-induced benign prostatic hyperplasia in Wistar rats. Phytother Res. 2017;31(12):1910–5.
69. Du GJ, Zhang Z, Wen XD, Yu C, Calway T, Yuan CS, et al. Epigallocatechin Gallate (EGCG) is the most effective cancer chemopreventive polyphenol in green tea. Nutrients. 2012;4(11):1679–91.
70. Chen BH, Hsieh CH, Tsai SY, Wang CY, Wang CC. Anticancer effects of epigallocatechin-3-gallate nanoemulsion on lung cancer cells through the activation of AMP-activated protein kinase signaling pathway. Sci Rep. 2020;10(1):5163.
71. Spagnuolo C, Russo GL, Orhan IE, Habtemariam S, Daglia M, Sureda A, et al. Genistein and cancer: current status, challenges, and future directions. Adv Nutr. 2015;6(4):408–19.
72. Perabo FG, Von Löw EC, Ellinger J, von Rücker A, Müller SC, Bastian PJ. Soy isoflavone genistein in prevention and treatment of prostate cancer. Prostate Cancer Prostatic Dis. 2008;11(1):6–12.
73. Meeran SM, Katiyar SK. Cell cycle control as a basis for cancer chemoprevention through dietary agents. Front Biosci. 2008;13:2191–202.
74. Sarkar FH, Adsule S, Padhye S, Kulkarni S, Li Y. The role of genistein and synthetic derivatives of isoflavone in cancer prevention and therapy. Mini Rev Med Chem. 2006;6(4):401–7.
75. Shafiee G, Saidijam M, Tayebinia H, Khodadadi I. Beneficial effects of genistein in suppression of proliferation, inhibition of metastasis, and induction of apoptosis in PC3 prostate cancer cells. Arch Physiol Biochem. 2022;128(3):694–702.
76. Mukund V, Mukund D, Sharma V, Mannarapu M, Alam A. Genistein: its role in metabolic diseases and cancer. Crit Rev Oncol Hematol. 2017;119:13–22.
77. Gong L, Li Y, Nedeljkovic-Kurepa A, Sarkar FH. Inactivation of NF-kappaB by genistein is mediated via Akt signaling pathway in breast cancer cells. Oncogene. 2003;22(30):4702–9.
78. Oh HY, Leem J, Yoon SJ, Yoon S, Hong SJ. Lipid raft cholesterol and genistein inhibit the cell viability of prostate cancer cells via the partial contribution of EGFR-Akt/p70S6k pathway and down-regulation of androgen receptor. Biochem Biophys Res Commun. 2010;393(2):319–24.

79. Basak S, Pookot D, Noonan EJ, Dahiya R. Genistein down-regulates androgen receptor by modulating HDAC6-Hsp90 chaperone function. Mol Cancer Ther. 2008;7(10):3195–202.
80. Williams B, Lees F, Tsangari H, Hutchinson MR, Perilli E, Crotti TN. Assessing the effects of Parthenolide on inflammation, bone loss, and glial cells within a collagen antibody-induced arthritis mouse model. Mediat Inflamm. 2020;2020:6245798.
81. Talib WH, Al Kury LT. Parthenolide inhibits tumor-promoting effects of nicotine in lung cancer by inducing P53—dependent apoptosis and inhibiting VEGF expression. Biomed Pharmacother. 2018;107:1488–95.
82. Talib WH, Mahmod AI, Abuarab SF, Hasen E, Munaim AA, Haif SK, et al. Diabetes and cancer: metabolic association, therapeutic challenges, and the role of natural products. Molecules. 2021;26(8):2179.
83. Zhou JZ, Kou X, Stevenson D. Rapid extraction and high-performance liquid chromatographic determination of parthenolide in feverfew (Tanacetum parthenium). J Agric Food Chem. 1999;47(3):1018–22.
84. Liu Q, Manzano D, Tanić N, Pesic M, Bankovic J, Pateraki I, et al. Elucidation and in planta reconstitution of the parthenolide biosynthetic pathway. Metab Eng. 2014;23:145–53.
85. Che ST, Bie L, Li X, Qi H, Yu P, Zuo L. Parthenolide inhibits the proliferation and induces the apoptosis of human uveal melanoma cells. Int J Ophthalmol. 2019;12(10):1531–8.
86. Neelakantan S, Nasim S, Guzman ML, Jordan CT, Crooks PA. Aminoparthenolides as novel anti-leukemic agents: discovery of the NF-kappaB inhibitor, DMAPT (LC-1). Bioorg Med Chem Lett. 2009;19(15):4346–9.
87. Paço A, Brás T, Santos JO, Sampaio P, Gomes AC, Duarte MF. Anti-inflammatory and immunoregulatory action of sesquiterpene lactones. Molecules. 2022;27(3):1142.
88. Pourianezhad F, Tahmasebi S, Abdusi V, Nikfar S, Mirhoseini M. Review on feverfew, a valuable medicinal plant. J Herbmed Pharmacol. 2016;5(2):45–9.
89. Carlisi D, D'Anneo A, Angileri L, Lauricella M, Emanuele S, Santulli A, et al. Parthenolide sensitizes hepatocellular carcinoma cells to TRAIL by inducing the expression of death receptors through inhibition of STAT3 activation. J Cell Physiol. 2011;226(6):1632–41.
90. Tadic V, Živković J, Bigovic D, Žugić A. Variation of parthenolide and phenolic compounds content in different parts of Tanacetum parthenium (L.) Schulz Bip., Asteraceae during 18 months storage. Lek Sirovine. 2019;39:35–9.
91. Laurella LC, Mirakian NT, Garcia MN, Grasso DH, Sülsen VP, Papademetrio DL. Sesquiterpene lactones as promising candidates for Cancer therapy: focus on pancreatic cancer. Molecules. 2022;27(11):3492.
92. Duan D, Zhang J, Yao J, Liu Y, Fang J. Targeting Thioredoxin reductase by Parthenolide contributes to inducing apoptosis of HeLa cells. J Biol Chem. 2016;291(19):10021–31.
93. Fonrose X, Ausseil F, Soleilhac E, Masson V, David B, Pouny I, et al. Parthenolide inhibits tubulin carboxypeptidase activity. Cancer Res. 2007;67(7):3371–8.
94. Sahler J, Bernard JJ, Spinelli SL, Blumberg N, Phipps RP. The feverfew plant-derived compound, parthenolide enhances platelet production and attenuates platelet activation through NF-κB inhibition. Thromb Res. 2011;127(5):426–34.
95. Berdan CA, Ho R, Lehtola HS, To M, Hu X, Huffman TR, et al. Parthenolide covalently targets and inhibits focal adhesion kinase in breast Cancer cells. Cell Chem Biol. 2019;26(7):1027–35.e22.
96. Pajak B, Gajkowska B, Orzechowski A. Molecular basis of parthenolide-dependent proapoptotic activity in cancer cells. Folia Histochem Cytobiol. 2008;46(2):129–35.
97. Morel KL, Ormsby RJ, Bezak E, Sweeney CJ, Sykes PJ. Parthenolide selectively sensitizes prostate tumor tissue to radiotherapy while protecting healthy tissues in vivo. Radiat Res. 2017;187(5):501–12.
98. Kletecka-Pulker M, Mondal H, Wang D, Parra RG, Maigoro AY, Lee S, et al. Impacts of biomedical hashtag-based twitter campaign: #DHPSP utilization for promotion of open innovation in digital health, patient safety, and personalized medicine. Curr Res Biotechnol. 2021;3:146–53.

Chapter 13
Gene Therapy as a New Emerging Strategy for Prostate Cancer

Samaneh Adelian, Amin Soltani, and Michael R. Hamblin

Abstract Therapeutic gene modification has emerged as a prominent topic in both public discourse and scholarly investigations in the fields of fundamental and clinical research, garnering significant attention over the course of many decades. The usage of CRISPR–Cas9-based technologies in both basic and clinical investigations, as well as the current clinical trials, have shown the promising prospects of genome editing in the treatment of human diseases. The examination of studies and clinical trials in the field of gene therapy indicates a notable focus on prostate cancer studies and its use in clinical practice. There are several factors that contribute to the attractiveness of gene therapy as a potential treatment for prostate cancer. These factors include the ability to directly inject and sample tumors due to anatomical considerations, the existence of preclinical models that mimic the immune system, and the identification of tumor-specific antigens that can be targeted to stimulate an immune response. These aspects collectively enhance the potential of gene therapy as a viable approach for managing this prevalent form of cancer. Vaccine-based treatments that elicit an immune response and novel technologies using CRISPR–Cas9-assisted methodologies, such as chimeric antigen receptor (CAR) T cell therapies, have significant potential and are now being examined in both laboratory and clinical settings. Despite the lack of oncologically significant effects in clinical settings, laboratory and preclinical advancements in gene therapy for PCa hold considerable possibilities for future investigations.

Keywords Chimeric antigen receptor (CAR) T cell therapies · CRISPR–Cas9 · Vaccine-based treatments · Viral vectors · Prostate-specific antigen (PSA)

Samaneh Adelian and Michael R. Hamblin contributed equally with all other contributors.

S. Adelian · A. Soltani
Cellular and Molecular Research Center, Basic Health Sciences Institute, Shahrekord University of Medical Sciences, Shahrekord, Iran

M. R. Hamblin (✉)
Laser Research Centre, Faculty of Health Science, University of Johannesburg, Doornfontein, South Africa

G. Sethi et al. (eds.), *Prostate Cancer: Molecular Events and Therapeutic Modalities*, https://doi.org/10.1007/978-981-97-4612-5_13

13.1 Introduction

The advancement of gene therapy has elicited enthusiasm throughout various scientific fields and society as a whole. Progress in both fundamental and clinical research has played a crucial role in propelling and directing this inventive and imaginative endeavor. The first uses of gene therapy were mostly centered on addressing genetic illnesses of a simpler kind, including severe combined immunodeficiency [1]. In these cases, the primary objective was frequently to substitute the defective gene responsible for the ailment [2]. Nevertheless, the emergence of cancer gene therapy has brought out novel concepts and methodologies, supported by the understanding that cancer originates from genetic changes occurring in both germline and somatic cells [3]. Gene treatments have shown promise in the therapy of prostate cancer due to their ability to diagnose early stage PCa via a blood test for prostate-specific antigen (PSA) and their potential to target primary prostate cancer lesions by intraprostatic injection [4]. The capacity to precisely guide intraprostatic administration of gene therapy carriers is of great use for the implementation of immunotherapy-based gene therapy and cytotoxic strategies. Furthermore, because of the often slow-growing nature of prostate cancer, there has been a significant emphasis on developing non-aggressive therapy options for individuals with early stage and localized illnesses [5]. This objective has been and continues to be of utmost importance. The initiation of the first clinical trial for in situ gene therapy in PCa in 1999, as well as subsequent studies, was a result of clinical and preclinical investigations that focused on the unique features of PCa and advancements in cancer gene therapy [6, 7]. These studies laid the groundwork for the implementation of this clinical strategy. The introduction of gene therapy in the salvage context after initial radiation was a result of advancements in the improvement of novel ways for PCa therapy [6, 7]. In addition, the first advancements in gene therapy for PCa prompted the emergence of novel gene delivery methods using viral vectors and liposomes, alongside the creation of innovative preclinical models for evaluating these advancements [8]. These early investigations also contributed to an enhanced comprehension of the bystander impact of immunostimulatory genes and cytotoxic transfer into PCa tissues [9]. The fundamental comprehension of the bystander consequence has influenced the examination of interactions between PCa and the tumor microenvironment. This topic is now being extensively explored based on the idea of systemic immuno-oncology and cytotoxic combination treatment regimens [10–12]. While the implementation of gene therapy for PCa in clinical settings has not progressed as rapidly as it has for hematological malignancies, there have been notable advancements in PCa imaging techniques that are bringing gene therapy functions closer to clinical use [2].

A variety of gene therapy approaches have been established, including the activation of tumor suppressor genes, direct inhibition or reduction of tumor cell growth, prodrug-induced cell death, radionuclide imaging, modification of the immune milieu, and vaccine-based techniques. While this compilation is not comprehensive, it highlights key ways by which gene therapy may be used to modify

PCa cells in both laboratory and clinical settings, showcasing its potential for significant effect. Ongoing research is being conducted to explore these pathways, with a specific focus on vaccine-based treatments and the application of oncolytic viruses to enhance the effectiveness of antitumor treatments when used in conjunction with other systemic medicines. The usage of the CRISPR–Cas9 technology with chimeric antigen receptor (CAR) T cell therapy is seeing significant growth [13].

This chapter begins by providing a description of non-viral vectors and viral-based vectors, both replicating and non-replicating, that are used for gene delivery. The focus is placed on their application in preclinical investigations involving prostate cancer animals. Subsequently, our attention is directed toward concluded investigations pertaining to gene therapy in human PCa, specifically examining the utilization of CAR T cells and the CRISPR–Cas9 system. In conclusion, we proceed to elucidate the current status of clinical studies in the field of gene therapy and provide a concise overview of the outcomes achieved so far. In the context of this chapter, gene therapy is operationally described as a therapeutic approach encompassing the transfer of genetic material, either through direct injection into tumors or systemic administration. This genetic material has the capacity to elicit cytotoxic effects on tumor cells by directly activating prodrugs, or by modulating specific biochemical processes and/or gene expression [13].

13.2 The Applicable Vectors in Direction of Gene Delivery

The usage of vectors for the purpose of gene delivery is a well-explored area of research in the field of molecular biology. Gene therapy for genetic illnesses entails the use of a vector to transport an adequate amount of genetic material to the specific site with a level of accuracy that allows for the activation of a transgene, hence inducing a therapeutic reaction [2]. Within this particular context, cancer is classified as a genetic ailment due to its attributes of modified gene expression, uncontrolled growth, and capacity to metastasize and inflict damage, all of which rely on somatic and/or germline gene mutations [14, 15]. In the realm of PCa gene therapy, several first endeavors included the direct introduction of DNA into tumors by physical injection, as opposed to using vectors as a means of gene delivery [16]. In a particular investigation employing both in vitro and in vivo models, the integration of DNA plasmids into cell lines occurred at a relatively low frequency, ranging from 2% to 12%. However, when coupled with focused ultrasonography, the expression of the transduced gene exhibited a substantial increase of 15-fold in a subcutaneous Dunning prostate tumor that was implanted in rats. Nonetheless, the process of cellular absorption of naked DNA is often characterized by low efficiency due to unique physiological conditions at the location. As a result, researchers have endeavored to address this issue by using gene vectors.

13.3 Viral Vectors in the Direction of Gene Therapy in PCa

Viruses have undergone evolutionary changes that enable them to effectively invade certain cells and facilitate the delivery of genetic materials, leading to the translation and transcription of viral proteins. Therefore, they provide a prospective approach for gene delivery [17]. The process of genetically modifying viral genomes allows for the alteration of viral infectivity, as well as the corresponding immunological response of the host, and facilitates the targeted delivery of certain genes to specific cells [18]. A variety of viruses have been chosen for use as possible vectors in the field of gene therapy, including those specifically targeted for PCa gene therapy. Adenoviruses, retroviruses, and adeno-associated virus (AAV) are often investigated as vectors for gene therapy in PCa. Each of these vectors has distinct benefits, drawbacks, and variations in connection with their replication competency [19].

Adenoviruses are a kind of DNA virus with a double-stranded structure. These viruses gain entry into cells by attaching to a particular receptor on the cell surface known as the coxsackievirus and adenovirus receptor [18]. After the process of internalization, the virus is able to evade the endosomes and move toward the nuclear pore. At the nuclear pore, the viral genome gains entry into the nucleus, facilitating the transcription of viral genes. One significant drawback associated with adenoviral vectors is their immunogenicity since around 70% of individuals possess neutralizing antibodies against the virus [19]. Due to the finding and the apprehension about the possible negative consequences associated with the use of a replicating virus, many modified adenoviruses have been created. These modified adenoviruses include the removal of the whole coding region from the adenovirus genome [20–22]. Adenoviruses have many notable benefits. First, they possess a rather big genome, roughly 7.5 kilobases in size. Additionally, these viruses have the capability to infect cells that are not actively dividing. Moreover, they exhibit gene transcription with no integration into the host DNA, hence reducing the potential hazards associated with mutational mutagenesis.

AAVs are a kind of DNA [23] virus characterized by their single-stranded nature [18]. These viruses have the ability to enter host cells via a process known as heparin sulfate binding. Nevertheless, the replication process of these viruses is contingent upon the assistance of machinery provided by a secondary virus, like adenovirus or herpesvirus. Therefore, an adeno-associated virus is a kind of virus that remains as integrated episomal DNA in the absence of a secondary infection. However, it should be noted that AAVs have been genetically engineered throughout their growth to produce proteins, eliminating the need for an extra viral infection [24]. There are many drawbacks associated with AAV vectors. First, they have a limited gene capacity of around 4.5 kb. Second, there is a potential for immunogenicity, since a significant portion (around 20–40%) of the population previously had antibodies against adeno-associated virus. Additionally, there is an insufficient immune reaction to the adeno-associated virus capsid, that typically manifests around 4–12 weeks after the introduction of the vector [25]. The first findings of a research conducted in 1995 demonstrated the successful transfer of IL2 to in vitro models, specifically using an AAV-based plasmid in conjunction with a lipid-based vector. These models included short-term cultures of primary human PCa cells obtained from prostatectomy tissues [26].

Retroviruses are a kind of RNA virus with a single-stranded genome that gains entry into host cells by attaching to envelope proteins on the cell surface [18]. The viral reverse transcriptase enzyme is responsible for transcribing the viral genome into DNA. This DNA is then qualified to enter the nucleus of multiplying cells and get integrated into the host genome. The utilization of retroviruses as vectors presents several drawbacks. One limitation is their small genome size, which restricts the amount of genetic material that is able to be accommodated. Additionally, there is a risk of insertional mutagenesis, particularly evident in human clinical trials involving individuals with immune disorders. This phenomenon has been observed in studies [1, 23, 27, 28]. Furthermore, retroviruses rely on cellular replication, although this characteristic can also be advantageous in the context of cancer gene therapy.

Additional viruses that have been examined as potential carriers for gene transfer consist of pox virus and herpes simplex virus (HSV). HSV is a substantial DNA virus with a double-stranded structure, capable of both replication and inducing illness in the human population [18]. While it is possible to render HSV replication poor, this procedure may inadvertently impact other intended viral characteristics. For instance, herpes simplex virus (HSV) mutants that lack thymidine kinase (TK) exhibit a preference for replicating in cells undergoing mitosis, thus showing potential for cancer treatment. Nevertheless, these mutants are no longer responsive to ganciclovir (GCV), which restricts the available therapy options due to the risk of unintended systemic infection and destruction of non-cancerous dividing cells [29]. Another genetically modified herpes simplex virus (HSV), known as G207, has revealed efficacy in treating malignant glioma [30] and bladder cancer [31], as well as in laboratory and animal models of prostate cancer [32]. Poxviruses are a category of double-stranded DNA viruses including some variations that exhibit the absence of a thymidine kinase gene. Consequently, these variants possess a propensity for selective replication inside tumor cells. Poxviruses have been used in several tumor models, such as those related to prostate cancer, for the purpose of administering genes encoding immunostimulatory cytokines and suicide genes, which may be utilized in combination with therapeutic interventions [33–35].

13.4 Non-viral Vectors in Direction of PCa Gene Therapy

Non-viral vectors contain several forms of vectors, such as lipid complexes, modified plasmids, and peptide vectors. Although viral vectors have shown efficacy in the field of gene therapy for PCa and other types of malignancies, they possess several inherent characteristics that impose limitations on their application in human cancer gene therapy. These limitations include the possibility of inducing mutagenesis in the host genome, the potential to trigger immune responses, a wide range of target cell tropism, restricted capacity for packaging nucleic acids, and difficulties in the production process [36, 37]. Novel gene therapy vectors that are not dependent on viral mechanisms have been created with the aim of addressing or surpassing these constraints. Non-viral vectors refer to artificially created carriers that are specifically intended for the transportation of nucleic acids and genes. In a broad sense, these vectors possess the capacity to transport bigger genetic payloads and encounter less significant obstacles in terms of production compared to viral vectors. Furthermore, it should be noted that they exhibit decreased immunogenicity, resulting in a considerable reduction in the likelihood of adverse effects [36]. Despite the persistent challenges affiliated with the effective delivery of payloads to specific target cells, the use of non-viral vectors in cancer therapy has been a subject of considerable investigation. Preliminary investigations using these gene therapy methods in the treatment of PCa have provided fundamental insights that have laid the groundwork for further advancements in this area of research.

In a study conducted in 2007, it was shown that the introduction of a degradable polymer (poly (butane diol diacrylate co amino pentanol) (C32)) combined with a diphtheria toxin suicide gene controlled by prostate-specific antigen expression directly into the prostates of mice with tumors led to a decrease in size by 33% or complete elimination by 13% of the injected prostatic lobes. This outcome was compared to the results of injecting naked diphtheria toxin gene DNA, which resulted in a reduction of 17% and no complete elimination in a TRAMP mouse model [38]. It is worth mentioning that the introduction of naked DNA through injection did not lead to apoptosis. In contrast, when the vector was combined with the diphtheria toxin suicide gene and injected at the initial site, tumor death was observed in 80% of cells. On the other hand, the administration of naked diphtheria toxin gene DNA resulted in less than 5% apoptotic cell death [38]. It is substantial to note that this vector is currently not utilized.

Lipid-based non-viral vectors have been widely recognized and utilized as a viable approach for facilitating gene transfer. In a research conducted in 1987, lipoplexes, which are lipid complexes used for the encapsulation of DNA, were recognized as promising non-viral vectors for transferring genes [39]. Previous investigations have revealed the effectiveness of lipid-based cationic particles in delivering DNA to human PCa cell lines and a nasopharyngeal cancer cell line [40]. Additionally, in vitro experiments using folate-linked lipid-based nanoparticles have shown a significant increase in transfection efficiency (~100-fold) compared to the commercially available vector Tfx20 in luciferase gene transfer assays. The study established the efficacy of using a folate-linked nanoparticle for the delivery of herpes simplex virus thymidine kinase (HSV-TK) by direct tumor injections, followed by the administration of ganciclovir (GCV). This treatment approach caused a significant decrease (>50%) in tumor volume, indicating the successful suppression of prostate cancer xenograft development [41]. In an alternative methodology, the implementation of systemic therapy with a cationic liposome-p53 gene complex targeted by human transferrin, in conjunction with radiation, resulted in the total regression of PCa xenograft tumors. Notably, no indications of tumor reversion were seen during the six-month treatment period, with statistical significance proven

($P < 0.001$) [42]. Various lipid formulations and targeting strategies have been explored in the laboratory for the delivery of macromolecules, such as DNA, to cancer cells using liposomes. These strategies include the use of pH-sensitive polymers like N-isopropylacrylamide copolymers and succinylated PEG, as well as fusogenic peptides and proteins like GALA peptide [41, 43, 44]. Nevertheless, there is a lack of clinical investigation about the usage of these techniques in PCa. In contrast, the utilization of a plasmid DNA expression vector harboring IL2 complexed with a cationic lipid vector known as leuvectin has been observed to facilitate in vivo transfection in phase I/II clinical trials conducted on patients with renal cell carcinoma. However, the clinical response to this approach has been varied, suggesting that its efficacy in treating kidney cancer or its translation to patients with prostate cancer is improbable [45]. Lipid-based non-viral vectors are now undergoing active development and continuous improvement in the realm of small-molecule medication delivery for cancer-related purposes. The ongoing progress in this field of study is likely to generate heightened attention toward the application of these delivery methods based on the idea of gene therapy applications for PCa.

Peptide-based vectors used for the delivery of gene consequences contain poly-arginine, a cationic cell-penetrating peptide that has revealed effective transportation of plasmid DNA to PCa cell lines [46]. The transfection efficacy of the final plasmid DNA complex was enhanced fourfold with the incorporation of poly-arginine, as compared to the control samples. Moreover, the synergistic use of aspartic acid and poly-arginine shows promising prospects for selective affinity toward hydroxyapatite, the predominant constituent of rigid connective tissue. This combination has promise as a viable bone-targeting vector [46]. Given the potential therapeutic benefit of delivering prostate transmembrane protein androgen induced 1 (PMEPA1), which has been linked to reduced tumor invasion and bone metastasis, making use of this vector in the context of metastasis is worth considering [46]. While the potential of poly-arginine is encouraging, it is considerable to note that alternative peptide-based vectors have not shown any discernible benefits in prostate cancer models, as far as our current understanding is concerned.

TA-MCs are truncated versions of plasmids that do not include prokaryotic elements and, if preferred, do not include antibiotic-resistance genes, resulting in the retention of only eukaryotic machinery [47]. In the year 2019, it was shown that a transcription activator-mediator complex has the capability to induce the expression of a reporter gene that is not naturally occurring inside an organism. This reporter gene has the potential to serve as a biomarker when detected in plasma samples [48]. The transfection effectiveness of TA-MCs is enhanced in comparison to plasmids, mostly due to decreased transcriptional silencing and their smaller size [49, 50]. Subsequent investigations employed the promoter region of survivin, a protein that exhibits heightened expression in various types of cancer (such as lung, prostate, and breast). This protein demonstrates low expression in normal prostate tissue but expands with the grade of PCa tumors. To induce the expression of embryonic alkaline phosphatase, a synthetically modified variant of human placental phosphatase, the aforementioned promoter region was utilized. The successful transfection of TA-MCs into various PCa cell lines resulted in the induction of detectable alkaline phosphatase expression in the blood of mouse models with subcutaneous PCa tumors. This expression was discovered to be correlated positively with survivin expression, recommending that alkaline phosphatase could serve as a potential marker for assessing the aggressiveness of PCa [48]. Despite being in its first phases of research, this technique has the potential to provide innovative approaches for estimating disease aggressiveness and may find use in screening for prostate cancer or other conditions characterized by high survivin expression. In conclusion, the administration of oligonucleotide antisense compounds by systemic injection represents a promising strategy for the control of gene products. Specifically, investigation attempts have been directed at suppressing the expression of STAT3, which has revealed potential in altering immunosuppressive myeloid cells in the context of PCa [51, 52].

13.5 CRISPR–Cas9 and CAR T in PCa Gene Therapy

The use of CRISPR and the CRISPR–Cas9 technology has significantly transformed the field of biological research [53]. In summary, this method allows accurate modifications of certain DNA sequences at any location inside the target DNA by inducing double-strand breaks [53]. The binding of a guide RNA to Cas9 facilitates its targeting to a complementary target sequence, resulting in the formation of a double-strand break [54]. Therefore, this technique facilitates genetic alteration by introducing single-stranded or double-stranded nucleotides into specific sites. The field of prostate cancer disease biology, along with other types of malignancies, has seen a significant transformation due to the advent of CRISPR–Cas9 technology. This breakthrough has paved the way for the emergence of a revolutionary therapeutic approach known as CAR T cell therapy.

The usage of CRISPR–Cas9 technology enables the expeditious and effective execution of many scientific procedures. The generation of activating and detrimental mutations in less time when compared to transgenic mice enables the production of novel genetic models for cancer. In previous studies, the targeted removal of phospholipase receptor A2 receptor 1 [55], the androgen receptor [56], and metabolically significant kinases [57] has been successfully achieved by the use of CRISPR–Cas9 technology in both PCa cell lines and xenograft models. The use of CRISPR–Cas9 technology allows for the generation of mouse models via the process of deletions, as shown by the production of a PTEN-knockout mouse [58]. Furthermore, the use of CRISPR technology has enabled the targeted removal of single-nucleotide polymorphisms linked to the risk of prostate cancer. This has provided valuable knowledge on the possible functional impacts of mutations in these specific risk alleles [59, 60]. The induction of phenotypes may be achieved by the use of a modified Cas9 protein in conjunction with a transcription-activating domain. This approach has been shown in research where the expression of RNA target genes, including DKK3, was raised in cell lines associated with prostate cancer [61]. In recent studies, researchers have successfully integrated CRISPR–Cas9 with other delivery mechanisms, including liposomes paired with an RNA aptamer targeting PSMA. This innovative approach enables the targeted delivery of precise genome-editing tools specifically to cancerous PCa cells in laboratory settings (in vitro) [62]. This work effectively demonstrated the specific targeting of PSMA-expressing PCa cell lines and xenograft models by the method. Furthermore, the editing of PLK1 mRNA levels resulted in disrupted proliferation of both cell lines and tumors.

The use of CRISPR–Cas9 may also facilitate the conduction of high-throughput screenings targeting biological components that play a crucial role in the proliferation of cancer cells [63]. From a methodological perspective, the construction of a gene library consisting of single-guide sequences facilitates the targeted suppression of a substantial number of genes within a single experimental setup. The gene library was subjected to incubation together with the required equipment, leading to the integration of the single-guide sequences into the cells and the targeted suppression of a significant percentage of them. After a phase of expansion, the procedure of DNA sequencing is carried out for the purpose of ascertaining the proportional occurrence of sequences that match those present in the sequence library. In contrast to the baseline controls, a reduction in the abundance of a certain gene sequence signifies genes that have undergone negative selection and are hence crucial for the survival of cells [63]. Numerous research endeavors using this technological approach have explored a wide range of gene-associated results, including medication resistance [64], cancer metastasis [65], and immune response [66]. A comprehensive screening of the LNCaP cell line has been conducted in the context of prostate cancer, using a single-guide RNA library that specifically targets over 19,000 genes. The findings from this study, in conjunction with further mechanistic investigations, have shown that a cluster of genes encoding RNA-binding proteins, including those involved in alternative splicing and the regulation of the androgen receptor, plays a crucial role in the proliferation of LNCaP PCa cells [67]. In addition, a recent study using a CRISPR screen identified novel pathways of resistance to inhibition of PARP, which may have implications for the therapy of metastatic PCa [68].

CAR T cells are a kind of genetically modified receptors that have the ability to attach to particular antigens and also activate T cells [69]. Over the course of many generations, CAR T cells have undergone engineering that incorporates double or multiple costimulatory signals. These modifications have been aimed at enhancing the immune response by promoting the activation of cytotoxic T cells [69]. CAR T cells are created by the manipulation of T cells obtained from patients, wherein a virus, often lentiviral in nature, is used as a means of introducing the desired genetic information. Significantly, CAR T cell technology exhibits independence from the major histocompatibility complex, hence allowing CAR T cells to recognize antigens in individuals with any human leukocyte antigen (HLA) lineage or in tumors where the major histocompatibility complex has been downregulated [69]. The efficacy of CAR T cell technology has been proven for the management of hematological malignancies [70], but its effectiveness in solid tumors has yet to be established. Several potential antigen targets for CAR T cell therapy in PCa have been discovered, including PSA, PAP, PSMA, and PSCA [71]. The research conducted in 2014 examined the effectiveness of several generations of anti-PSMA CAR T cells in an in vivo model that expressed PSMA [72]. One of the generations used CD28 as a costimulatory molecule, and it exhibited significant activity. A further investigation has shown that the manipulation of PD1, together with CD28 co-stimulation, successfully eradicates cancerous cells in animal models exhibiting various malignancies, such as prostate cancer [73]. In addition, a further investigation utilizing PCa cell lines and mouse models of PCa demonstrated that the inclusion of an intracellular 4-1BB costimulatory domain resulted in enhanced specificity toward PSCA+ tumor cells when compared to CAR T cells including a CD28 costimulatory domain [74]. Recent research conducted on patient-derived mCRPC cells has provided evidence suggesting that chimeric antigen receptor (CAR) T cells directed against PSMA might potentially exhibit efficacy when used in conjunction with the dominant-negative transforming growth factor beta (TGF-β) type II receptor. The aforementioned combination elicited a response in CD8+ T cells, causing them to exhibit reactivity toward PSMA and insensitivity toward TGF-β, which is a recognized consequence of resistance to CAR T cell treatment. To ensure safety, the T cell construct was engineered to be regulated by HSV-1-TK, enabling the elimination of cells with the administration of GCV. The in vitro use of GCV injection led to the successful eradication of castration-resistant cell lines [75].

Therefore, CAR T cells have potential in the management of metastatic PCa and, perhaps, non-metastatic PCa. Nevertheless, the presence of an immunosuppressive tumor microenvironment and the difficulty associated with directing cells to bone metastases are obstacles that still need to be addressed [76]. Patients with hematological malignancies who have undergone CAR T cell treatment have had adverse effects, including cytokine release syndrome and neurotoxicity [77]. Additionally, studies conducted on solid malignancies have shown modest response rates so far. The safety, practicality, and effectiveness of this intriguing technique will be determined via ongoing experiments.

13.6 Perspective of Gene Therapy in PCa

While gene therapy has demonstrated promise as an emerging modality for addressing PCa, the limited number of therapies available in clinical settings may be attributed to the underwhelming outcomes seen in early clinical studies with vector-based systems. The absence of achievement may be attributed to several factors. In investigations pertaining to direct injection therapies, it has been regularly shown that both replication-incompetent and replication-competent vectors have not been successful in achieving comprehensive eradication of tumors. Despite the promising substantiation of tumor cell death and immune response, the overarching objective of preventing cancer has yet to be achieved. Similar to previous endeavors in focal therapy utilizing ablation devices, which have persistently demonstrated a high recurrence rate beyond the targeted treatment area [78], direct injection therapy is additionally hindered by the prevalent heterogeneity observed in localized prostate cancer [79]. This heterogeneity poses a challenge to direct oncolytic injection treatments, as they are vulnerable to potential inadequacy beyond the intended treatment zone, particularly when the objective is the complete eradication of cancer.

The emergence of the CRISPR–Cas9 system, CAR T cell treatment, and advancements in laboratory research have stimulated a renewed enthusiasm for the function of gene therapy in the management of PCa. The promise of gene editing in the context of PCa treatment seems to be vast, and the enthusiasm around the clinical implementation of these strategies is well-founded. Nevertheless, despite the increasing impetus, the development of new or enhanced treatments will encounter similar challenges as those encountered in the past when attempting to translate promising oncolytic and vaccine-based findings into outcomes that are clinically significant. The efficacy of presently promising medicines in significantly ameliorating the trajectory of disease development in males diagnosed with prostate cancer has to be determined and will be revealed over time [13].

13.7 Conclusion

Prostate cancer possesses favorable characteristics for the application of gene therapy as a treatment modality. These include its physiological availability for biopsy and treatment, the relatively protracted disease progression observed in men with both localized and metastatic forms of the disease, and the extensive prior research conducted on therapies using both immune-incompetent and immune-competent models. Nevertheless, regardless of the promising outcomes shown in preclinical studies including immune material administration by direct injection and vaccine-based approaches, gene therapy has not yet been included in the therapy protocol for individuals diagnosed with PCa. Future research endeavors exploring the potential of gene therapy-based approaches, in conjunction with other therapeutic modalities, as well as innovative strategies for gene delivery and immune activation, hold promise in enhancing the longevity and overall well-being of those afflicted with PCa [13].

References

1. Hacein-Bey-Abina S, Von Kalle C, Schmidt M, McCormack MP, Wulffraat N, Leboulch P, et al. LMO2-associated clonal T cell proliferation in two patients after gene therapy for SCID-X1. Science (New York, NY). 2003;302(5644):415–9. Epub 2003/10/18. eng
2. High KA, Roncarolo MG. Gene therapy. N Engl J Med. 2019;381(5):455–64. Epub 2019/08/01. eng.
3. Stratton MR, Campbell PJ, Futreal PA. The cancer genome. Nature. 2009;458(7239):719–24. Pubmed Central PMCID: PMC2821689. Epub 2009/04/11. eng.

4. Catalona WJ, Smith DS, Ratliff TL, Dodds KM, Coplen DE, Yuan JJ, et al. Measurement of prostate-specific antigen in serum as a screening test for prostate cancer. N Engl J Med. 1991;324(17):1156–61. Epub 1991/04/25. eng.
5. Cooperberg MR, Broering JM, Carroll PR. Risk assessment for prostate cancer metastasis and mortality at the time of diagnosis. J Natl Cancer Inst. 2009;101(12):878–87. Pubmed Central PMCID: PMC2697208. Epub 2009/06/11. eng.
6. Herman JR, Adler HL, Aguilar-Cordova E, Rojas-Martinez A, Woo S, Timme TL, et al. In situ gene therapy for adenocarcinoma of the prostate: a phase I clinical trial. Hum Gene Ther. 1999;10(7):1239–49. Epub 1999/05/26. eng.
7. Miles BJ, Shalev M, Aguilar-Cordova E, Timme TL, Lee HM, Yang G, et al. Prostate-specific antigen response and systemic T cell activation after in situ gene therapy in prostate cancer patients failing radiotherapy. Hum Gene Ther. 2001;12(16):1955–67. Epub 2001/11/01. eng.
8. Shalev M, Thompson TC, Kadmon D, Ayala G, Kernen K, Miles BJ. Gene therapy for prostate cancer. Urology. 2001;57(1):8–16. Epub 2001/02/13. eng.
9. Thompson TC, Timme TL, Ebara S, Satoh T, Yang G, Wang J, et al. In situ gene therapy for prostate cancer: immunomodulatory approaches. Expert Opin Biol Ther. 2001;1(3):481–95. Epub 2001/12/01. eng.
10. Stewart RA, Pilié PG, Yap TA. Development of PARP and immune-checkpoint inhibitor combinations. Cancer Res. 2018;78(24):6717–25. Epub 2018/12/01. eng.
11. Pilié PG, Tang C, Mills GB, Yap TA. State-of-the-art strategies for targeting the DNA damage response in cancer. Nat Rev Clin Oncol. 2019;16(2):81–104. Pubmed Central PMCID: PMC8327299.Epub 2018/10/26. eng.
12. Pilié PG, Gay CM, Byers LA, O'Connor MJ, Yap TA. PARP inhibitors: extending benefit beyond BRCA-mutant cancers. Clin Cancer Res. 2019;25(13):3759–71. Epub 2019/02/15. eng.
13. Gregg JR, Thompson TC. Considering the potential for gene-based therapy in prostate cancer. Nat Rev Urol. 2021;18(3):170–84. Epub 2021/02/28. eng.
14. Akagi K, Suzuki T, Stephens RM, Jenkins NA, Copeland NG. RTCGD: retroviral tagged cancer gene database. Nucleic Acids Res. 2004;32(Database issue):D523–7. Pubmed Central PMCID: PMC308748. Epub 2003/12/19. eng.
15. Sadelain M, Papapetrou EP, Bushman FD. Safe harbours for the integration of new DNA in the human genome. Nat Rev Cancer. 2011;12(1):51–8. Epub 2011/12/02. eng.
16. Huber PE, Pfisterer P. In vitro and in vivo transfection of plasmid DNA in the dunning prostate tumor R3327-AT1 is enhanced by focused ultrasound. Gene Ther. 2000;7(17):1516–25. Epub 2000/09/23. eng.
17. Chen YH, Keiser MS, Davidson BL. Viral vectors for gene transfer. Curr Protocols Mouse Biol. 2018;8(4):e58. Epub 2018/11/30. eng.
18. Warnock JN, Daigre C, Al-Rubeai M. Introduction to viral vectors. Method Mol Biol (Clifton, NJ). 2011;737:1–25. Epub 2011/05/19. eng.
19. Harrington KJ, Spitzweg C, Bateman AR, Morris JC, Vile RG. Gene therapy for prostate cancer: current status and future prospects. J Urol. 2001;166(4):1220–33. Epub 2001/09/08. eng.
20. Hay RT. The origin of adenovirus DNA replication: minimal DNA sequence requirement in vivo. EMBO J. 1985;4(2):421–6. Pubmed Central PMCID: PMC554202. Epub 1985/02/01. eng.
21. Berkner KL. Development of adenovirus vectors for the expression of heterologous genes. BioTechniques. 1988;6(7):616–29. Epub 1988/07/01. eng.
22. Kovesdi I, Brough DE, Bruder JT, Wickham TJ. Adenoviral vectors for gene transfer. Curr Opin Biotechnol. 1997;8(5):583–9.
23. Ott MG, Schmidt M, Schwarzwaelder K, Stein S, Siler U, Koehl U, et al. Correction of X-linked chronic granulomatous disease by gene therapy, augmented by insertional activation of MDS1-EVI1, PRDM16 or SETBP1. Nat Med. 2006;12(4):401–9. Epub 2006/04/04. eng.
24. Gonçalves MA. Adeno-associated virus: from defective virus to effective vector. Virol J. 2005;2:43. Pubmed Central PMCID: PMC1131931. Epub 2005/05/10. eng.

25. Manno CS, Pierce GF, Arruda VR, Glader B, Ragni M, Rasko JJ, et al. Successful transduction of liver in hemophilia by AAV-factor IX and limitations imposed by the host immune response. Nat Med. 2006;12(3):342–7. Epub 2006/02/14. eng.
26. Vieweg J, Boczkowski D, Roberson KM, Edwards DW, Philip M, Philip R, et al. Efficient gene transfer with adeno-associated virus-based plasmids complexed to cationic liposomes for gene therapy of human prostate cancer. Cancer Res. 1995;55(11):2366–72. Epub 1995/06/01. eng.
27. Howe SJ, Mansour MR, Schwarzwaelder K, Bartholomae C, Hubank M, Kempski H, et al. Insertional mutagenesis combined with acquired somatic mutations causes leukemogenesis following gene therapy of SCID-X1 patients. J Clin Invest. 2008;118(9):3143–50. Pubmed Central PMCID: PMC2496964. Epub 2008/08/09. eng.
28. Braun CJ, Boztug K, Paruzynski A, Witzel M, Schwarzer A, Rothe M, et al. Gene therapy for Wiskott-Aldrich syndrome—long-term efficacy and genotoxicity. Sci Transl Med. 2014;6(227):227ra33. Epub 2014/03/14. eng.
29. Martuza RL, Malick A, Markert JM, Ruffner KL, Coen DM. Experimental therapy of human glioma by means of a genetically engineered virus mutant. Science (New York, NY). 1991;252(5007):854–6. Epub 1991/05/10. eng.
30. Mineta T, Rabkin SD, Yazaki T, Hunter WD, Martuza RL. Attenuated multi-mutated herpes simplex virus-1 for the treatment of malignant gliomas. Nat Med. 1995;1(9):938–43. Epub 1995/09/01. eng.
31. Oyama M, Ohigashi T, Hoshi M, Nakashima J, Tachibana M, Murai M, et al. Intravesical and intravenous therapy of human bladder cancer by the herpes vector G207. Hum Gene Ther. 2000;11(12):1683–93. Epub 2000/08/24. eng.
32. Walker JR, McGeagh KG, Sundaresan P, Jorgensen TJ, Rabkin SD, Martuza RL. Local and systemic therapy of human prostate adenocarcinoma with the conditionally replicating herpes simplex virus vector G207. Hum Gene Ther. 1999;10(13):2237–43. Epub 1999/09/25. eng.
33. Puhlmann M, Gnant M, Brown CK, Alexander HR, Bartlett DL. Thymidine kinase-deleted vaccinia virus expressing purine nucleoside phosphorylase as a vector for tumor-directed gene therapy. Hum Gene Ther. 1999;10(4):649–57. Epub 1999/03/27. eng.
34. Kawakita M, Rao GS, Ritchey JK, Ornstein DK, Hudson MA, Tartaglia J, et al. Effect of canarypox virus (ALVAC)-mediated cytokine expression on murine prostate tumor growth. J Natl Cancer Inst. 1997;89(6):428–36. Epub 1997/03/19. eng.
35. Gnant MF, Puhlmann M, Alexander HR Jr, Bartlett DL. Systemic administration of a recombinant vaccinia virus expressing the cytosine deaminase gene and subsequent treatment with 5 fluorocytosine leads to tumor-specific gene expression and prolongation of survival in mice. Cancer Res. 1999;59(14):3396–403. Epub 1999/07/23. eng.
36. Yin H, Kanasty RL, Eltoukhy AA, Vegas AJ, Dorkin JR, Anderson DG. Non-viral vectors for gene-based therapy. Nat Rev Genet. 2014;15(8):541–55. Epub 2014/07/16. eng.
37. Kotterman MA, Chalberg TW, Schaffer DV. Viral vectors for gene therapy: translational and clinical outlook. Annu Rev Biomed Eng. 2015;17:63–89. Epub 2015/12/09. eng.
38. Peng W, Anderson DG, Bao Y, Padera RF Jr, Langer R, Sawicki JA. Nanoparticulate delivery of suicide DNA to murine prostate and prostate tumors. Prostate. 2007;67(8):855–62. Epub 2007/04/12. eng.
39. Felgner PL, Gadek TR, Holm M, Roman R, Chan HW, Wenz M, et al. Lipofection: a highly efficient, lipid-mediated DNA-transfection procedure. Proc Natl Acad Sci USA. 1987;84(21):7413–7. Pubmed Central PMCID: PMC299306. Epub 1987/11/01. eng.
40. Hattori Y, Maitani Y. Folate-linked nanoparticle-mediated suicide gene therapy in human prostate cancer and nasopharyngeal cancer with herpes simplex virus thymidine kinase. Cancer Gene Ther. 2005;12(10):796–809. Epub 2005/05/14. eng.
41. Samad A, Sultana Y, Aqil M. Liposomal drug delivery systems: an update review. Curr Drug Deliv. 2007;4(4):297–305. Epub 2007/11/06. eng.
42. Xu L, Frederik P, Pirollo KF, Tang WH, Rait A, Xiang LM, et al. Self-assembly of a virus-mimicking nanostructure system for efficient tumor-targeted gene delivery. Hum Gene Ther. 2002;13(3):469–81. Epub 2002/02/28. eng.

43. Dorraj G, Carreras JJ, Nunez H, Abushammala I, Melero A. Lipid nanoparticles as potential gene therapeutic delivery Systems for Oral Administration. Curr Gene Ther. 2017;17(2):89–104. Epub 2017/05/13. eng.
44. Tila D, Ghasemi S, Yazdani-Arazi SN, Ghanbarzadeh S. Functional liposomes in the cancer-targeted drug delivery. J Biomater Appl. 2015;30(1):3–16. Epub 2015/04/01. eng.
45. Galanis E, Hersh EM, Stopeck AT, Gonzalez R, Burch P, Spier C, et al. Immunotherapy of advanced malignancy by direct gene transfer of an interleukin-2 DNA/DMRIE/DOPE lipid complex: phase I/II experience. J Clin Oncol. 1999;17(10):3313–23. Epub 1999/10/03. eng.
46. Lu Y, Jiang W, Wu X, Huang S, Huang Z, Shi Y, et al. Peptide T7-modified polypeptide with disulfide bonds for targeted delivery of plasmid DNA for gene therapy of prostate cancer. Int J Nanomedicine. 2018;13:6913–27. Pubmed Central PMCID: PMC6214593. Epub 2018/11/23. eng.
47. Darquet AM, Cameron B, Wils P, Scherman D, Crouzet J. A new DNA vehicle for nonviral gene delivery: supercoiled minicircle. Gene Ther. 1997;4(12):1341.
48. Wang T, Chen Y, Ronald JA. A novel approach for assessment of prostate cancer aggressiveness using survivin-driven tumour-activatable minicircles. Gene Ther. 2019;26(5):177–86. Epub 2019/03/15. eng.
49. Chen ZY, He CY, Ehrhardt A, Kay MA. Minicircle DNA vectors devoid of bacterial DNA result in persistent and high-level transgene expression in vivo. Mol Ther. 2003;8(3):495–500. Epub 2003/08/30. eng.
50. Chen ZY, Riu E, He CY, Xu H, Kay MA. Silencing of episomal transgene expression in liver by plasmid bacterial backbone DNA is independent of CpG methylation. Mol Ther. 2008;16(3):548–56. Epub 2008/02/07. eng.
51. Yu H, Pardoll D, Jove R. STATs in cancer inflammation and immunity: a leading role for STAT3. Nat Rev Cancer. 2009;9(11):798–809. Pubmed Central PMCID: PMC4856025. Epub 2009/10/24. eng.
52. Su YL, Banerjee S, White SV, Kortylewski M. STAT3 in tumor-associated myeloid cells: multitasking to disrupt immunity. Int J Mol Sci. 2018;19(6):1803. Pubmed Central PMCID: PMC6032252. Epub 2018/06/21. eng.
53. Doudna JA, Charpentier E. Genome editing. The new frontier of genome engineering with CRISPR-Cas9. Science (New York, NY). 2014;346(6213):1258096. Epub 2014/11/29. eng
54. Sánchez-Rivera FJ, Jacks T. Applications of the CRISPR-Cas9 system in cancer biology. Nat Rev Cancer. 2015;15(7):387–95. Pubmed Central PMCID: PMC4530801. Epub 2015/06/05. eng.
55. Friedemann M, Nacke B, Hagelgans A, Jandeck C, Bechmann N, Ullrich M, et al. Diverse effects of phospholipase A2 receptor expression on LNCaP and PC-3 prostate cancer cell growth in vitro and in vivo. Oncotarget. 2018;9(89):35983–96. Pubmed Central PMCID: PMC6267604. Epub 2018/12/14. eng.
56. Wei C, Wang F, Liu W, Zhao W, Yang Y, Li K, et al. CRISPR/Cas9 targeting of the androgen receptor suppresses the growth of LNCaP human prostate cancer cells. Mol Med Rep. 2018;17(2):2901–6. Pubmed Central PMCID: PMC5783506. Epub 2017/12/20. eng.
57. Yu G, Cheng CJ, Lin SC, Lee YC, Frigo DE, Yu-Lee LY, et al. Organelle-derived acetyl-CoA promotes prostate cancer cell survival, migration, and metastasis via activation of calmodulin kinase II. Cancer Res. 2018;78(10):2490–502. Pubmed Central PMCID: PMC6556391. Epub 2018/03/15. eng.
58. Takao A, Yoshikawa K, Karnan S, Ota A, Uemura H, De Velasco MA, et al. Generation of PTEN-knockout (−/−) murine prostate cancer cells using the CRISPR/Cas9 system and comprehensive gene expression profiling. Oncol Rep. 2018;40(5):2455–66. Epub 2018/09/19. eng.
59. Guo H, Ahmed M, Zhang F, Yao CQ, Li S, Liang Y, et al. Modulation of long noncoding RNAs by risk SNPs underlying genetic predispositions to prostate cancer. Nat Genet. 2016;48(10):1142–50. Epub 2016/08/16. eng.

60. Gao P, Xia JH, Sipeky C, Dong XM, Zhang Q, Yang Y, et al. Biology and clinical implications of the 19q13 aggressive prostate cancer susceptibility locus. Cell. 2018;174(3):576–89. Pubmed Central PMCID: PMC6091222. Epub 2018/07/24. eng.
61. Kardooni H, Gonzalez-Gualda E, Stylianakis E, Saffaran S, Waxman J, Kypta RM. CRISPR-mediated reactivation of DKK3 expression attenuates TGF-β signaling in prostate cancer. Cancers. 2018;10(6):165. Pubmed Central PMCID: PMC6025141. Epub 2018/05/31. eng.
62. Zhen S, Takahashi Y, Narita S, Yang YC, Li X. Targeted delivery of CRISPR/Cas9 to prostate cancer by modified gRNA using a flexible aptamer-cationic liposome. Oncotarget. 2017;8(6):9375–87. Pubmed Central PMCID: PMC5354738.Epub 2016/12/29. eng.
63. Wang T, Wei JJ, Sabatini DM, Lander ES. Genetic screens in human cells using the CRISPR-Cas9 system. Science (New York, NY). 2014;343(6166):80–4. Pubmed Central PMCID: PMC3972032. Epub 2013/12/18. eng.
64. Shalem O, Sanjana NE, Hartenian E, Shi X, Scott DA, Mikkelson T, et al. Genome-scale CRISPR-Cas9 knockout screening in human cells. Science (New York, NY). 2014;343(6166):84–7. Pubmed Central PMCID: PMC4089965. Epub 2013/12/18. eng.
65. Chen S, Sanjana NE, Zheng K, Shalem O, Lee K, Shi X, et al. Genome-wide CRISPR screen in a mouse model of tumor growth and metastasis. Cell. 2015;160(6):1246–60. Pubmed Central PMCID: PMC4380877. Epub 2015/03/10. eng.
66. Parnas O, Jovanovic M, Eisenhaure TM, Herbst RH, Dixit A, Ye CJ, et al. A genome-wide CRISPR screen in primary immune cells to dissect regulatory networks. Cell. 2015;162(3):675–86. Pubmed Central PMCID: PMC4522370. Epub 2015/07/21. eng.
67. Fei T, Chen Y, Xiao T, Li W, Cato L, Zhang P, et al. Genome-wide CRISPR screen identifies HNRNPL as a prostate cancer dependency regulating RNA splicing. Proc Natl Acad Sci USA. 2017;114(26):E5207–E15. Pubmed Central PMCID: PMC5495225.Epub 2017/06/15. eng.
68. Zimmermann M, Murina O, Reijns MAM, Agathanggelou A, Challis R, Tarnauskaitė Ž, et al. CRISPR screens identify genomic ribonucleotides as a source of PARP-trapping lesions. Nature. 2018;559(7713):285–9. Pubmed Central PMCID: PMC6071917. Epub 2018/07/06. eng.
69. Sadelain M, Brentjens R, Rivière I. The basic principles of chimeric antigen receptor design. Cancer Discov. 2013;3(4):388–98. Pubmed Central PMCID: PMC3667586. Epub 2013/04/04. eng.
70. Gill S, June CH. Going viral: chimeric antigen receptor T-cell therapy for hematological malignancies. Immunol Rev. 2015;263(1):68–89. Epub 2014/12/17. eng.
71. Yu H, Pan J, Guo Z, Yang C, Mao L. CART cell therapy for prostate cancer: status and promise. Onco Targets Ther. 2019;12:391–5. Pubmed Central PMCID: PMC6322708. Epub 2019/01/19.eng.
72. Ma Q, Gomes EM, Lo AS, Junghans RP. Advanced generation anti-prostate specific membrane antigen designer T cells for prostate cancer immunotherapy. Prostate. 2014;74(3):286–96. Epub 2013/11/01. eng.
73. Liu X, Ranganathan R, Jiang S, Fang C, Sun J, Kim S, et al. A chimeric switch-receptor targeting PD1 augments the efficacy of second-generation CAR T cells in advanced solid tumors. Cancer Res. 2016;76(6):1578–90. Pubmed Central PMCID: PMC4800826. Epub 2016/03/17. eng.
74. Priceman SJ, Gerdts EA, Tilakawardane D, Kennewick KT, Murad JP, Park AK, et al. Co-stimulatory signaling determines tumor antigen sensitivity and persistence of CAR T cells targeting PSCA+ metastatic prostate cancer. Onco Targets Ther. 2018;7(2):e1380764. Pubmed Central PMCID: PMC5749625. Epub 2018/01/09. eng.
75. Zhang Q, Helfand BT, Carneiro BA, Qin W, Yang XJ, Lee C, et al. Efficacy against human prostate cancer by prostate-specific membrane antigen-specific, transforming growth factor-β insensitive genetically targeted CD8(+) T-cells derived from patients with metastatic castrate-resistant disease. Eur Urol. 2018;73(5):648–52. Pubmed Central PMCID: PMC6682506. Epub 2017/12/26. eng.

76. Hillerdal V, Essand M. Chimeric antigen receptor-engineered T cells for the treatment of metastatic prostate cancer. BioDrugs. 2015;29(2):75–89. Pubmed Central PMCID: PMC4544486. Epub 2015/04/11. eng.
77. Grigor EJM, Fergusson D, Kekre N, Montroy J, Atkins H, Seftel MD, et al. Risks and benefits of chimeric antigen receptor T-cell (CAR-T) therapy in cancer: a systematic review and meta-analysis. Transfus Med Rev. 2019;33(2):98–110. Epub 2019/04/06. eng
78. Valerio M, Cerantola Y, Eggener SE, Lepor H, Polascik TJ, Villers A, et al. New and established technology in focal Ablation of the prostate: a systematic review. Eur Urol. 2017;71(1):17–34. Epub 2016/09/07. eng.
79. Boutros PC, Fraser M, Harding NJ, de Borja R, Trudel D, Lalonde E, et al. Spatial genomic heterogeneity within localized, multifocal prostate cancer. Nat Genet. 2015;47(7):736–45. Epub 2015/05/26. eng.

Chapter 14
Nanoparticle-Based Therapeutic Strategies in Prostate Cancer Suppression

Samaneh Adelian, Amin Soltani, and Michael R. Hamblin

Abstract The use of a combination of cytotoxic medications and hormone therapy/gene therapy has been widely acknowledged as an established approach to treating metastatic prostate cancer. Nevertheless, the effectiveness of this approach is limited by the inadequate ability of the chemotherapy to reach tumor sites, leading to a higher occurrence of collateral damage and multidrug resistance (MDR). The use of nanovectorization techniques has developed into a successful method for achieving excellent therapeutic results. This technology has the potential to increase the targeted and less hazardous targeting mechanisms for anticancer action, as well as provide diagnostic imaging using theragnostic. While research on nanomedicine is prevalent in several cancer types, there has been less emphasis on its use specifically in prostate cancer. This study offers a comprehensive understanding of the fundamental concepts behind nanotherapeutics and nanotheranostics, as well as their potential clinical implications in the treatment of prostate cancer. This study focuses on the clinical and preclinical data on the use of nanovectors in prostate cancer therapy techniques. Specifically, we examine the possibilities and prospects of using homing nanovectorization in these tactics.

Keywords Non-AR therapeutic targets · Multidrug resistance (MDR) · Nanotheranostics · Permeability and retention (EPR) effect · Liposomal nanoparticles

Samaneh Adelian and Amin Soltani contributed equally with all other contributors.

S. Adelian (✉) · A. Soltani
Cellular and Molecular Research Center, Basic Health Sciences Institute, Shahrekord University of Medical Sciences, Shahrekord, Iran

M. R. Hamblin (✉)
Laser Research Centre, Faculty of Health Science, University of Johannesburg, Doornfontein, South Africa

G. Sethi et al. (eds.), *Prostate Cancer: Molecular Events and Therapeutic Modalities*, https://doi.org/10.1007/978-981-97-4612-5_14

14.1 Introduction

In contemporary times, a multitude of therapeutic techniques have undergone development and refinement for the management of PC over the course of many years. Nevertheless, the efficacy of combining any of the therapeutic choices with chemotherapy has been notably higher compared to using single treatments [1]. Consequently, there has been a notable rise in the quantity of chemotherapy treatments authorized by the Food and Drug Administration (FDA) for the treatment of prostate cancer in recent years. There is no doubt that the therapeutic potential of these agents is indisputable. Nevertheless, it is important to acknowledge that there are some constraints that often impede the clinical efficacy of pharmaceuticals. These restrictions may either originate from intrinsic characteristics of the drugs themselves, known as pharmacodynamics, or arise during the process of drug administration and metabolism inside patients, referred to as pharmacokinetics.

To begin with, there are several biological obstacles that significantly impede the effectiveness of cancer treatments. As a result, there has been a rise in the occurrence of nonspecific distribution inside the tissue or cellular compartments that are of therapeutic significance. The difficulties that may be encountered include the infiltration of cellular membranes, assaults by humoral factors, eviction facilitated by efflux pumps, and trapping inside endosomes [2]. Ultimately, a few 0.01% of medicine molecules are capable of reaching the intended destination, resulting in diminished effectiveness [3]. To enhance bioavailability and hence deliver a sufficient quantity of medication to the targeted disease site for desired therapeutic outcomes, greater dosages are often delivered. However, this practice is associated with elevated rates of collateral toxicity and the development of multidrug resistance (MDR) [4]. The administration of paclitaxel in molecular form is primarily limited by its physicochemical characteristics. The low solubility value (0.0015 mg/mL) of the compound has a detrimental impact on its polycyclic chemistry when dissolved in an aqueous solution [5], making it unsuitable for intravenous administration [6].

In recent times, the implementation of combination treatment, which incorporates the use of cytotoxic medicines and antiandrogen regimens, has emerged as a potent technique for addressing castration-resistant prostate cancer (CRPC). The use of docetaxel (Doc), in conjunction with prednisone, has been shown to be correlated with improved clinical results [7]. Docetaxel exerts its inhibitory effects on cell replication by impeding the depolymerization process of the mitotic spindles. Nevertheless, the administration of this substance is marked by a significant level of toxicity, which mostly impacts cells that undergo fast division, including but not limited to those in the bone marrow, hair follicles, germ cells, and blood cells [8]. Prominent adverse effects include neutropenia, hypersensitivity responses, stomatitis, peripheral neuropathy, and fluid retention [9]. Despite the development of premedication regimens and prolonged delivery schemes, the incidence of hypersensitivity reactions related to paclitaxel or docetaxel has significantly decreased [10]. Nevertheless, there have been recent studies suggesting a potential association between docetaxel and deadly interstitial pneumonitis in individuals with castration-resistant prostate cancer. Indeed, the research conducted on 2045 patients revealed that approximately 2% of the population had toxicity resulting in mortality due to docetaxel treatment [11].

Moreover, the simultaneous administration of various medicines is seen as a promising approach in the treatment of castration-resistant prostate cancer. Nevertheless, this methodology is constrained by the disparities in the independent pharmacokinetics, biodistribution, and clearance rate of the distinct agents. This poses challenges in achieving a harmonious operational alignment of the separate efficacies of these agents, thus undermining the fundamental principle of synergism. Due to these factors, there exists a significant need for a drug delivery method that may provide enhanced stability, solubility, safety, and specificity of various chemotherapeutic drugs from a pharmacological standpoint. One potential approach to achieve this objective is the use of nanotherapeutics, a field that enables the incorporation of medicinal molecules into delivery platforms at the nanoscale. This allows for tailored delivery, using both passive and active targeting mechanisms while minimizing toxicity and enhancing the therapeutic index. This chapter offers a comprehensive understanding of the fundamental concepts behind nanotherapeutics and nanotheranostics, as well as their potential clinical implications in the context of prostate cancer therapy. This study focuses on the clinical and preclinical information regarding nanovectors, specifically in relation to their potential and prospects in the context of prostate cancer therapy techniques.

14.2 The Potential of Nanotherapy in Prostate Cancer

Due to the issues associated with collateral toxicity and nonspecific distribution of conventional administration techniques for PC treatments, which ultimately result in limited effectiveness, researchers have undertaken the quest for a viable alternative to address these obstacles. Nanotechnology has intrinsic attributes that ensure the safety, specificity, and therapeutic effectiveness of modern medicines for prostate cancer. The nanoparticles (NPs) described in this study are composed of biodevices and materials that possess functional ductility and exhibit a range of structural characteristics, including polymers, lipids, inorganic carriers, and biological scaffolds. These nanoparticles are designed to serve as nanoscale drug carrier systems, specifically engineered for the targeted delivery of cancer therapeutics [12].

With the emergence of nanovectors and the application of nanovectorization in the field of personalized cancer therapies, several advancements have been made. These include the ability to administer a concentrated dosage of anticancer agents, the simultaneous delivery of multiple therapeutic molecules within a single nanoformulation, the successful delivery of drug agents to their intended targets, the mitigation of toxicity associated with treatment, and the enhancement of therapeutic efficacy. For example, the use of functionalized nanovectors allows for the integration of the distinct pharmacokinetics and pharmacodynamics of therapeutic agents inside a single carrier, hence enhancing the probability of administering each agent to the tumor cells at a certain dosage ratio [13]. Furthermore, our research team, together with other researchers, has recently provided evidence of the feasibility of simultaneously delivering a combination of chemotherapy and gene-based therapy, known as chemogene, inside a single nanoconstruct. This approach has shown promising results in enhancing the effectiveness of suppressing genes and cytotoxicity for the treatment of CRPC [14]. Nanoparticles have emerged as a very effective drug delivery method that offers improved targeted drug delivery abilities via both passive and active processes. Previous studies have shown the ability of these agents to reduce drug toxicity, enhance drug accumulation at specific disease locations, extend the overall circulation time of the medication, and provide protection against humoral assaults [15]. The field of nanomedicine has not given enough attention to treatment approaches for prostate cancer. However, existing research suggests a bright outlook for the future. As an example, the utilization of near-infrared fluorescence (NIRF) imaging in mice harboring PC-3 xenografts showed that polyethylene glycol (PEG)-micelles exhibited a discernible accumulation at the tumor site while displaying limited dispersion in vital organs such as the liver and spleen [16]. In a study conducted by researchers, it was shown that the administration of paclitaxel using PEG5K-embelin2 micelles resulted in more effective suppression of tumor growth in breast and prostate cancer mouse models, as compared to the use of Taxol [17]. Xang et al. have published a study detailing the effects of oxygenation generated by perfluorocarbon nanodroplets on the formation of these droplets in xenograft prostate cancers. The researchers noted a deposition of particles in the tumor of mice within a 24-h timeframe, resulting in a decrease in tumor hypoxia without any concurrent improvement in oxygen inhalation [18]. Based on the existing testimonies and more evidence about the potential benefits of nanoparticles in the treatment of castration-resistant prostate cancer, it can be reasonably argued that nanovectorization has significant potential to transform the approach to CRPC therapy.

14.3 Various Types of Nanoparticles for Prostate Cancer Therapy

Nanotechnology is now a leading area of focus in the field of anticancer medication research, whereby nanoparticles (NPs) are used to enhance the efficacy of cancer detection and therapy. The field of cancer treatment has seen significant interest and intensive research in the development of nanodrug delivery methods. Various forms of nanocarriers are often used in the field, such as liposomes, polymeric nanoparticles, magnetic nanoparticles, gold nanoparticles (AuNPs), mesoporous silica nanoparticles (MSNs), quantum dots (QDs), micelles, and dendritic polymers, among other options. The biological dispersion of nanoparticles in vivo is significantly influenced by their size, surface characteristics, and shape [19]. Nanotechnology offers potential optimization for various issues, such as the utilization of nanodelivery systems to prevent renal elimination by leveraging their optimal size, employing nanodelivery systems to extend drug circulation time in vivo through sustained release and targeting capabilities, thereby enhancing the efficacy of chemotherapeutic drugs while minimizing side effects, and capitalizing on the presence of abnormal blood vessels in cancer tissues to exploit the enhanced permeability and retention (EPR) effects of nanodelivery systems, thereby augmenting the level of small molecule drugs at the tumor site. Drug-loaded nanoparticles, also known as nano-drugs, have the ability to utilize passive targeting mechanisms like the enhanced permeability and retention effect. This allows them to accumulate in pathological sites, extend their presence in the bloodstream, and regulate the release of drugs. Additionally, nano-drugs can effectively employ various ligands such as hormones, antibodies, vitamins, modified carbohydrates, aptamers, oligopeptides, and more. These ligands play a crucial role in accurately identifying specific organs or cell receptors at different levels, ranging from the macrostructure of tumors to microscopic organelles [20]. Active targeting offers further benefits. The prostate cancer surface is known to be targeted by particular expression substances such as mannose 6-phosphate receptor (M6PR), CD44, folic acid receptor (FR), and prostate-specific membrane antigen (PSMA) [21, 22] (Fig. 14.1).

14.3.1 Polymer-Based Nanoparticles

Polymeric nanoparticles, with a diameter of less than 1 μm, may be synthesized using either synthetic or natural polymers [24]. Not only do they possess the capacity to modulate the pharmacokinetic properties of diverse active compounds, but they also have an influence on the biodegradability and biocompatibility of polymers used in the synthesis of nanoparticles. Polymer nanoparticles may be further categorized based on their interior structure into two main types: nanospheres (NSs) and nanocapsules (NCs) [24, 25]. Polymer nanocapsules are composed of a nucleus that may be either liquid or solid, which is enveloped by a polymer shell. Typically, the medicine is dissolved inside the core of the nanocapsules; however, it can also be found on the surface of these structures. Polymer nanospheres often exhibit a uniform spherical morphology and are composed of a solid polymer matrix devoid of a polymer shell. The medication may be either kept inside or adsorbed onto the matrix [26].

Shitole and colleagues conducted a study whereby they synthesized chemically modified polymeric NCs that contained a combination of the chemotherapeutic medicines doxorubicin (DTX) and quercetin (QU). The purpose of this study was to investigate the potential of these nanocapsules for actively targeting prostate cancer. Active targeting is accomplished by the attachment of luteinizing hormone-releasing hormone (LHRH) ligands to poly(propyleneglycol-co-glycolide) (PLGA) by means of polyethylene glycol (PEG) as a carrier. The results of in vitro investigations demonstrated a significant increase in the cellular absorption of LHRH-targeted NCs,

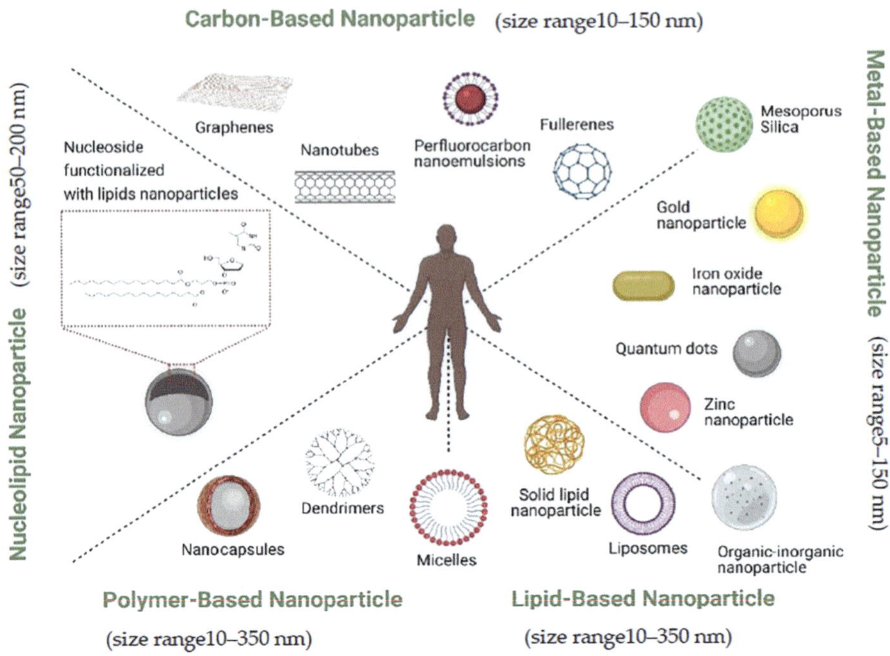

Fig. 14.1 Various types of nanoparticles [23]

leading to greater cellular inhibitory action. The findings from in vivo investigations on tumor location and anticancer activity align with and reinforce the in vitro results, which highlight the advantageous impacts of nanoparticles containing a combination of DTX and QU in combating prostate cancer [27]. The physicochemical features of polymeric nanoparticles have been thoroughly examined since they exhibit a stable core-shell structure and possess a homogeneous size distribution within the necessary nanometer range. These characteristics make them well-suited for the delivery of drugs to tumor sites, either by passive or active means.

14.3.2 Liposomes

Liposomes emerged as the pioneering nanodrug delivery method that achieved effective translation into real-time clinical usage, therefore bringing about a revolutionary transformation in the pharmaceutical domain [28]. Liposomes were first reported by Alec Bangham in 1961 [29]. Since then, much study has been conducted on the subject of liposomes, leading to their widespread use in diverse areas like medication administration, biomolecules, and gene transport [28]. A liposome is a versatile carrier material that undergoes self-assembly and consists of one or more lipid bilayers composed primarily of phospholipids and/or cholesterol. This structure enables the encapsulation of hydrophilic drugs within the internal aqueous compartments, while more hydrophobic drugs may interact with the lipid bilayers [30]. In comparison to other nanocarriers, lipid carriers exhibit comparatively straightforward preparation methods, biodegradability, and non-toxicity [31]. At present, liposomal doxorubicin has received clinical approval for the therapeutic management of several medical conditions, including breast cancer, advanced breast cancer, Kaposi's sarcoma, multiple myeloma, and ovarian cancer [32]. Zhang et al. devised a drug delivery method to concurrently administer docetaxel (Doc) and resveratrol (Res) using liposomes. The experimental results show that liposomes can effectively maintain the simultaneous release of both medicines and efficiently transport them to the specific prostate PC-3 cells. The results of the animal trials indicated that the administration of Doc/Res containing liposomes led to little toxicity and extended life in nude mice with PC-3 tumors in comparison to the control group that was subjected to Doc/Res without liposomes [33]. A significant proportion of clinical investigations in the domain of liposome-mediated tumor targeting have mostly concentrated on examining the efficacy of liposomes in addressing various types of cancer, with little attention given to exploring their potential in treating prostate cancer. Furthermore, clinical research pertaining to prostate cancer has predominantly centered on the utilization of liposome doxorubicin as the primary therapeutic agent. Furthermore, the studies conducted have given comparatively less consideration to CRPC due to its status as the most perilous kind of advanced cancer, along with the limited availability of efficient treatment options [34].

14.3.3 Gold Nanoparticles

Gold nanoparticles (AuNPs) have garnered significant interest in recent years owing to their distinctive physical and chemical characteristics, such as surface plasmon resonance (SPR) and fluorescence amplification. These traits render them well-suited for applications in drug administration and targeting [35]. The material's distinct characteristics, including its inertness, non-toxicity, and biocompatibility, render it highly valuable and appealing to researchers in the fields of biology and biomedicine. It finds utility in various applications, such as serving as leads for pacemakers and functioning as intravenous contrast agents for imaging purposes. Additionally, it has shown promise in the non-invasive detection of lung cancer [36]. In their study, Luo et al. developed a novel approach for magnetic resonance (MR)-guided treatment targeting prostate cancer. This included the use of gold nanoparticles as carriers, which were functionalized with gadolinium (Gd) Gd (III) complexes and PSMA-targeted ligands, enabling precise targeting of prostate cancer cells. The application of this surface alteration led to a four-fold increase in the r1 relaxation rate and therefore resulted in a greater level of binding affinity. The findings of the study indicated an increased absorption of gold nanoparticles by prostate cancer cells expressing PSMA, as well as favorable magnetic resonance imaging (MRI) contrast both in laboratory settings and in living organisms. Furthermore, the binding of gold and Gd (III) demonstrated superior suppression of prostate cancer after radiation [37]. The confirmation of the remarkable specificity of Au-Gd (III)-PSMA nanoparticles in targeting prostate cancer cells expressing PSMA, together with their ability to improve cellular magnetic resonance contrast and sensitize cells to radiation in laboratory settings, has been shown in previous studies [37, 38]. The use of PSMA-targeted gold nanoparticles has shown a notable ability to selectively target tumors, enabling the administration of radiation treatment with enhanced precision, lower irradiation dosage, and minimum harm to surrounding healthy tissues [37].

14.3.4 Quantum Dots (QDs)

Quantum dots (QDs) refer to semiconductor crystals that fall within the nanometer range of 2–10 nm. These crystals are mostly formed of semiconductor elements from periodic groups II-VI or III-V. QDs possess distinctive photoluminescent and electrical features [39]. The phenomenon is distinguished by a symmetrical and narrow emission spectrum, accompanied by a large absorption spectrum. The material exhibits high light absorption over a broad range of wavelengths, spanning from ultraviolet to near-infrared (NIR), and subsequently generates fluorescence within a distinct and symmetrical spectral band. The positioning of the nanocrystals is contingent upon the dimensions of the nanocrystals themselves as well as the specific semiconductor material used [40]. The optical characteristics of quantum dots are determined by their composition. These nanoparticles consist of a core made of semiconductor material, such as cadmium selenide (CdSe), lead selenide (PbSe), or indium arsenide (InAs), which is then coated or enveloped by a shell layer composed of the same semiconductor material [41]. Quantum dot (QD)-based nanotechnology has shown the ability to effectively monitor several aspects of cell activity, including adhesion, motility, and invasion. This technology has also shown promise in tracking therapeutic responses via both in vitro and in vivo imaging. Consequently, it presents novel opportunities for the fields of diagnosis and therapy [41, 42].

Ncapayi and colleagues successfully synthesized ternary AgInSe/ZnS QDs that emit near infrared light. The synthesis process included using a commercially available home pressure cooker. These QDs have potential use in cancer imaging. The produced quantum dots (QDs) have a spherical morphology, characterized by a particle diameter of 4.5 ± 0.5 nm. Additionally, these QDs demonstrate strong fluorescence, with a photoluminescence peak occurring at a wavelength of 705 nm. The quantum dots exhibited little cytotoxicity toward mouse prostate cancer cells and demonstrated efficient internalization inside prostate cancer cells. The aforementioned study represents a significant advancement in the use of ternary quantum dots for the purpose of diagnosing and providing targeted therapy for prostate cancer [43]. Jiang et al. have successfully created a graphene oxide nanosystem that is loaded with enzalutamide and has multifunctional properties. This nanosystem has been specifically designed for intravenous treatment in patients with castration-resistant prostate cancer. The process included the initial cross-linking of graphene quantum dots via disulfide bonds, resulting in the formation of graphene quantum dot derivatives measuring around 200 nm. Subsequently, enzalutamide was loaded into these derivatives. Subsequently, the graphene quantum nano-drug system was subjected to further functionalization by the incorporation of tumor-targeting peptides and polyethylene glycol (PEG). The achievement of high drug-loading efficiency was shown by both in vitro and in vivo investigations, wherein it was observed that π-π electron interaction played a significant role. The nano-drug carrier shows a notable capacity for targeting prostate cancer, specifically in cells with castration-resistant prostate cancer, by means of efficient internalization by endocytosis. This internalization process resulted in the inhibition of prostate cancer cell development and the mitigation of enzalutamide's adverse effects in vivo [44]. The considerable obstacles to the medical applications of quantum dot probes arise from their inherent toxicity concerns and prolonged retention period in vivo, notwithstanding the promising potential of quantum dots in clinical settings [45]. Consequently, scholars are diligently endeavoring to address the aforementioned challenges related to quantum dots by applying a protective and stable shell to the surface of QDs. This approach aims to ensure the safe utilization of QDs for further bioconjugation with macromolecules or other chemical elements [39].

14.3.5 Magnetic Nanoparticles (MNPs)

The growing interest in magnetic nanoparticles (MNPs) may be attributed to their distinct physical features, biocompatibility, stability, and several other characteristics [46]. Metal nanoparticles have been extensively used in the production of nanomedicine and nanosensors for a considerable duration. The regulated interaction between magnetic nanoparticles and an external magnetic field, created by a permanent magnet, is a well-established phenomenon. As a result, the precise position of MNPs may be used to accurately identify the presence of a medical condition [47]. Hence, the distinctive magnetic response characteristics shown by magnetic nanoparticles may be used to achieve accurate localization inside an organism and then trigger the release of the encapsulated medication under the influence of an externally applied magnetic field. This approach enables the development of a highly targeted drug delivery system. Furthermore, the utilization of magnetic nanomaterials as contrast agents in magnetic resonance imaging (MRI) exhibits enhanced capabilities in terms of expedited and accurate targeting of tumor tissues, surpassing the performance of conventional contrast agents. Additionally, the application of magnetic nanomaterials as contrast agents contributes to the enhancement of specificity and sensitivity in the early diagnosis of tumors by augmenting the contrast, thereby facilitating the detection of minute lesions [48].

Currently, there is a growing use of superparamagnetic iron oxide nanoparticles (SPION) coated with a biocompatible shell in the field of personalized medicine, namely for the detection and therapy of certain cancerous conditions. The real-time monitoring of therapy may be facilitated by the use of superparamagnetic iron oxide nanoparticles. This can be achieved by mixing SPION with various medications and afterward observing the alterations in T1 or T2 relaxation parameters [49]. In addition, MNPs possess several advantageous characteristics that render them highly suitable for various disease treatments. These benefits include a substantial surface area-to-volume ratio, optimal pore size, functionalized surfaces, multiple interaction or binding sites, and little mass transfer resistance [47]. The researchers Ngen et al. devised a magnetic nanoparticle with a particular affinity for the prostate-specific membrane antigen (PSMA). This nanoparticle was subsequently assessed in a mouse model utilizing T2-weighted magnetic resonance imaging after intravenous injection of 50 mg/kg of the nanoparticle at the dose necessary for thermotherapy. The study found that nanoparticles had a higher tendency to collect toward the outer edges of tumors, specifically in comparison to tumors that lacked prostate-specific membrane antigen. Additionally, tumors that expressed PSMA showed noticeable elevation in contrast at both 24 and 48 h after nanoparticle delivery [50]. While some magnetic nanoparticles and superparamagnetic iron oxide nanoparticles have received FDA approval, excessive quantities of these substances may pose risks to human health. These risks include adverse effects on several organs such as the liver, brain, skin, gastrointestinal function, and potential neurological impairment [35]. Hence, in the context of clinical investigations, it is imperative to take into account the physicochemical characteristics and potential toxicity of MNPs. Moreover, to ensure their safe and effective use in treatment, it is essential to implement appropriate control measures and functionalize their surfaces by the incorporation of diverse inorganic or organic chemicals, leading to the attainment of passivated surfaces [47].

14.3.6 Mesoporous Silica Nanoparticles (MSNs)

Mesoporous silica nanoparticles (MSNs) are characterized as silica-based materials that possess nanopores within the nanometer scale. Based on the categorization established by the International Union of Pure and Applied Chemistry (IUPAC), the mesoporous silica nanoparticles have a pore size that falls within the range of 2–50 nm [51]. The unique qualities of this substance make it very valuable in nano-drug delivery systems. These properties include the capacity to adjust particle and pore size, a large surface area and pore volume, ease of functionalization and modification of the surface, exceptional stability, and efficient trapping of cargo molecules [52]. The high drug-loading capacity of mesoporous silica nanoparticle is attributed to their surface area and pore volume. This characteristic enables them to adsorb a wide range of molecules, which can be conveniently modified with targeting and visualizing agents. Consequently, the incorporation of MSNs in drug delivery systems enhances their therapeutic efficiency and contributes to their diagnostic capabilities [53].

Vallet-Regi et al. (2001) were the first to demonstrate the effective use of mesoporous silica nanoparticles as drug carriers for the encapsulation of ibuprofen. This pioneering study marked the first application of MSNs as drug delivery agents in the field of nanomaterials. The FDA has determined that mesoporous silica nanodelivery systems are safe. Additionally, the FDA has cleared tiny silica nanoparticles to be employed as visualizers in clinical studies on humans. These findings highlight the potential of silica nanoparticles as potential nanoplatforms for clinical applications [54]. In their study, Du et al. introduced a novel approach including the use of manganese oxide-Msns that are targeted toward the prostate-specific membrane antigen. Through the application of optical imaging and magnetic resonance imaging techniques in preclinical models, the researchers demonstrated the selective accumulation of these nanoparticles in both prostate cancer cells and tumor tissue. The use of fluorescent and magnetic resonance (MR) bifunctional nanoparticles that specifically target prostate-specific antigens has shown the ability to see prostate cancer. In vitro and in vivo imaging findings have indicated that the PSA-targeted Mn-Msn-Cy7 nanoprobe has significant potential for the detection of prostate cancer [55]. Although the promise of mesoporous silica nanoparticles as agents for delivering anticancer drugs is recognized, there remains a limited knowledge of their application in clinical investigations. In future periods, it will be essential to comprehend and execute an assessment of the cytotoxicity of mesoporous silica nanoparticles (MSNs) as vehicles in human subjects, as well as evaluate their efficacy in human delivery. Further research is required to thoroughly investigate the potential anticancer activities of MSN. Nevertheless, via the passage of time and further enhancements, it is reasonable to assert that MSNs will undoubtedly realize their considerable potential.

14.3.7 Dendritic Polymers

Dendritic polymers are characterized by their intricate three-dimensional branching structure, making them a distinct and significant kind of polymer structure alongside linear, cross-linked, and branched architectures [56]. Dendrimers may be synthesized by two distinct methods: divergent and convergent approaches. In the divergent approach, dendrimers are grown either from the core nucleus or from the peripheral toward the inside, ultimately forming the nucleus [57]. In contrast to linear polymers, dendrimers have a significant abundance of terminal functional groups, possess a reduced solution or melt viscosity, and demonstrate favorable solubility [58]. The aforementioned features render them very promising for diverse biological applications, such as medication delivery, gene therapy, and bioimaging [59]. Dendrimer-based nano-drugs have shown use in facilitating accurate detection of cancers in their early stages, as well as in monitoring and gathering pertinent information on tumor characteristics, aggressiveness, metastasis, and prognosis

[60]. The highly branching three-dimensional structure and presence of several functional groups in in vitro cancer diagnostics contribute to an increased capture density per unit area and improved capacity to bind cancer markers. Regarding in vivo cancer diagnostics, the excellent biocompatibility and low viscosity of nanoparticles serve as the fundamental factors for their potential use in in vivo settings [61].

The manufacture of PSMA-targeted polyamidoamine (PAMAM) dendrimer nanocarriers was described by Lesniak et al. in their study [1547]. One of the methods used was a straightforward single-step synthesis to produce dendritic nanoparticles that were electrically neutral, had a limited variation in particle size, and possessed a diameter of around 5 nm. The findings from positron emission tomography (PET) and biodistribution studies using 64Cu-labeled dendrimer nanocarriers, both in vitro and in vivo, demonstrated a significant accumulation of these nanocarriers in PSMA+PC3 PIP tumors within 24 hours post-injection. This observation further substantiated the specific uptake of dendrimer nanocarriers by PSMA+ tumors [62]. Significant advancements have been achieved so far in the application of dendritic polymers in the field of therapeutic diagnostics. Nevertheless, the use of dendritic macromolecules in clinical practice is hindered by factors such as possible toxicity, bio-elimination, and long-term impacts, which are attributed to the intricate production process [63]. Nonetheless, ongoing endeavors are being made to advance the translation of dendritic polymer nanosystem-based diagnostic therapeutics from the experimental stage to practical use in clinical settings. These efforts primarily focus on enhancing the design of synthetic methods, refining procedures, and implementing precise characterization processes.

14.4 Micelles

Micelles are nanostructures composed of amphiphilic polymers that undergo self-assembly. These structures typically vary in size from 5 to 100 nm. Within the micelles, there exists a hydrophobic core that serves to accommodate water-insoluble pharmaceuticals, while an outer hydrophilic shell acts as a barrier, isolating the encapsulated drug from the surrounding environment [64]. The process of micelle structure creation involves the contact between the polar head group and the surrounding water. This interaction may cause a segregation between hydrophobic and hydrophilic regions, ultimately leading to the production of micelles that are flexible and porous [65]. The morphologies of micelles, such as spheres and rods, may vary depending on many factors, including the quality of the solvent, the length of the blocker chain, the type of blocker, and the temperature. Previous studies have used the micellar structure in a range of experimental methods, including nuclear magnetic resonance (NMR), X-ray diffraction (XRD), and fluorescence spectroscopy [66]. The core-shell structure is the primary characteristic of micelles. Hence, micelles have the ability to encapsulate and solubilize hydrophobic medicines inside their hydrophobic regions, safeguarding them from clearance by the mononuclear phagocyte systems (MPS) [67]. The encapsulation of medicine inside a polymeric micelle fraction has the potential to significantly enhance the drug's water solubility. This increase in solubility may range from ten-fold to 500-fold, therefore enabling the intravenous delivery of hydrophobic drugs that are encased within micelles. For instance, the water solubility of paclitaxel, a medication that is typically insoluble in water, may be significantly increased by its encapsulation inside micelles [68].

In their study, Barve et al. devised a polymeric micelle that is both biodegradable and enzyme-responsive, with the specific purpose of delivering cabazitaxel. The formation of micelles was facilitated by the presence of two amphiphilic block copolymers. The first block copolymer was composed of polyethylene glycol (PEG), an enzyme-responsive peptide, and cholesterol. In contrast, the subsequent block copolymer included a targeting ligand (DUPA), PEG, and cholesterol. The formation of micelles was facilitated by the presence of two amphiphilic block copolymers. The micelles demonstrated a significantly reduced critical micelle concentration (CMC), along with a high drug-loading capacity and a high level of encapsulation efficiency. The liberation of cabazitaxel from the micelles was contingent upon the enzymatic cleavage of the peptide with reactivity. In vitro, there was a notable enhancement in the internalization of micelles by prostate cancer cells as compared to the unencapsulated form of cabazitaxel. Additionally, it is noteworthy that ligand-coupled polymer micelles demonstrated enhanced efficacy in suppressing tumor development in mice with prostate cancer xenografts [69]. Micelles have been extensively used as nanosystems for the delivery of anticancer drugs. Nevertheless, the stability of micelles in the circulation may be compromised by hemodilution, leading to a reduction in the critical micelle concentration. Consequently, achieving efficient drug delivery to the tumor remains a formidable task [70].

14.5 Use of Nanoparticles in siRNA-Based Prostate Cancer Therapy

The advent of gene therapy interventions, such as RNA interference (RNAi) or antisense oligonucleotides (ASO), elicits a multitude of optimistic expectations. Nevertheless, recent research indicates that the effectiveness of these technologies is hindered by the cells' restricted capacity to allow nucleic acids to pass through their membranes, as well as the poor stability of nucleic acids in the presence of serum proteins and degradation enzymes. This is particularly true for small interfering RNAs (siRNA) [71]. One potential approach to address these challenges is the use of efficient vector systems that may safeguard nucleic acids from nucleases found in bodily fluids while also enhancing the permeability of the plasma membrane to facilitate the delivery of these therapeutic agents. Viral vectors have been recognized as a viable method for delivering nucleic acids, but their effectiveness is hindered by their ability to cause inflammation, immune responses, and mutations. Consequently, there is a pressing need for alternative nonviral vectors. Cationic polymers and lipids are widely recognized as the predominant nonviral vectors used in gene therapy. The capacity to form stable compounds with them via electrostatic interactions has been shown [72, 73].

Chitosan is a positively charged polymer that demonstrates little toxicity to cells, has excellent compatibility with biological systems, and allows for great cellular permeability. Therapeutic nucleic acid delivery is a commonly used practice. However, it is important to note that current chitosan-based vectors exhibit in vivo toxicity and limited efficacy in releasing nucleic acids. To address these limitations, ongoing research is focused on the synthesis of a nanocomplex including the unmodified version of this polymer, together with protamine, lecithin, and thiamine pyrophosphate. This nanocomplex is being investigated for its potential as a vector for delivering siRNA molecules that target the survivin (SVN) gene. The gene in question is responsible for encoding an inhibitor of apoptosis known as SVN, which has been identified as a promising target for therapeutic interventions aimed at addressing prostate cancer. In an in vitro setting, it has been shown that the GP-L-CT vector is capable of decreasing the expression of SVN by a maximum of 22 percent in human prostate cancer cells. In vivo studies conducted on mice bearing a GP-L-CT tumor have similarly shown the observed efficiency of tumor development and targeted inhibition. The inclusion of PC-3 xenograft in this vector renders it a favorable option for other formulations using polymer nanoparticles. The potential use of this technology as a therapeutic and theragnostic tool for prostate cancer is plausible [74].

Lipid vectors are hypothesized to facilitate the delivery of nucleic acid release through a process involving membrane fusion. On the other hand, polymeric vectors use the proton sponge impact to evade the endosome, where the acidic pH ultimately leads to the denaturation of the endosome. The cell internalizes therapeutic nucleic acids. The use of an amphiphilic Dendron dendrimer composed of PANAM has the potential to synergistically include the benefits associated with both vector types [73]. The dendrimer under consideration is a hybrid compound that combines lipid and dendrimer components. It is composed of a lengthy alkyl chain and a dendrimer moiety. The vector has undergone testing as a means of delivering siRNA to inhibit the translation of Hsp27, a gene responsible for encoding a chaperone protein that significantly contributes to the growth of CRPC. The induction of apoptosis and inhibition of cell growth in vitro are seen with the inhibition of translation [75]. The administration of this medication to mice resulted in a considerable reduction in the translation of Hsp27, leading to a robust anticancer impact. This approach presents a novel option for the management of castration-resistant prostate cancer, a condition that currently lacks viable therapeutic interventions.

Nanovectors composed of nucleic acids, which have the potential for combating prostate cancer, have reached a somewhat advanced level of research. The aforementioned scenario pertains specifically to the SGT-53 system, an innovation by SynerGene Therapeutics. This method involves the vectorization of the tumor suppressor gene p53 inside a liposome. The aforementioned therapy is now undergoing a Phase 1 clinical investigation. The TCTP-LASO system, designed for targeting castration-resistant prostate cancers, operates by the self-assembly of micellar nanoparticles composed of antisense nucleotides conjugated with a lipid chain. The therapeutic approach in question involves the use of an antisense oligonucleotide that specifically targets the TCTP protein, also known as translationally controlled tumor protein. This protein plays a crucial part in the cytoprotection function of Hsp27. The submission of a patent by a partnership of many French labs was documented [23].

14.6 Conclusion

In contemporary times, the dynamic interaction between technology and biology has had a profound influence on the fields of drug design, medication delivery, and illness management. The emergence of nanotherapeutics in recent decades has revitalized and transformed the field of cancer therapy. This advancement enables the precise administration of anticancer medicines via the use of nanovectors, leading to reduced negative impacts and improved therapeutic outcomes. Consequently, the use of nanovectorization is growing as a compelling approach in the field of cancer treatment. While the discovery of novel nanovectors is still in progress, micelles, liposomes, and dendrimers have been extensively researched and widely used for the treatment of many medical situations, including cancer. Despite the significant advancements in research, which have facilitated the use of nanotechnology for the medical management of many cancer types, there remain a limited number of preclinical studies that have specifically investigated the use of nanovectorization-based therapy for prostate cancer.

This chapter aims to provide an overview of the nanovectors now utilized as drug delivery systems in cancer treatment, focusing on their potential application in transforming prostate cancer therapy. The review commenced by providing a comprehensive depiction and categorization of nanovectors. It then proceeded to elucidate how these vectors are tailored to facilitate the delivery of antitumor agents, with a particular emphasis on their structural attributes that make them highly suitable for transporting drugs for the treatment of prostate cancer. Additionally, the review explored the utilization of gene delivery strategies, specifically targeting the refractory subtypes of prostate cancer. The benefits and potential of nanovectorization in the setting of diseases such as prostate cancer have been extensively studied and supported by both clinical and preclinical evidence. While a significant number of first nanovectors have shown considerable therapeutic advantages by using the passive targeting mechanism for delivering cancer medicines, nanovectors employing an active targeting approach are still facing obstacles in their journey toward clinical use. In the current era, gene therapy has emerged as a prominent approach in cancer treatment, either used along with chemotherapeutic agents or as a standalone treatment. It has demonstrated significant potential for addressing castration-resistant prostate cancer by targeting genes that are triggered when androgen levels are reduced. However, challenges related to limited cellular uptake, lack of specificity, and systemic instability have proven to be difficult to overcome. Nanovectorization provides a durable resolution to the three-fold challenges connected not just with gene therapy for prostate cancer, but also with several other forms of cancer. It is anticipated that nanotherapeutics will revolutionize cancer therapy by shifting the paradigm from traditional delivery methods to tumor-specific, active targeting delivery. This optimism is supported by the growing interest and rapid research progress in nanovectorization across various laboratories. Additionally, the potential of nanovectorization in cancer therapy has generated considerable excitement, further fueling the exploration of nanovectorization strategies for diverse pharmacological applications by numerous pharmaceutical companies. The integration of real-time in vivo imaging with nanotherapeutics is expected to have a transformative impact on both oncological and non-oncological therapies.

References

1. Galsky MD, Vogelzang NJ. Docetaxel-based combination therapy for castration-resistant prostate cancer. Ann Oncol. 2010;21(11):2135–44.
2. Sriraman SK, Aryasomayajula B, Torchilin VP. Barriers to drug delivery in solid tumors. Tissue Barriers. 2014;2:e29528.
3. Zhou M, et al. Overcoming chemotherapy resistance via simultaneous drug-efflux circumvention and mitochondrial targeting. Acta Pharm Sin B. 2019;9(3):615–25.
4. Gillet JP, Gottesman MM. Mechanisms of multidrug resistance in cancer. Methods Mol Biol. 2010;596:47–76.
5. Narvekar M, et al. Nanocarrier for poorly water-soluble anticancer drugs—barriers of translation and solutions. AAPS PharmSciTech. 2014;15(4):822–33.
6. Ma P, Mumper RJ. Paclitaxel Nano-delivery systems: a comprehensive review. J Nanomed Nanotechnol. 2013;4(2):1000164.
7. Teply BA, et al. The influence of prednisone on the efficacy of docetaxel in men with metastatic castration-resistant prostate cancer. Prostate Cancer Prostatic Dis. 2016;19(1):72–8.
8. Zheng R, et al. Role of taxane and anthracycline combination regimens in the management of advanced breast cancer: a meta-analysis of randomized trials. Medicine (Baltimore). 2015;94(17):e803.
9. Elm'hadi C, et al. Toxicities of docetaxel: original drug versus generics-a comparative study about 81 cases. Springerplus. 2016;5(1):732.
10. Picard M. Management of Hypersensitivity Reactions to Taxanes. Immunol Allergy Clin N Am. 2017;37(4):679–93.
11. Min BD, et al. Docetaxel-induced fatal interstitial pneumonitis in a patient with castration-resistant prostate cancer. Korean J Urol. 2012;53(5):371–4.
12. Sakamoto JH, et al. Enabling individualized therapy through nanotechnology. Pharmacol Res. 2010;62(2):57–89.
13. Miao L, et al. Nanoparticles with precise Ratiometric co-loading and co-delivery of gemcitabine monophosphate and cisplatin for treatment of bladder cancer. Adv Funct Mater. 2014;24(42):6601–11.
14. Mou Q, et al. Two-in-one Chemogene assembled from drug-integrated antisense oligonucleotides to reverse Chemoresistance. J Am Chem Soc. 2019;141(17):6955–66.
15. Senapati S, et al. Controlled drug delivery vehicles for cancer treatment and their performance. Signal Transduct Target Ther. 2018;3:7.

16. Zhang Y, Huang Y, Li S. Polymeric micelles: nanocarriers for cancer-targeted drug delivery. AAPS PharmSciTech. 2014;15(4):862–71.
17. Omabe K, Paris C, Rocchi P. Nanovectorization of prostate cancer treatment strategies: a new approach to improved outcomes. Pharmaceutics. 2021;13:591.
18. Xiang Y, et al. Perfluorocarbon nanodroplets can reoxygenate hypoxic tumors in vivo without carbogen breathing. Nano. 2019;3(2):135–44.
19. Ahmed A, et al. Surface-modified polymeric nanoparticles for drug delivery to cancer cells. Expert Opin Drug Deliv. 2021;18(1):1–24.
20. Gupta S, et al. Current prospects and challenges of nanomedicine delivery in prostate cancer therapy. Nanomedicine (Lond). 2017;12(23):2675–92.
21. Lakshmanan VK. Therapeutic efficacy of nanomedicines for prostate cancer: an update. Investig Clin Urol. 2016;57(1):21–9.
22. Moles E, Kavallaris M. A potent targeted cancer nanotherapeutic. Nat Biomed Eng. 2019;3(4):248–50.
23. Omabe K, et al. Nanovectorization of prostate cancer treatment strategies: a new approach to improved outcomes. Pharmaceutics. 2021;13(5):591.
24. Karlsson J, Vaughan HJ, Green JJ. Biodegradable polymeric nanoparticles for therapeutic cancer treatments. Annu Rev Chem Biomol Eng. 2018;9:105–27.
25. Łukasiewicz S, et al. Encapsulation of clozapine in polymeric nanocapsules and its biological effects. Colloids Surf B Biointerfaces. 2016;140:342–52.
26. Deng S, et al. Polymeric Nanocapsules as Nanotechnological alternative for drug delivery system: current status, challenges and opportunities. Nanomaterials (Basel). 2020;10(5):847.
27. Shitole AA, et al. LHRH-conjugated, PEGylated, poly-lactide-co-glycolide nanocapsules for targeted delivery of combinational chemotherapeutic drugs docetaxel and quercetin for prostate cancer. Mater Sci Eng C Mater Biol Appl. 2020;114:111035.
28. Bulbake U, et al. Liposomal formulations in clinical use: an updated review. Pharmaceutics. 2017;9(2):12.
29. Bangham AD, Standish MM, Watkins JC. Diffusion of univalent ions across the lamellae of swollen phospholipids. J Mol Biol. 1965;13(1):238–52.
30. Apolinário AC, et al. Lipid nanovesicles for biomedical applications: 'What is in a name'? Prog Lipid Res. 2021;82:101096.
31. Moosavian SA, et al. Challenges and pitfalls in the development of liposomal delivery systems for cancer therapy. Semin Cancer Biol. 2021;69:337–48.
32. Ko MS. The comparison in daily intake of nutrients, dietary habits and body composition of female college students by body mass index. Nutr Res Pract. 2007;1(2):131–42.
33. Zhang L, et al. Co-delivery of docetaxel and resveratrol by liposomes synergistically boosts antitumor efficiency against prostate cancer. Eur J Pharm Sci. 2022;174:106199.
34. Kroon J, et al. Liposomal nanomedicines in the treatment of prostate cancer. Cancer Treat Rev. 2014;40(4):578–84.
35. Chen X, et al. Broadening horizons: the role of ferroptosis in cancer. Nat Rev Clin Oncol. 2021;18(5):280–96.
36. Anker JN, et al. Biosensing with plasmonic nanosensors. Nat Mater. 2008;7(6):442–53.
37. Luo D, et al. Targeted Chemoradiotherapy of prostate cancer using gold nanoclusters with protease Activatable monomethyl Auristatin E. ACS Appl Mater Interfaces. 2022;14(13):14916–27.
38. Bouché M, et al. Recent advances in molecular imaging with gold nanoparticles. Bioconjug Chem. 2020;31(2):303–14.
39. He Y, et al. Functionalized nanoparticles targeting tumor-associated macrophages as cancer therapy. Pharmaceutics. 2021;13(10):1670.
40. Zhang J, et al. Fluorescent oxygen-doped g-C(3)N(4) quantum dots for selective detection Fe(3+) ions in cell imaging. Nanomaterials (Basel). 2022;12(11):1826.
41. Kargozar S, et al. Quantum dots: a review from concept to clinic. Biotechnol J. 2020;15(12):e2000117.

42. Wang ZG, Liu SL, Pang DW. Quantum dots: a promising fluorescent label for probing virus trafficking. Acc Chem Res. 2021;54(14):2991–3002.
43. Uysal A, et al. Prostatitis, the great mimicker of prostate cancer: can we differentiate them quantitatively with multiparametric MRI? AJR Am J Roentgenol. 2020;215(5):1104–12.
44. Jiang W, et al. Intravenous delivery of enzalutamide based on high drug loading multifunctional graphene oxide nanoparticles for castration-resistant prostate cancer therapy. J Nanobiotechnol. 2020;18(1):50.
45. Yang H-L, et al. Carbon quantum dots: preparation, optical properties, and biomedical applications. Mater Today Adv. 2023;18:100376.
46. Lima-Tenório MK, et al. Magnetic nanoparticles: in vivo cancer diagnosis and therapy. Int J Pharm. 2015;493(1–2):313–27.
47. Manescu Paltanea V, et al. Magnetic nanoparticles used in oncology. Materials (Basel). 2021;14(20):5948.
48. Dhavale RP, et al. Monolayer grafting of aminosilane on magnetic nanoparticles: an efficient approach for targeted drug delivery system. J Colloid Interface Sci. 2018;529:415–25.
49. Caspani S, et al. Magnetic nanomaterials as contrast agents for MRI. Materials (Basel). 2020;13(11):2586.
50. Ngen EJ, et al. MRI assessment of prostate-specific membrane antigen (PSMA) targeting by a PSMA-targeted magnetic nanoparticle: potential for image-guided therapy. Mol Pharm. 2019;16(5):2060–8.
51. Isa EDM, et al. Optimization of synthesis parameters of mesoporous silica nanoparticles based on ionic liquid by experimental design and its application as a drug delivery agent. J Nanomaterials. 2019;2019:8.
52. Frickenstein AN, et al. Mesoporous silica nanoparticles: properties and strategies for enhancing clinical effect. Pharmaceutics. 2021;13(4):570.
53. Hu J-J, Xiao D, Zhang X-Z. Advances in peptide functionalization on mesoporous silica nanoparticles for controlled drug release. Small. 2016;12(25):3344–59.
54. Bradbury MS, et al. Intraoperative mapping of sentinel lymph node metastases using a clinically translated ultrasmall silica nanoparticle. Wiley Interdiscip Rev Nanomed Nanobiotechnol. 2016;8(4):535–53.
55. Du D, et al. PSA targeted dual-modality manganese oxide-mesoporous silica nanoparticles for prostate cancer imaging. Biomed Pharmacother. 2020;121:109614.
56. Qu Y, et al. Linear and Core-crosslinked Glycopolymer-gadolinium conjugates: preparation and their behaviors as nanoscale magnetic resonance imaging contrast agents. J Biomed Nanotechnol. 2019;15(8):1637–53.
57. Sandoval-Yañez C, Castro Rodriguez C. Dendrimers: amazing platforms for bioactive molecule delivery systems. Materials (Basel). 2020;13(3):570.
58. Zhou Y, et al. Self-assembly of hyperbranched polymers and its biomedical applications. Adv Mater. 2010;22(41):4567–90.
59. El-Betany AMM, et al. Auto-fluorescent PAMAM-based dendritic molecules and their potential application in pharmaceutical sciences. Int J Pharm. 2020;579:119187.
60. Li C, et al. Hydrogen peroxide-response nanoprobe for CD44-targeted circulating tumor cell detection and H(2)O(2) analysis. Biomaterials. 2020;255:120071.
61. Wang S, Farnood R, Yan N. Corn-derived dendrimer-like carbohydrate phytoglycogen nanoparticles as selective fluorescent sensor for silver ions. Carbohydr Polym. 2019;223:115095.
62. Lesniak WG, et al. Evaluation of PSMA-targeted PAMAM dendrimer nanoparticles in a murine model of prostate cancer. Mol Pharm. 2019;16(6):2590–604.
63. Li X, et al. Safety challenges and application strategies for the use of dendrimers in medicine. Pharmaceutics. 2022;14(6):1292.
64. Kabanov AV, Batrakova EV, Alakhov VY. Pluronic block copolymers as novel polymer therapeutics for drug and gene delivery. J Control Release. 2002;82(2–3):189–212.
65. Raval N, et al. Multifunctional polymeric micellar nanomedicine in the diagnosis and treatment of cancer. Mater Sci Eng C Mater Biol Appl. 2021;126:112186.

66. Hanafy NAN, El-Kemary M, Leporatti S. Micelles structure development as a strategy to improve smart cancer therapy. Cancers (Basel). 2018;10(7):238.
67. Wang N, et al. Biodegradable polymeric micelles coencapsulating paclitaxel and honokiol: a strategy for breast cancer therapy in vitro and in vivo. Int J Nanomedicine. 2017;12:1499–514.
68. Han Y, et al. A chitosan-based micellar system as Nanocarrier for the delivery of paclitaxel. Polymers (Basel). 2020;12(2):380.
69. Barve A, et al. Enzyme-responsive polymeric micelles of cabazitaxel for prostate cancer targeted therapy. Acta Biomater. 2020;113:501–11.
70. Biswas S. Polymeric micelles as drug-delivery systems in cancer: challenges and opportunities. Nanomedicine (Lond). 2021;16(18):1541–4.
71. Zhang W, et al. A supramolecular self-assembling Nanoagent by inducing intracellular aggregation of PSMA for prostate cancer molecularly targeted Theranostics. Small. 2022;18(38):e2203325.
72. Almowalad J, et al. Lactoferrin—and dendrimer-bearing gold Nanocages for stimulus-free DNA delivery to prostate cancer cells. Int J Nanomedicine. 2022;17:1409–21.
73. Yu T, et al. An amphiphilic dendrimer for effective delivery of small interfering RNA and gene silencing in vitro and in vivo. Angew Chem Int Ed Engl. 2012;51(34):8478–84.
74. Ki MH, et al. Chitosan-based hybrid nanocomplex for siRNA delivery and its application for cancer therapy. Pharm Res. 2014;31(12):3323–34.
75. Liu XX, et al. PAMAM dendrimers mediate siRNA delivery to target Hsp27 and produce potent antiproliferative effects on prostate cancer cells. ChemMedChem. 2009;4(8):1302–10.

Correction to: Prostate Cancer: Molecular Events and Therapeutic Modalities

Gautam Sethi, Milad Ashrafizadeh, and Nasim Ebrahimi

Correction to:
G. Sethi et al. (eds.), *Prostate Cancer: Molecular Events and Therapeutic Modalities*, https://doi.org/10.1007/978-981-97-4612-5

The original version of this book was inadvertently published with errors. Chapters 1, 3, 8, and 9 have been updated with the following changes:

1. Chapters 1 and 3: The last name of Vahid Tavakolipour was unfortunately published with a spelling error. The initially published version has now been corrected.
2. Chapter 8: Owing to an oversight on the production, the author name "Nasim Ebrahimi" was omitted. The correct authorship is given here.

Mahshid Seyed Karimi, Ferdos Faghihkhorasani, Al-Hasnawi Rasool Riyadh Abdulwahid, Sahar Mohammadi, Atiyeh Tavakoli, Parisa Osati, Nasim Ebrahimi*, Mostafa Haji-Fatahaliha, and Amir Reza Aref**Corresponding author*

3. Chapter 9: The corresponding authorship has been updated. Nasim Ebrahimi and Amir Reza Aref are the corresponding authors of this chapter.

The updated versions of these chapters can be found at
https://doi.org/10.1007/978-981-97-4612-5_1
https://doi.org/10.1007/978-981-97-4612-5_3
https://doi.org/10.1007/978-981-97-4612-5_8
https://doi.org/10.1007/978-981-97-4612-5_9

G. Sethi et al. (eds.), *Prostate Cancer: Molecular Events and Therapeutic Modalities*, https://doi.org/10.1007/978-981-97-4612-5_15

MIX
Papier aus verantwortungsvollen Quellen
Paper from responsible sources
FSC® C105338

If you have any concerns about our products,
you can contact us on
ProductSafety@springernature.com

In case Publisher is established outside the EU,
the EU authorized representative is:
Springer Nature Customer Service Center GmbH
Europaplatz 3, 69115 Heidelberg, Germany

Printed by Libri Plureos GmbH
in Hamburg, Germany